Oral Health: Care and Treatment

Oral Health: Care and Treatment

Editor: Timothy Campbell

AMERICAN
MEDICAL PUBLISHERS
www.americanmedicalpublishers.com

AMERICAN
MEDICAL PUBLISHERS
www.americanmedicalpublishers.com

Cataloging-in-Publication Data

Oral health : care and treatment / edited by Timothy Campbell.
p. cm.
Includes bibliographical references and index.
ISBN 978-1-63927-772-8
1. Mouth--Care and hygiene. 2. Dental hygiene. 3. Oral medicine.
4. Mouth--Diseases--Treatment. 5. Dental therapeutics. I. Campbell, Timothy.
RK60.7 .O73 2023
617.601--dc23

American Medical Publishers,
41 Flatbush Avenue,
1st Floor, New York,
NY 11217, USA

ISBN 978-1-63927-772-8 (Hardback)

Contents

Preface

Every book is initially just a concept; it takes months of research and hard work to give it the final shape in which the readers receive it. In its early stages, this book also went through rigorous reviewing. The notable contributions made by experts from across the globe were first molded into patterned chapters and then arranged in a sensibly sequential manner to bring out the best results.

Oral health is an indicator of quality of life, well-being and overall health. It incorporates a wide variety of conditions and diseases, which include tooth loss, dental caries, periodontal disease, oro-dental trauma, noma, oral cancer, and birth defects, like palate and cleft lip. Majority of the oral conditions and diseases share changeable risk factors with major non communicable diseases, such as diabetes, cancer, cardiovascular diseases and severe respiratory diseases. The risk factors consist of alcohol consumption, tobacco use, and unhealthy diets having high sugars. Poor oral health causes devastating pain and can affect the effectiveness of the individuals in various formal settings, which can result in personal and social problems. Furthermore, the psychological effect of the oral diseases can substantially decrease the quality of life. The topics included in this book on oral health are of utmost significance and bound to provide incredible insights to readers. Also included herein is a detailed explanation of the care and treatment required for good oral health. Those in search of information to further their knowledge will be greatly assisted by this book.

It has been my immense pleasure to be a part of this project and to contribute my years of learning in such a meaningful form. I would like to take this opportunity to thank all the people who have been associated with the completion of this book at any step.

Editor

1

Analysis of Chronic Periodontitis in Tonsillectomy Patients: A Longitudinal Follow-Up Study Using a National Health Screening Cohort

Soo Hwan Byun [1], Chanyang Min [2,3], Yong Bok Kim [4], Heejin Kim [4], Sung Hun Kang [5], Bum Jung Park [6], Ji Hye Wee [6], Hyo Geun Choi [2,6,*] and Seok Jin Hong [4,*]

1 Department of Oral & Maxillofacial Surgery, Dentistry, Sacred Heart Hospital, Hallym University College of Medicine, Anyang 14068, Korea; purheit@daum.net
2 Hallym Data Science Laboratory, Hallym University College of Medicine, 14068 Anyang, Korea; joicemin@naver.com
3 Graduate School of Public Health, Seoul National University, Seoul 03080, Korea
4 Department of Otorhinolaryngology-Head & Neck Surgery, Dongtan Sacred Heart Hospital, Hallym University College of Medicine, Dongtan 18450, Korea; yongbok@hallym.or.kr (Y.B.K.); mir5020@hallym.or.kr (H.K.)
5 Department of Biomedical Sciences, College of Medicine, Hallym University, Chuncheon 24252, Korea; malice23@nate.com
6 Department of Otorhinolaryngology-Head & Neck Surgery, Sacred Heart Hospital, Hallym University College of Medicine, Anyang 14068, Korea; bumjung426@gmail.com (B.J.P.); weejh07@gmail.com (J.H.W.)
* Correspondence: pupen@naver.com (H.G.C.); enthsj@hanmail.net (S.J.H.)

Abstract: This study aimed to compare the risk of chronic periodontitis (CP) between participants who underwent tonsillectomy and those who did not (control participants) using a national cohort dataset. Patients who underwent tonsillectomy were selected from a total of 514,866 participants. A control group was included if participants had not undergone tonsillectomy from 2002 to 2015. The number of CP treatments was counted from the date of the tonsillectomy treatment. Patients who underwent tonsillectomy were matched 1:4 with control participants who were categorized based on age, sex, income, and region of residence. Finally, 1044 patients who underwent tonsillectomy were matched 1:4 with 4176 control participants. The adjusted estimated value of the number of post-index date (ID) CP did not reach statistical significance in any post-ID year (each of $p > 0.05$). In another subgroup analysis according to the number of pre- ID CP, it did not show statistical significance. This study revealed that tonsillectomy was not strongly associated with reducing the risk of CP. Even though the tonsils and periodontium are located adjacently, and tonsillectomy and CP may be related to bacterial inflammation, there was no significant risk of CP in patients undergoing tonsillectomy.

Keywords: tonsillectomy; chronic periodontitis; cohort; Korea

1. Introduction

Periodontitis is inflammation around the teeth and alveolar bone that causes destruction of the surrounding structures [1]. Bacterial microorganisms in the subgingival area are generally thought to be the main etiological factor in the development of periodontitis [2]. Bacterial microorganisms— such as *Tanerella forsythia*, *Treponema denticola*, and *Porphyromonas gingivalis*—are related to chronic periodontitis [3,4]. Socransky et al. reported that bacteria such as *Fusobacterium nucleatum*, *Peptostreptococcus micros*, *Campylobacter rectus*, and *Eubacterium nodatum* could be factors for periodontitis [3]. Periodontal inflammation could be worsened by systemic factors such as general diseases and tobacco use [5–9]. Previous studies have shown that periodontitis can cause reactions in the immune system and a variety of diseases, including IgA nephropathy and glycosylated haemoglobin leading to diabetes onset [10–12]. Isola et al. reported that patients with chronic periodontitis (CP) exhibited significantly lower serum levels of vitamin D compared to the healthy controls [13]. The study showed that low serum vitamin D levels correlated with tooth loss and periodontitis, especially in CP patients. Evaluation of vitamin D levels should be recommended at the beginning of periodontal treatment as it can predict and decrease the risk of CP aggravation [13,14].

Periodontitis is difficult to control and can be managed with periodontal treatment to maintain the present condition and prevent further deterioration. Biofilms should be removed, and oral hygiene training should be conducted to reduce the production of new biofilms [15]. Regeneration for the loss of the alveolar bone and gingiva has been attempted with various types of surgical flaps, bone grafting, guided generation, enamel matrix protein, and laser treatment [16]. However, the attempts have not been satisfactory; therefore, many studies have been conducted from various perspectives attempting to assist with regeneration.

Several studies have been conducted that focus on periodontal treatment, including the use of pharmaceutics, such as the application of topical antiseptics (povidone-iodine or chlorhexidine) [15,17]. Quirynen et al. proposed Full Mouth Disinfection (FMD), a treatment that focuses on the disinfection of all the intraoral niches including the periodontal pockets, dorsum of the tongue, and palatine tonsils [18]. According to the FMD proposal, it is vital to prevent microbial reinfection of the previously treated periodontium and niches. Therefore, meticulous scaling within 24 h was proposed, followed by repeated disinfection of all the intraoral niches [18].

A tonsillectomy is usually performed for the treatment of chronic tonsillitis or sleep apnea [19]. It is also recommended for periodic fever, peritonsillar abscess, guttate psoriasis, aphthous stomatitis, and tonsil cancer. There is sufficient evidence that tonsillectomy does not have a significant negative effect on the immune system [19,20]. The majority of studies have reported that the procedure does not appear to affect the long-term risk of infection [21]. On the contrary, some studies have demonstrated changes in immunoglobulin concentrations following tonsillectomy [19]. Bacterial activity determines the level of inflammation, ulceration, or necrosis of the palatine tonsils. These inflammatory or pathologic disorders related to the tonsils are common causes of tonsillectomy.

The palatine tonsils are located in the oropharynx, close to the intraoral area, and it is assumed that the transmission of bacteria can occur between these areas [22]. The relationship between the anatomic position of the tonsils and the intraoral area is believed to explain why tonsillectomy and periodontitis may exhibit similar bacteriologic and clinical properties. In a previous study, periodontal pathogens were detected in the tonsillar area of periodontitis patients [23]. The palatine tonsils have already been suggested as the source of reinfection for previously treated periodontal areas [17]. Biofilms in the subgingival area and saliva exhibited the highest similarity to that of the tonsils in the study [23]. Anaerobic bacteria of the intraoral area—such as *Porphyromonas gingivalis* and *Fusobacterium nucleatum*—was found to be similar to the bacteria of the oropharyngeal area in previous studies [8]. *Prevotella intermedia* and *Treponema denticola* were also found more frequently in infected subgingival pockets [24,25]. While these bacteria are rarely found in a normal periodontium, they are usually present in periodontitis. Similarly, these anaerobic bacteria were found in tonsils with recurrent inflammation [25]. The present study was designed based on the anatomic nearness and bacterial similarity indicated in previous studies, suggesting the possibility of an association between the palatine tonsil area and periodontitis [18,22,24–26].

Despite the validity of those previous studies, the clinical association between tonsillectomy and periodontitis has not been evaluated in detail. Due to these reasons, this study was designed to evaluate whether tonsillectomy significantly influenced CP. Based on these pivotal observations, we designed the present study to assess whether periodontal parameters significantly influenced serum vitamin D levels.

The purpose of this study was to compare the risk of CP between participants who underwent tonsillectomy and those who did not (control participants) using a national cohort dataset. It was hypothesized that tonsillectomy would decrease the risk of CP. In this study, those who underwent tonsillectomy and the control participants were matched using a 1:4 ratio, adjusting for age, sex, region of residence, pre-index date CP treatment, obesity, smoking, alcohol consumption, and Charlson comorbidity index (CCI) score.

2. Materials and Methods

2.1. Study Population

The ethics committee of Hallym University (2019-01-003) approved this study. Written informed consent was waived by the Institutional Review Board. All analyses adhered to the guidelines and regulations of the ethics committee of Hallym University. A detailed description of The Korean National Health Insurance Service-Health Screening Cohort data is given elsewhere [27].

2.2. Tonsillectomy

Tonsillectomy was defined using operation code Q2300.

2.3. Chronic Periodontitis

Patients with CP were diagnosed based on ICD-10 codes (K05.3) and were treated by dentists. The number of CP treatments was counted from the date of tonsillectomy treatment (index date [ID]) to the date before the two-year period (pre-ID CP for 2 y). The number of CP treatments was also counted from the index date to the date after the first-year period (post-ID 1 y CP, post-operative 1–365 days), second-year period (post-ID 2 y CP, post-operative 366–730 days), third-year period (post-ID 3 y CP, post-operative 731–1095 days), fourth-year period (post-ID 4 y CP, post-operative 1096–1460 days), and fifth-year period (post-ID 5 y CP, post-operative 1461–1825 days).

2.4. Participant Selection

Patients who underwent tonsillectomy were selected from 514,866 participants with 497,931,549 medical claim codes (n = 1321). A control group was included if participants had not undergone tonsillectomy between 2002 and 2015 (n = 513,545). To select tonsillectomy patients who were diagnosed for the first time, we excluded those who were diagnosed from 2002 to 2003 (washout periods, n = 228). Patients who underwent tonsillectomy were matched 1:4 with control participants based on age, sex, income, and region of residence. To analyze the subgroups according to pre-ID CP for 2 y, tonsillectomy patients were additionally matched with pre-ID CP for 2 y with a categorical variable (0 times, 1 time, and ≥2 times). To minimize the selection bias, the control participants were selected in random number order. The index date of each tonsillectomy patient was set as the time of the tonsillectomy treatment. The index date of control participants was set as the index date of their matched tonsillectomy. Therefore, each tonsillectomy patient that was subsequently matched with the control participants had the same index date. During the 1:4 matching process, 509,173 un-matched control participants were excluded. Participants who were recorded in 2015 were excluded to calculate post-ID 1 y CP (n = 49 for tonsillectomy patients, n = 196 for control participants). Finally, 1044 patients who underwent tonsillectomy were matched 1:4 with 4176 control participants; see Figure 1.

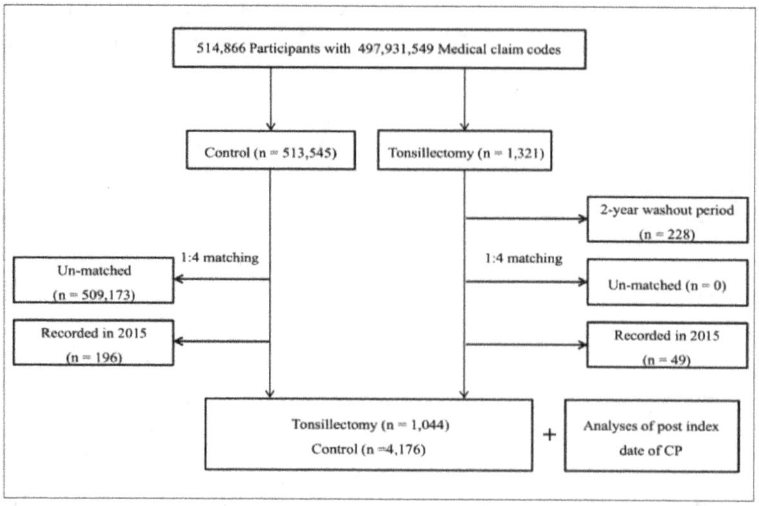

Figure 1. A schematic illustration of the participant selection process that was used in the present study. Of a total of 514,866 participants, 1044 of tonsillectomy participants were matched with 4176 control participants based on age, sex, income, region of residence, and pre-index date (ID) chronic periodontitis (CP) for 2 y.

2.5. Covariates

The age groups were divided by the following 5-year intervals: 40–44, 45–49, 50–54 ... , and 85+ years old. Income groups were organized into five classes (class 1 [lowest income] to 5 [highest income]). The region of residence was classed as either urban (Seoul, Busan, Daegu, Incheon, Gwangju, Daejeon, and Ulsan) or rural (Gyeonggi, Gangwon, Chungcheongbuk, Chungcheongnam, Jeollabuk, Jeollanam, Gyeongsangbuk, Gyeongsangnam, and Jeju).

Tobacco smoking was categorized based on the current smoking status of the participant (nonsmoker, past smoker, or current smoker). Alcohol consumption was categorized on the basis of the frequency of alcohol consumption (<1 time a week or ≥1 time a week). Obesity was measured using body mass index (BMI, kg/m^2). Missing BMI variables were replaced by mean BMI from final selected participants. BMI was categorized as <18.5 (underweight), ≥18.5 to <23 (normal), ≥23 to <25 (overweight), ≥25 to <30 (obese I), or ≥30 (obese II) based on the Asia-Pacific criteria following the Western Pacific Regional Office (WPRO) 2000.

The Charlson Comorbidity Index (CCI) has been widely used to measure disease burden using 17 comorbidities. A score was given to each participant depending on the severity and number of diseases they presented with. CCI was measured as a continuous variable (0 [no comorbidities] through 29 [multiple comorbidities]) [28]. The scores were calculated and the final CCI score was used as a covariate in the analyses.

2.6. Statistical Analyses

The general characteristics between the tonsillectomy and control groups were compared using a Chi-square test.

A simple linear regression and a multiple linear regression were used to calculate the estimated values and 95% of the confidence intervals (CI) for post-ID 1 y CP, post-ID 2 y CP, post-ID 3 y CP, post-ID 4 y CP, and post-ID 5 y CP in the tonsillectomy group compared to the control group. Both the simple linear regression and the multiple linear regression were stratified by age, sex, income, and region of residence. In the multiple linear regression, the model was adjusted for obesity, smoking status, alcohol consumption, CCI score, and pre-ID CP for 2 y as a continuous variable.

For the subgroup analyses, we divided participants by age (<60 years old and ≥60 years old), sex (male or female), and pre-ID CP for 2 y (0 times, 1 time, and ≥2 times) using a crude model and an adjusted model.

Two-tailed analyses were performed, and significance was defined as p-value less than 0.05. The SAS version 9.4 (SAS Institute Inc., Cary, NC, USA) was used for statistical analysis.

3. Results

Age, sex, income, and region of residence were matched between tonsillectomy and control participants exactly ($p = 1.000$), while obesity, smoking, and CCI were different ($p < 0.05$, Table 1). The number of CP treatments prior to the index date were matched as the categorical variable.

Table 1. General Characteristics of Participants.

Characteristics	**Total Participants**		
	Tonsillectomy (n, %)	**Control (n, %)**	**p-Value**
Age (years old)			1.000
40–44	74 (7.1)	296 (7.1)	
45–49	252 (24.1)	1008 (24.1)	
50–54	324 (31.0)	1296 (31.0)	
55–59	226 (21.7)	904 (21.7)	
60–64	100 (9.6)	400 (9.6)	
65–69	46 (4.4)	184 (4.4)	
70–74	13 (1.3)	52 (1.3)	
75–79	6 (0.6)	24 (0.6)	
80–84	3 (0.3)	12 (0.3)	
Sex			1.000
Male	720 (69.0)	2880 (69.0)	
Female	324 (31.0)	1296 (31.0)	
Income			1.000
1 (lowest)	114 (10.9)	456 (10.9)	
2	105 (10.1)	420 (10.1)	
3	127 (12.2)	508 (12.2)	
4	216 (20.7)	864 (20.7)	
5 (highest)	482 (46.2)	1928 (46.2)	
Region of residence			1.000
Urban	527 (50.5)	2108 (50.5)	
Rural	517 (49.5)	2068 (49.5)	
Pre index date of CP			1.000
0 time	701 (67.2)	2804 (67.2)	
1 time	145 (13.9)	580 (13.9)	
≥2 times	198 (19.0)	792 (19.0)	
Obesity †			<0.001 *
Underweight	6 (0.6)	61 (1.5)	
Normal	245 (23.5)	1436 (34.4)	
Overweight	286 (27.4)	1143 (27.4)	
Obese I	442 (42.3)	1427 (34.2)	
Obese II	65 (6.2)	109 (2.6)	
Smoking status			0.019 *
Nonsmoker	611 (58.5)	2483 (59.5)	
Past smoker	193 (18.5)	633 (15.2)	
Current smoker	240 (23.0)	1060 (25.4)	
Alcohol consumption			0.219
<1 time a week	647 (62.0)	2501 (59.9)	
≥1 time a week	397 (38.0)	1675 (40.1)	
CCI score			<0.001 *
0	713 (68.3)	3,275 (78.4)	
1	168 (16.1)	448 (10.7)	
2	85 (8.1)	240 (5.8)	
3	29 (2.8)	91 (2.2)	
≥4	49 (4.7)	122 (2.9)	

Abbreviations: CCI, Charlson comorbidity index; CP, chronic periodontitis. * Chi-square test. Significance at $p < 0.05$. † Obesity (BMI, body mass index, kg/m^2) was categorized as <18.5 (underweight), ≥18.5 to <23 (normal), ≥23 to <25 (overweight), ≥25 to <30 (obese I), and ≥30 (obese II).

The adjusted estimated value (EV) of the number of post-ID CP did not reach statistical significance in any post-ID year (each of $p > 0.05$, Table 2). In the subgroup analyses according to age and sex, statistical significance was only reached in ≥60-year-old men in post ID 2 y (EV = 0.561, 95% CI = 0.156–0.967, $p = 0.007$, Figure 2). In another subgroup analysis according to the number of pre-ID CP, statistical significance was not found in any analysis, see Figure 3.

Table 2. Simple and multiple linear regression model (estimated value [95% confidence interval]) for post-index date of CP (post-ID CP) periods in tonsillectomy group compared to control group.

Characteristics	Linear Regression			
	Simple †	*p*-Value	Multiple †,‡	*p*-Value
	Post ID 1 y CP (n = 5220)			
Tonsillectomy	−0.068 (−0.153 to 0.018)	0.123	−0.073 (−0.158 to 0.012)	0.091
	Post ID 2 y CP (n = 4920)			
Tonsillectomy	0.009 (−0.083 to 0.100)	0.853	0.021 (−0.069 to 0.111)	0.649
	Post ID 3 y CP (n = 4610)			
Tonsillectomy	−0.055 (−0.163 to 0.052)	0.313	−0.040 (−0.148 to 0.067)	0.459
	Post ID 4 y CP (n = 4245)			
Tonsillectomy	0.052 (−0.064 to 0.169)	0.377	0.059 (−0.058 to 0.176)	0.325
	Post ID 5 y CP (n = 3825)			
Tonsillectomy	0.031 (−0.092 to 0.153)	0.623	0.054 (−0.069 to 0.177)	0.388

Abbreviations: CCI, Charlson comorbidity index; CP, chronic periodontitis. Linear regression model, Significance at $p < 0.05$. † Models stratified by age, sex, income, and region of residence. ‡ A model adjusted for obesity, smoking, alcohol consumption, CCI scores, and pre-index date of CP (pre-ID CP) for 2 y.

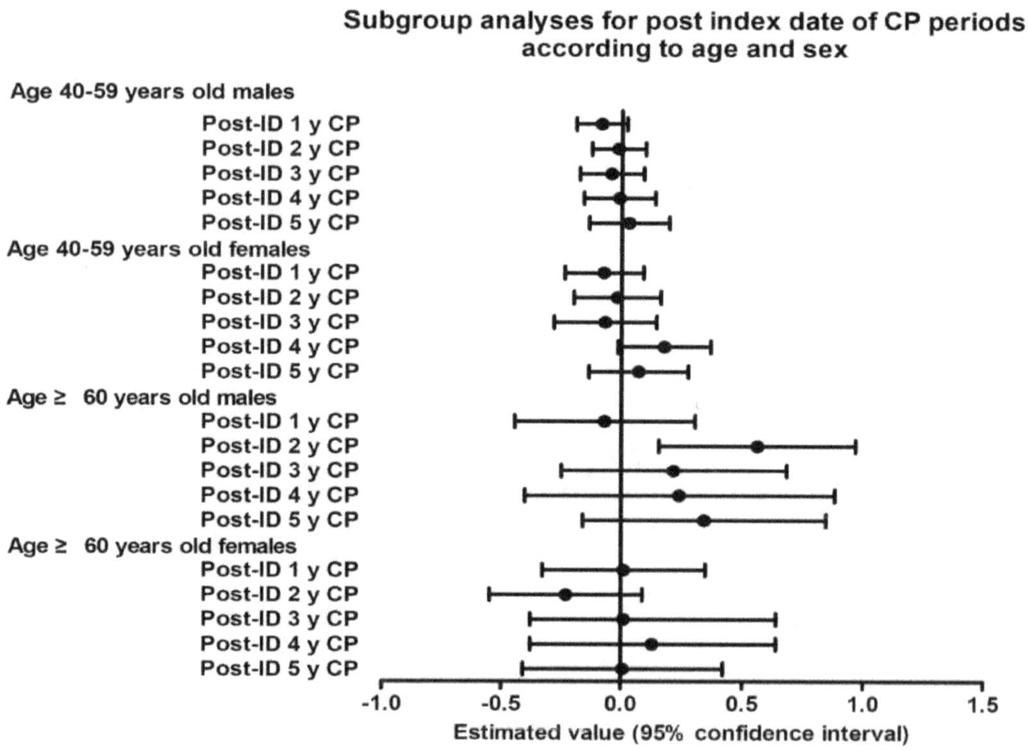

Figure 2. Subgroup analyses of simple and multiple linear regression models (estimated value [95% confidence interval]) for post-index date of CP (post-ID CP) periods in tonsillectomy group compared to control group according to age and sex.

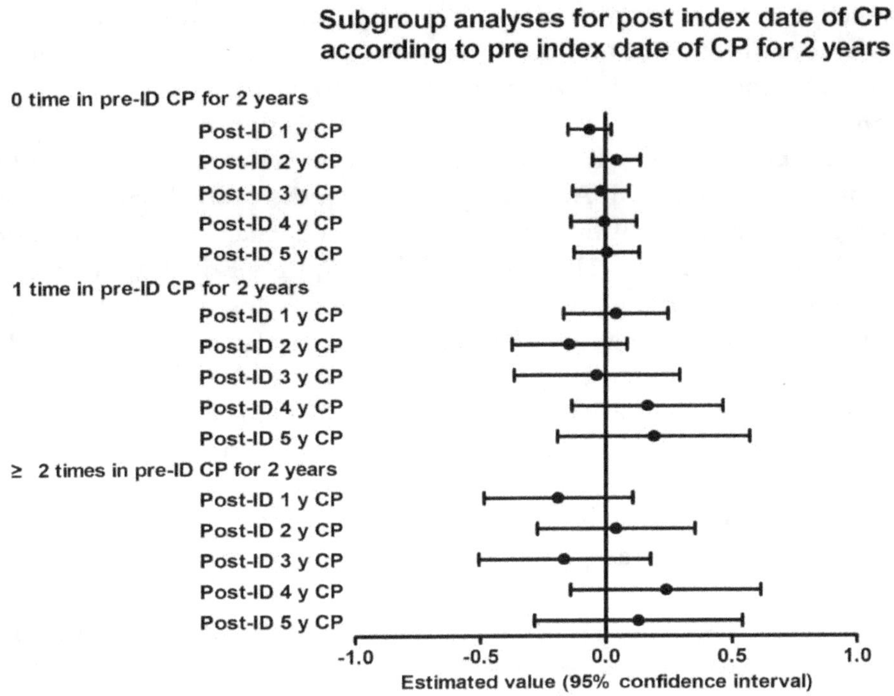

Figure 3. Subgroup analyses of simple and multiple linear regression models (estimated value [95% confidence interval]) for post-index date of CP (post-ID CP) periods in tonsillectomy and control groups according to pre-index date of CP (pre-ID CP) for 2 years.

4. Discussion

The hypothesis of this study, based on previous research that suggests a link between peritonsillar infection and periodontitis, was that the bacteriological and clinical outcomes of tonsillectomy could influence the diagnosis and treatment of CP [29]. It has previously been suggested that the niches around the palatine tonsils are the sources of bacterial infection for the periodontal area [18,23].

Unexpectedly, this study revealed that the adjusted EV of the number of post-ID CP did not reach statistical significance in any post-ID year. In another subgroup analysis according to the number of pre-ID CP, statistical significance was not found in any analysis. These findings oppose the assumption made by Quiryinen et al., although limitations of this study should be further discussed [18].

Tonsillectomy, including removal of the biofilm, has a positive effect on the intraoral areas such as the gingiva and tongue. A previous study reported that the microorganisms in the tongue area were altered following tonsillectomy [26]. The study showed that *Tannerella forsythia* and *Porphyromonas gingivalis* levels decreased in samples taken from the tongue after tonsillectomy [26]. This result could be explained by how anatomically close the tongue and tonsils are, and the fact that saliva is exchanged between them while speaking and swallowing. On the contrary, the same study reported that lesser changes occurred in other bacteria levels in the periodontal pocket following tonsillectomy [26]. They suggested that, with regards to the tonsillar area, the periodontal pocket would be more distant and difficult to access than the tongue area. As such, other bacteria in the periodontal pocket may be less affected. We also believe that the risk of developing CP after tonsillectomy was not reduced in our study for this reason.

Another reason for the discrepancy between the diagnosis and treatment of CP and tonsillectomy is that the major bacteria in culture-dependent studies of tonsils and the microbiome in culture-independent 16 s sequencing studies are *Streptococcus* and *Haemophilus influenzae* [8,30]. However, the essential microbiome in CP was *Porpyromonas gingivalis*, which can increase the activity of biofilm bacteria by interrupting homeostasis in the host.

Our findings could be explained by the improvements that occur with regards to mouth breathing following tonsillectomy. Tonsillectomy can eliminate breathing problems such as snoring or mouth breathing [31], which is likely to increase the risk of periodontitis. Kaur et al. have reported that a patient's periodontal condition is influenced by mouth breathing even after periodontal treatment such as scaling and root planning [32]. Mouth breathing also induces a dry condition in the intraoral area, which could increase the possibility of periodontitis. This hypothesis was explained in another study, suggesting that the salivary substitute had a positive effect on the periodontal condition in mouth breathing patients with CP [33]. According to these studies, tonsillectomy might reduce mouth breathing, and improved mouth breathing could have a beneficial effect on periodontitis.

This study has four advantages. The first is the large number of study participants (n = 5220). Participants were followed up for a maximum of 13 years following tonsillectomy, whereas a similar study only conducted a 3-year follow-up [29]. Secondly, the Korean National Health Insurance Service-Health Screening Cohort dataset is a large national survey that is representative of the Korean population. These cohort records were available for each participant, and the records used in our study were not distorted by the memory of participants. The data are also inclusive of all Koreans without exception; therefore, no participants were missed during the follow-up period. Thirdly, well-trained clinicians documented general health examinations and laboratory evaluations. Finally, adjusting factors showed a statistically significant independent association with tonsillectomy in our data, thus confirming the reliability of our study.

This study used a large population dataset; nevertheless, the findings have limitations. Firstly, the dataset included many factors such as alcohol consumption, obesity, smoking, and age. However, it was impossible to adjust for all systemic factors that were not included in the dataset. Secondly, this study could have been subject to surveillance bias. Tonsillectomy was more likely to be diagnosed for possibly unrelated CP, based on a higher number of visits to medical institutions. However, it is very unlikely that increased participant visits would induce the detection of CP. Dental examinations were conducted during regular visits that were covered by the Korean National Health Service (KNHS), which has exclusive characteristics, including low payment, widespread coverage, and easy access to medical institutions in Korea. In addition to these advantages, most Koreans undergo regular dental check-ups. Additionally, the large population dataset of this study was adjusted for many factors; thus, the surveillance bias was minimized by this adjustment. Therefore, this study prevented surveillance bias by adjusting the characteristics of the KNHS system. Furthermore, the present study analyzed the association using only code from data of the Korean National Health Service (KNHS), and thus the data did not indicate periodontitis severity. There may also be confounders that were not adjusted for. Finally, data were collected from individuals over the age of 40 years. Therefore, considering these limitations, further studies are required to validate our findings.

5. Conclusions

This study revealed that tonsillectomy was not significantly associated with reducing CP. Though the tonsils and periodontium are close in location, and tonsillectomy and CP may be related with regards to bacterial inflammation, the risk of CP in patients undergoing tonsillectomy was not statistically significant. However, further studies with a larger population should be considered to confirm, with greater plausibility, the influence of tonsillectomy on periodontal conditions in patients affected by CP.

Author Contributions: Conceptualization, S.H.B. and H.G.C.; Data curation, C.M. and H.G.C.; Formal analysis, B.J.P. and H.G.C.; Funding acquisition, S.J.H.; Investigation, S.H.B., H.K., S.H.K., B.J.P., and H.G.C.; Methodology, C.M., B.J.P., and H.G.C.; Resources, S.J.H.; Supervision, S.H.B., Y.B.K., and S.J.H.; Visualization, S.H.B. and J.H.W.; Writing—Original draft, S.H.B. and S.J.H.; Writing—Review and editing, S.H.B., H.K., and S.J.H. All authors have read and agreed to the published version of the manuscript.

References

1. Dentino, A.; Lee, S.; Mailhot, J.; Hefti, A.F. Principles of periodontology. *Periodontology 2000* **2013**, *61*, 16–53. [CrossRef] [PubMed]
2. Socransky, S.S. Microbiology of periodontal disease—Present status and future considerations. *J. Periodontol.* **1977**, *48*, 497–504. [CrossRef] [PubMed]

3. Stingu, C.S.; Jentsch, H.; Eick, S.; Schaumann, R.; Knofler, G.; Rodloff, A. Microbial profile of patients with periodontitis compared with healthy subjects. *Quintessence Int.* **2012**, *43*, e23–e31. [PubMed]
4. Socransky, S.S.; Haffajee, A.D.; Cugini, M.A.; Smith, C.; Kent, R.L., Jr. Microbial complexes in subgingival plaque. *J. Clin. Periodontol.* **1998**, *25*, 134–144. [CrossRef] [PubMed]
5. Persic Bukmir, R.; Jurcevic Grgic, M.; Brumini, G.; Spalj, S.; Pezelj-Ribaric, S.; Brekalo Prso, I. Influence of tobacco smoking on dental periapical condition in a sample of Croatian adults. *Wien. Klin. Wochenschr.* **2016**, *128*, 260–265. [CrossRef] [PubMed]
6. Dietrich, T.; Walter, C.; Oluwagbemigun, K.; Bergmann, M.; Pischon, T.; Pischon, N.; Boeing, H. Smoking, Smoking Cessation, and Risk of Tooth Loss: The EPIC-Potsdam Study. *J. Dent. Res.* **2015**, *94*, 1369–1375. [CrossRef]
7. Chavarry, N.G.; Vettore, M.V.; Sansone, C.; Sheiham, A. The relationship between diabetes mellitus and destructive periodontal disease: A meta-analysis. *Oral Health Prev. Dent.* **2009**, *7*, 107–127.
8. Jensen, A.; Fago-Olsen, H.; Sorensen, C.H.; Kilian, M. Molecular mapping to species level of the tonsillar crypt microbiota associated with health and recurrent tonsillitis. *PLoS ONE* **2013**, *8*, e56418. [CrossRef]
9. Kim, E.K.; Lee, S.G.; Choi, Y.H.; Won, K.C.; Moon, J.S.; Merchant, A.T.; Lee, H.-K. Association between diabetes-related factors and clinical periodontal parameters in type-2 diabetes mellitus. *BMC Oral Health* **2013**, *13*, 64. [CrossRef]
10. Nagasawa, Y.; Iio, K.; Fukuda, S.; Date, Y.; Iwatani, H.; Yamamoto, R.; Horii, A.; Inohara, H.; Imai, E.; Nakanishi, T.; et al. Periodontal disease bacteria specific to tonsil in IgA nephropathy patients predicts the remission by the treatment. *PLoS ONE* **2014**, *9*, e81636. [CrossRef]
11. Isola, G.; Matarese, G.; Ramaglia, L.; Pedulla, E.; Rapisarda, E.; Iorio-Siciliano, V. Association between periodontitis and glycosylated haemoglobin before diabetes onset: A cross-sectional study. *Clin. Oral Investig.* **2019**. [CrossRef] [PubMed]
12. Isola, G.; Alibrandi, A.; Curro, M.; Matarese, M.; Ricca, S.; Matarese, G.; Ientile, R.; Kocher, T. Evaluation of salivary and serum ADMA levels in patients with periodontal and cardiovascular disease as subclinical marker of cardiovascular risk. *J. Periodontol.* **2020**. [CrossRef] [PubMed]
13. Isola, G.; Alibrandi, A.; Rapisarda, E.; Matarese, G.; Williams, R.C.; Leonardi, R. Association of vitamin D in patients with periodontitis: A cross-sectional study. *J. Periodontal Res.* **2020**. [CrossRef]
14. Isola, G. Current Evidence of Natural Agents in Oral and Periodontal Health. *Nutrients* **2020**, *12*, 585. [CrossRef] [PubMed]
15. Slots, J. Low-cost periodontal therapy. *Periodontology 2000* **2012**, *60*, 110–137. [CrossRef] [PubMed]
16. Ramseier, C.A.; Warnakulasuriya, S.; Needleman, I.G.; Gallagher, J.E.; Lahtinen, A.; Ainamo, A.; Alajbeg, I.; Albert, D.; Al-Hazmi, N.; Antohe, M.E.; et al. Consensus Report: 2nd European Workshop on Tobacco Use Prevention and Cessation for Oral Health Professionals. *Int. Dent. J.* **2010**, *60*, 3–6. [PubMed]
17. Sahrmann, P.; Puhan, M.A.; Attin, T.; Schmidlin, P.R. Systematic review on the effect of rinsing with povidone-iodine during nonsurgical periodontal therapy. *J. Periodontal Res.* **2010**, *45*, 153–164. [CrossRef]
18. Quirynen, M.; Bollen, C.M.; Vandekerckhove, B.N.; Dekeyser, C.; Papaioannou, W.; Eyssen, H. Full- vs. partial-mouth disinfection in the treatment of periodontal infections: Short-term clinical and microbiological observations. *J. Dent. Res.* **1995**, *74*, 1459–1467. [CrossRef]
19. Mitchell, R.B.; Archer, S.M.; Ishman, S.L.; Rosenfeld, R.M.; Coles, S.; Finestone, S.A.; Friedman, N.R.; Giordano, T.; Hildrew, D.M.; Kim, T.W.; et al. Clinical Practice Guideline: Tonsillectomy in Children (Update). *Otolaryngol. Head Neck Surg.* **2019**, *160* (Suppl. 1), S1–S42. [CrossRef]
20. Bitar, M.A.; Dowli, A.; Mourad, M. The effect of tonsillectomy on the immune system: A systematic review and meta-analysis. *Int. J. Pediatr. Otorhinolaryngol.* **2015**, *79*, 1184–1191. [CrossRef]
21. Ingram, D.G.; Friedman, N.R. Toward Adenotonsillectomy in Children: A Review for the General Pediatrician. *JAMA Pediatr.* **2015**, *169*, 1155–1161. [CrossRef] [PubMed]
22. Quirynen, M.; De Soete, M.; Dierickx, K.; van Steenberghe, D. The intra-oral translocation of periodontopathogens jeopardises the outcome of periodontal therapy. A review of the literature. *J. Clin. Periodontol.* **2001**, *28*, 499–507. [CrossRef] [PubMed]
23. Cieplik, F.; Zaura, E.; Brandt, B.W.; Buijs, M.J.; Buchalla, W.; Crielaard, W.; Laine, M.L.; Deng, D.M.; Exterkate, R.A.M. Microcosm biofilms cultured from different oral niches in periodontitis patients. *J. Oral Microbiol.* **2019**, *11*, 1551596. [CrossRef] [PubMed]

24. Sakalauskiene, J.; Kubilius, R.; Gleiznys, A.; Vitkauskiene, A.; Ivanauskiene, E.; Saferis, V. Relationship of clinical and microbiological variables in patients with type 1 diabetes mellitus and periodontitis. *Med. Sci. Monit.* **2014**, *20*, 1871–1877. [CrossRef]
25. Develioglu, O.N.; Ipek, H.D.; Bahar, H.; Can, G.; Kulekci, M.; Aygun, G. Bacteriological evaluation of tonsillar microbial flora according to age and tonsillar size in recurrent tonsillitis. *Eur. Arch. Otorhinolaryngol.* **2014**, *271*, 1661–1665. [CrossRef]
26. Diener, V.N.; Gay, A.; Soyka, M.B.; Attin, T.; Schmidlin, P.R.; Sahrmann, P. What is the influence of tonsillectomy on the level of periodontal pathogens on the tongue dorsum and in periodontal pockets. *BMC Oral Health* **2018**, *18*, 62. [CrossRef]
27. Kim, S.Y.; Min, C.; Oh, D.J.; Choi, H.G. Tobacco Smoking and Alcohol Consumption Are Related to Benign Parotid Tumor: A Nested Case-Control Study Using a National Health Screening Cohort. *Clin. Exp. Otorhinolaryngol.* **2019**, *12*, 412–419. [CrossRef]
28. Quan, H.; Li, B.; Couris, C.M.; Fushimi, K.; Graham, P.; Hider, P.; Januel, J.-M.; Sundararajan, V. Updating and validating the Charlson comorbidity index and score for risk adjustment in hospital discharge abstracts using data from 6 countries. *Am. J. Epidemiol.* **2011**, *173*, 676–682. [CrossRef]
29. Georgalas, C.; Kanagalingam, J.; Zainal, A.; Ahmed, H.; Singh, A.; Patel, K.S. The association between periodontal disease and peritonsillar infection: A prospective study. *Otolaryngol. Head Neck Surg.* **2002**, *126*, 91–94. [CrossRef]
30. Liu, C.M.; Cosetti, M.K.; Aziz, M.; Buchhagen, J.L.; Contente-Cuomo, T.L.; Price, L.B.; Keim, P.S.; Lalwani, A.K. The otologic microbiome: A study of the bacterial microbiota in a pediatric patient with chronic serous otitis media using 16SrRNA gene-based pyrosequencing. *Arch. Otolaryngol. Head Neck Surg.* **2011**, *137*, 664–668. [CrossRef]
31. Zhang, L.Y.; Zhong, L.; David, M.; Cervin, A. Tonsillectomy or tonsillotomy? A systematic review for paediatric sleep-disordered breathing. *Int. J. Pediatr. Otorhinolaryngol.* **2017**, *103*, 41–50. [CrossRef] [PubMed]
32. Kaur, M.; Sharma, R.K.; Tewari, S.; Narula, S.C. Influence of mouth breathing on outcome of scaling and root planing in chronic periodontitis. *BDJ Open* **2018**, *4*, 17039. [CrossRef] [PubMed]
33. Bhatia, A.; Sharma, R.K.; Tewari, S.; Narula, S.C. A randomized clinical trial of salivary substitute as an adjunct to scaling and root planing for management of periodontal inflammation in mouth breathing patients. *J. Oral Sci.* **2015**, *57*, 241–247. [CrossRef] [PubMed]

2

Monitoring of Bactericidal Effects of Silver Nanoparticles Based on Protein Signatures and VOC Emissions from *Escherichia coli* and Selected Salivary Bacteria

Fernanda Monedeiro [1,2,3,†], Paweł Pomastowski [1,2,†], Maciej Milanowski [1,2], Tomasz Ligor [1,2] and Bogusław Buszewski [1,2,*]

1 Department of Environmental Chemistry and Bioanalytics, Faculty of Chemistry, Nicolaus Copernicus University, 87-100 Toruń, Poland; fernandamonedeiro@usp.br (F.M.); pawel_pomastowski@wp.pl (P.P.); milanowski.maciej@gmail.com (M.M.); msd2501@chem.uni.torun.pl (T.L.)

2 Interdisciplinary Centre of Modern Technologies, Nicolaus Copernicus University, 87-100 Toruń, Poland

3 Department of Chemistry, Faculty of Philosophy, Science and Letters of Ribeirão Preto, University of São Paulo, Ribeirão Preto CEP 14040-901, Brazil

* Correspondence: bbusz@chem.uni.torun.pl

† Those authors contributed equally to this work.

Abstract: *Escherichia coli* and salivary *Klebsiella oxytoca* and *Staphylococcus saccharolyticus* were subjected to different concentrations of silver nanoparticles (AgNPs), namely: 12.5, 50, and 100 μg mL^{-1}. Matrix-assisted laser desorption/ionization–time-of-flight mass spectrometry (MALDI-TOF MS) spectra were acquired after specified periods: 0, 1, 4, and 12 h. For study of volatile metabolites, headspace solid-phase microextraction coupled to gas chromatography/mass spectrometry (HS-SPME-GC-MS) was employed—AgNPs were added to bacteria cultures and the headspace was analyzed immediately and after 12 h of incubation. Principal components analysis provided discrimination between clusters of protein profiles belonging to different strains. Canonical correlation, network analysis, and multiple linear regression approach revealed that dimethyl disulfide, dimethyl trisulfide, 2-heptanone, and dodecanal (related to the metabolism of sulfur-containing amino acids and fatty acids synthesis) are exemplary molecular indicators, whose response variation deeply correlated to the interaction with bacteria. Therefore, such species can serve as biomarkers of the agent's effectiveness. The present investigation pointed out that the used approaches can be useful in the monitoring of response to therapeutic treatment based on AgNPs. Furthermore, biochemical mechanisms enrolled in the bactericidal action of nanoparticles can be applied in the development of new agents with enhanced properties.

Keywords: bacteria; HS-SPME-GC-MS; MALDI-TOF MS; silver nanoparticles; VOCs

---

1. Introduction

Silver nanoparticles (AgNPs) are widely used in a growing number of industrial and medical applications, such as electronics, food industry, paints, clothing, cosmetics, and medical devices [1,2]. They are well-known antimicrobial agents and their antimicrobial activity against bacteria is attributed to their high reactivity with proteins and initiation of structural changes in the cell wall and membrane. Silver nanoparticles can interact with SH-groups of amino acids and hence inhibit protein synthesis and function. Also, uptake of free silver ions followed by disruption of ATP production and DNA replication is one possible mechanism of toxicity. As a consequence, it leads to inhibition of vital functions and cell death [3,4]. Possible mechanisms of function of silver nanoparticles are described in many publications, however, there are still gaps in the understanding of this phenomenon [4]. Effectiveness of function of AgNPs was investigated by means of various techniques including well and disc diffusion methods and flow cytometry [5–9]. In the current study, we employed matrix-assisted laser desorption/ionization–time-of-flight mass spectrometry (MALDI-TOF MS), which has emerged as a powerful technique for identification of microorganisms [10,11] and for investigation of, for instance, bacterial drug resistance [12]. Protein profiles obtained within the mass range of 2000 to 20,000 Da using MALDI-TOF MS can reflect many physiological states of bacteria [10]. Ag nanoparticles have a dual function in MALDI-TOF MS analyzes, they can serve as a MALDI matrix for enhanced detection of bacteria or as a bactericidal agent. A critical limiting threshold concentration, which governs whether AgNPs would function as an affinity probe or would express bactericidal property, was investigated in the study of Gopal et al. (2011) [13]. Authors conducted their studies using two model bacterial strains: *Escherichia coli* and *Serratia marcescens*. They stated that critical concentration of affinity probes (CCAP) for silver nanoparticles was 1 mL L^{-1} in the case of *E. coli* and 0.5 mL L^{-1} for *S. marcescens*. Above these concentrations, AgNPs became bactericidal for tested bacteria.

Saliva is a biological matrix with promising applications in clinical settings. Its rapid, non-invasive, and cost-effective collection, easy storage and transportation are advantages over other specimens [14,15]. Like serum, saliva contains hormones, antibodies, growth factors, enzymes, microbes, and their products. Consequently, saliva can be considered as a "mirror" of the body for diagnostic purposes of (inter alia) oral diseases [16]. Volatile organic compounds (VOCs) are one of salivary constituents that can indicate various oral conditions, such as halitosis, periodontal disease, lung cancer, and celiac disease [17]. Gas chromatography–mass spectrometry (GC-MS) is a technique which allows detection of VOCs from different niches, including breath, tissues, saliva, or bacteria [18–23]. Solid phase microextraction (SPME) in headspace (HS) variant is a commonly used method for extraction and enrichment of VOCs from many biological matrices [24–26]. Also, VOCs from bacterial strains were analyzed using gas chromatography–mass spectrometry technique. For example, the effect of applied growth medium on emission of volatiles from *E. coli* was investigated in the work of Ratiu et al. (2017) [27]. *Streptococcus pneumoniae* and *Haemophilus influenzae* cultures were identified to find characteristic volatile biomarkers of these bacteria associated with community-acquired pneumonia (CAP) [28]. *Staphylococcus aureus* and *Pseudomonas aeruginosa* were investigated by Filipiak et al. (2012) [29] to find volatile organic compounds from bacteria most frequently found in ventilator-associated pneumonia (VAP) patients. Headspace samples from bacteria were collected and preconcentrated on multibed sorption tubes and analyzed by GC-MS. Once the investigation of bacterial profiles of molecular species can be related with the presence of a specific strain and its metabolic behavior, the features regarding the activity of bactericidal agents can be measured and thoroughly investigated employing the comprehensive evaluation of these profiles.

The aim of the present work is to provide correlated relationships between expressed proteins and volatile metabolites, as a form to assess bactericidal agent performance. Moreover, such knowledge can contribute for elucidation of action mechanism of silver nanoparticles and how they can influence the physiological state of selected bacteria. Growth curves of *E. coli*, *Klebsiella oxytoca*, and *Staphylococcus saccharolyticus* were prepared, then, MALDI-TOF MS technique was employed to obtain proteins profiles of these bacteria and to investigate the addition of selected levels of AgNPs on them. Furthermore, in order to assess alterations in the produced bacterial volatile metabolites, VOCs were investigated by means of HS-SPME-GC-MS, for strains in the unstressed form and after their treatment with silver nanoparticles.

2. Experimental Section

2.1. Instruments

The ultrafleXtreme MALDI-TOF/TOF mass spectrometer (Bruker Daltonik, Bremen, Germany) equipped with a modified Nd:YAG laser (Smartbeam IITM) operating at the wavelength of 355 nm and the frequency of 2 kHz was used to acquire spectra from strains of bacteria by means of two methods and to investigate the interactions between silver nanoparticles and bacterial cells. Optical density (OD) measurements were performed with a DEN-1B Densitometer (Biosan, Riga, Latvia). VITEK® 2 Compact system (bioMérieux, Marcy l'Etoile, France) was employed for identification of salivary bacteria. The GC-MS analyses were carried out using an Agilent 6890A gas chromatograph coupled to an Agilent 5975 Inert XL MSD mass spectrometer (both from Agilent Technologies, Santa Clara, CA, USA). The system was equipped with a Rtx®-5MS w/Integra Guard 30 m × 0.25 mm × 0.25 μm column (Restek Corporation, Bellefonte, PA, USA). Extractions of volatile organic compounds were performed using 65 μm polydimethylsiloxane (PDMS)/divinylbenzene (DVB) fiber (Supelco, Bellefonte, PA, USA). Incubating Microplate Shaker (VWR International, Radnor, PA, USA) was used for incubation of headspace vials with bacterial content.

2.2. Materials

Water LC-MS Chromasolv, ethanol, acetonitrile (ACN), trifluoroacetic acid (TFA), formic acid, and isopropanol were purchased from Sigma Aldrich (Steinheim, Germany). Ultra-pure water from a Milli-Q water system (Millipore, Bedford, MS, USA) was used throughout the work.

All chemicals for MALDI-MS analyses were supplied at the highest commercially available purity from Fluka Feinchemikalien GmbH (part of Sigma Aldrich). Polished steel targets (Bruker Daltonik) were used for sample deposition. α-cyano-4-hydroxycinnamic acid (HCCA; Sigma Aldrich) was employed as a matrix for MALDI analyses (dried droplet method). Bruker bacterial test standard (BTS) was used for external calibration (Bruker Daltonik).

Then, 15 mL sterile polypropylene tubes (ISOLAB, Wertheim, Germany) were used for collection of oral fluid. For identification of salivary bacteria strains, we used 0.45% saline and VITEK® 2 Compact ID Cards for Gram-negative (GN), Gram-positive (GP), and anaerobe corynbacteria (ANC) (bioMérieux). Headspace screw top 20 mL clear vials and magnetic polytetrafluoroethylene (PTFE)/Sil screw caps for headspace vials, 18 mm thread, were purchased from Agilent Technologies.

Three media were used for bacteria cultivation: tryptic soy broth (TSB; Soybean-Casein Digest Medium; Bacto, Sydney, Australia), Mueller Hinton (MH) broth, and M9 (both from Sigma Aldrich). Glucose used as an additive to the minimal medium M9 was purchased from Avantor Performance Materials (Gliwice, Poland). Detailed information regarding media technical aspects can be found elsewhere [30].

The silver nanoparticles used in this study were synthesized in our laboratory and physicochemical characterized previously by Railean-Plugaru et al. (2016) [31]. They were synthesized by the biological method. In comparison with the chemically synthesized one, it was found to be naturally coated with organic deposit, therefore, considered as a biocolloid. The biologically synthesized nanocomposites were tested against 7 different bacterial strains and the antimicrobial activity was found to be dependent on the silver nanocomposite concentrations [9,31].

Two bacterial strains used during investigations, namely: *Escherichia coli* ATCC 25922 and salivary *Klebsiella oxytoca* ATCC 13182 were obtained from POL-AURA (Dywity, Poland). The strain of *Staphylococcus saccharolyticus* was isolated from the saliva of a healthy human oral cavity and identified using VITEK® 2 Compact system, as described by Buszewski et al. (2017) [32].

2.3. Growth Curves of Bacteria

In order to draw the growth curves of the three bacteria, the OD of samples was measured using DEN-1B Densitometer, which provided results in the unit of McFarland (McF). First, three test tubes were filled with 4.8 mL of M9 medium and sterilized by autoclaving. Once the test tubes cooled down, 0.2 mL of prefiltered 10% (m/v) solution of glucose, which served as a source of carbon for bacteria, was added to each tube—the concentration of glucose in the obtained 5 mL of solution was 0.4% (m/v). The content of all test tubes was vortexed for 30 s and the OD of obtained blanks was measured using DEN-1B Densitometer. Then, three loopfuls of bacterial cells were suspended in 1 mL of saline solution to prepare inoculum. Bacterial suspension was thoroughly vortexed for 30 s and the test tubes were inoculated under sterile conditions using 100 μL of the obtained inoculum. Immediately after inoculation, OD at t_0 was determined. Subsequent measurements were performed at t_2, t_4, t_6, t_8, t_{23}, t_{25}, t_{27}, t_{29}, and t_{31}, corresponding to 2, 4, 6, 8, 23, 25, 27, 29, and 31 h of incubation at 37 °C. Growth profiles were assessed for selection of cultivation times to be used in further assays. Such cultivation periods were aimed to refer to the stationary phase of these bacteria, because in this stage the ratio alive/dead is rather constant, thus, the changes observed in the molecular profiles could be ascribed to a metabolic response to the added stressing agent, minimizing the contribution of metabolic alterations due to the growth process.

2.4. *MALDI-TOF MS Analysis*

MALDI-TOF MS spectra were recorded manually in linear positive mode within *m/z* range of 3000–30000 and applying the acceleration voltage of 25 kV. All mass spectra were acquired and processed with the dedicated software: flexControl and flexAnalysis, respectively (both from Bruker). Two following experiments with MALDI MS technique were conducted in triplicate during the study.

2.4.1. Comparison of Sample Preparation Methods

The first experiment concerned a comparison between two sample preparation protocols for microorganism profiling, according to the instructions of mass spectrometer manufacturer. The "DIRECT" procedure consists in direct smearing of a sample onto a MALDI target, whereas "EXTRACTION" involves extraction of proteins from a sample with ethanol and formic acid. The HCCA matrix (10 mg mL^{-1}) was prepared in a standard solvent (50% acetonitrile, 47.5% water, 2.5% trifluoroacetic acid). The "DIRECT" procedure was as follows: (i) direct smearing of a small amount of biological material (barely visible) using pipette tips onto a sample spot of a polished steel target, (ii) overlaying the biological material with 1 μL of HCCA matrix solution, (iii) allowing the sample spot to air dry before analysis. The above-mentioned biological material was a precentrifuged (13,000 rpm/RCF = 15,871× *g* for 2 min) bacterial pellet obtained from 1.5 mL of a liquid culture. For our purpose, we applied three different media (5 mL of TSB, MH, or M9) which were inoculated using a loopful with three bacterial strains and incubated at 37 °C for 24 h. Moreover, we performed OD measurements of a medium alone, a sample after inoculation, and a sample after incubation (next day in the morning). In addition, three types of media alone (TSB, MH, and M9) served as blanks. The "EXTRACTION" protocol was used in the following way: (i) 300 μL of water was transferred into an eppendorf tube containing the biological material and mixed; (ii) then 900 μL of 100% ethanol was added to the tube and mixed thoroughly; (iii) this was followed with centrifugation at 13,000 rpm/RCF = 15,871× *g* for 2 min and decanting the supernatant; (iv) centrifugation was continued for further 2 min and residual ethanol was removed from the pellet using a pipet; (v) subsequently, 5 μL of 70% formic acid was added to the pellet and mixed thoroughly by pipetting and by vortexing; (vi) 5 μL of acetonitrile was added to the tube and mixed carefully; (vii) the whole was centrifuged at 13,000 rpm/RCF = 15,871× *g* for 2 min and 1 μL of the supernatant was spotted onto a polished steel target; (viii) the sample was covered with 1 μL of HCCA matrix solution as soon as the sample spot had dried out; (ix) finally, the sample spot was allowed to air dry before analysis. The biological material for "EXTRACTION" method was a precentrifuged (13,000 rpm/RCF = 15,871× *g* for 2 min) bacterial pellet obtained from 1.5 mL of a liquid culture with MH medium. In this part of the experiment we used only MH medium (5 mL) inoculated using a loopful with three bacteria and incubated at 37 °C for 24 h. The samples were smeared onto a MALDI target in triplicate. Extract from pure MH was used as a blank in this step.

2.4.2. Influence of AgNPs on MALDI-TOF MS Profiles of the Selected Bacteria

A total of 150 mL of MH medium was prepared and shared between three Erlenmeyer flasks (50 mL in each). After sterilization, each portion of medium was inoculated with two loopfuls of bacterial cells (approximately 1×10^6 of cells) of *E. coli*, *K. oxytoca*, and *S. saccharolyticus* individual strains and placed into a shaker at 37 °C for 8, 15, or 18 h, depending on strain type (based on growth curves experiments). Then, under sterile conditions, nine sterilized test tubes received 10 mL of liquid culture each. Immediately, silver nanoparticles were added and vortexed to obtain the final silver concentration of 12.5, 50, and 100 μg mL^{-1}. After that, OD measurements were performed. Next, all test tubes with their content were placed into an incubator at 37 °C for a specified period of time, namely: 0, 1, 4, and 12 h, then 1.5 mL of each solution was transferred to an Eppendorf tube and centrifuged at 13,000 rpm/RCF = 15,871× *g* for 2 min. The supernatant was removed and the bacterial pellet was subjected to the "EXTRACTION" technique (treatment of a sample using ethanol and formic acid).

2.5. Gas Chromatography–Mass Spectrometry (GC-MS)

A total of 4 mL of sterilized MH broth was inoculated with 100 μL of a bacterial suspension (already cultured bacteria, under 37 °C for 8, 15, or 18 h, depending on strain type) of *E. coli*, *K. oxytoca*, and *S. saccharolyticus* in the medium (100 μL of pure medium was used as a blank). Before application of AgNPs, OD of the inoculum was always measured and was approximately 1.5 McF. Immediately, silver nanoparticles were added to obtain the final concentration of 12.5 and 50 μg mL^{-1}. All four headspace vials (three with bacteria and one with a blank) were placed into an incubator at 37 °C with continuous shaking. Then, the vials were taken out immediately (t = 0) and after 12 h (t = 12). VOCs were extracted at 37 °C for 45 min, using 65 μm PDMS/DVB fiber. All GC-MS experiments were done in triplicate. Helium with a flow rate of 1.1 mL min^{-1} was the carrier gas and temperature of the split–splitless injector was set at 240 °C. The oven temperature program was as follows: The initial temperature of 40 °C was kept for 3 min, then ramped at 10 °C min^{-1} to 300 °C and kept at this last temperature for 5 min. Spectra acquisition was performed within *m*/*z* range of 30–300 with electron ionization (EI) at 70 eV; both the ion source and the transfer line temperature was set at 250 °C.

2.6. Data Processing and Statistical Analysis

Part of the data processing and statistical analysis was performed in R environment, using RStudio v.1.1.463 console. GC-MS raw data (CDF format) was processed using the "xcms" package, peaks were detected in the shift region of 10 ppm, applying the "centWave" method. As result, a database displaying retention time and corresponding area for extracted ion chromatogram (EIC) was obtained. Peaks arising from medium blanks in different incubation times were subtracted from the related bacterial samples. Peak identification was performed using NIST11, for each peak detected belonging to the same retention time—a match factor of at least 750/1000 was considered. From MALDI-TOF MS data, the 100 most intense and corresponding signals were annotated and ion database was created manually.

A comparison between MALDI-TOF MS raw spectra (mzXML format) obtained from bacterial extract before and after AgNPs addition was performed by calculation of the spectrum similarity score (SSS), with usage of "OrgMassSpecR" package in default mode. Heatmaps based on the area of ions, associated with hierarchical cluster analysis using the Spearman method, were built employing "gplots" package.

Canonical correlation analysis (CCA) is a multivariate ordination analysis used to provide sample correlations between two sets of variables. This method was employed to relate the variation in the fold-change of VOCs and proteins ions after the treatment with nanoparticles. The analysis was conducted using representative features ($p < 0.05$, indicated by Mann–Whitney test), "vegan" package was applied to run CCA function.

Network analysis was performed using "igraph" package, in order to provide visualization of the connections between both sets of data. Spearman's coefficients were used to produce the edges between nodes representing protein ions and VOCs, which presented statistically relevant ($p < 0.05$) change in their response after the addition of nanoparticles.

With the usage of IBM SPSS Statistics v.24, Spearman correlation coefficient was calculated between triplicates to verify the reproducibility of the obtained profiles. Principal components analysis (PCA) was carried out to assess the distribution of MALDI-TOF MS profiles according to strain. Mann–Whitney U test was performed to indicate discriminating features. Linear regression was used to create a model able to predict the extension of AgNPs interaction with bacteria. Detailed information regarding used R packages and input formats, as well as employed databases are available in Supplementary Materials.

3. Results

3.1. Determination of Growth Curves

Figure S1 depicts growth curves of three selected bacteria grown in minimal medium M9 with glucose as a source of carbon. Based on the assessed curves, further experiments were conducted using 8, 15, or 18 h of cultivation of E. coli, K. oxytoca, and S. saccharolyticus, respectively. Bacteria at the given times were at the beginning of the stationary phase. Previous experiments reported growth profiles of the selected bacteria using MH medium [33–35].

3.2. Comparison of Procedures: Direct Smearing Versus Extraction and Medium Selection

Straight and clear baseline with negligible signals recorded in the acquired spectra were seen for all tested growth media (M9, MH, and TSB) after using "DIRECT" and "EXTRACTION" (MH only) protocols (Figure S2). Figure S3 demonstrates an exemplary comparison of MALDI-TOF MS spectra of *E. coli* cultured in M9, MH, and TSB media, obtained using "DIRECT" method. The presented observations for *E. coli* are typical for our selected bacterial strains. M9 was found to be the most effective medium among the used growth media. The number of peaks reached almost 100. Moreover, the number of signals with signal-to-noise ratio (S/N) greater than or equal to 10 was 77. Only 33 and 34 signals with such defined S/N were recorded for MH and TSB medium, respectively. However, for further MALDI-TOF MS investigations concerning addition of silver nanoparticles, we selected MH medium, since it provided the best results in the simultaneously conducted GC-MS study (Figure 1).

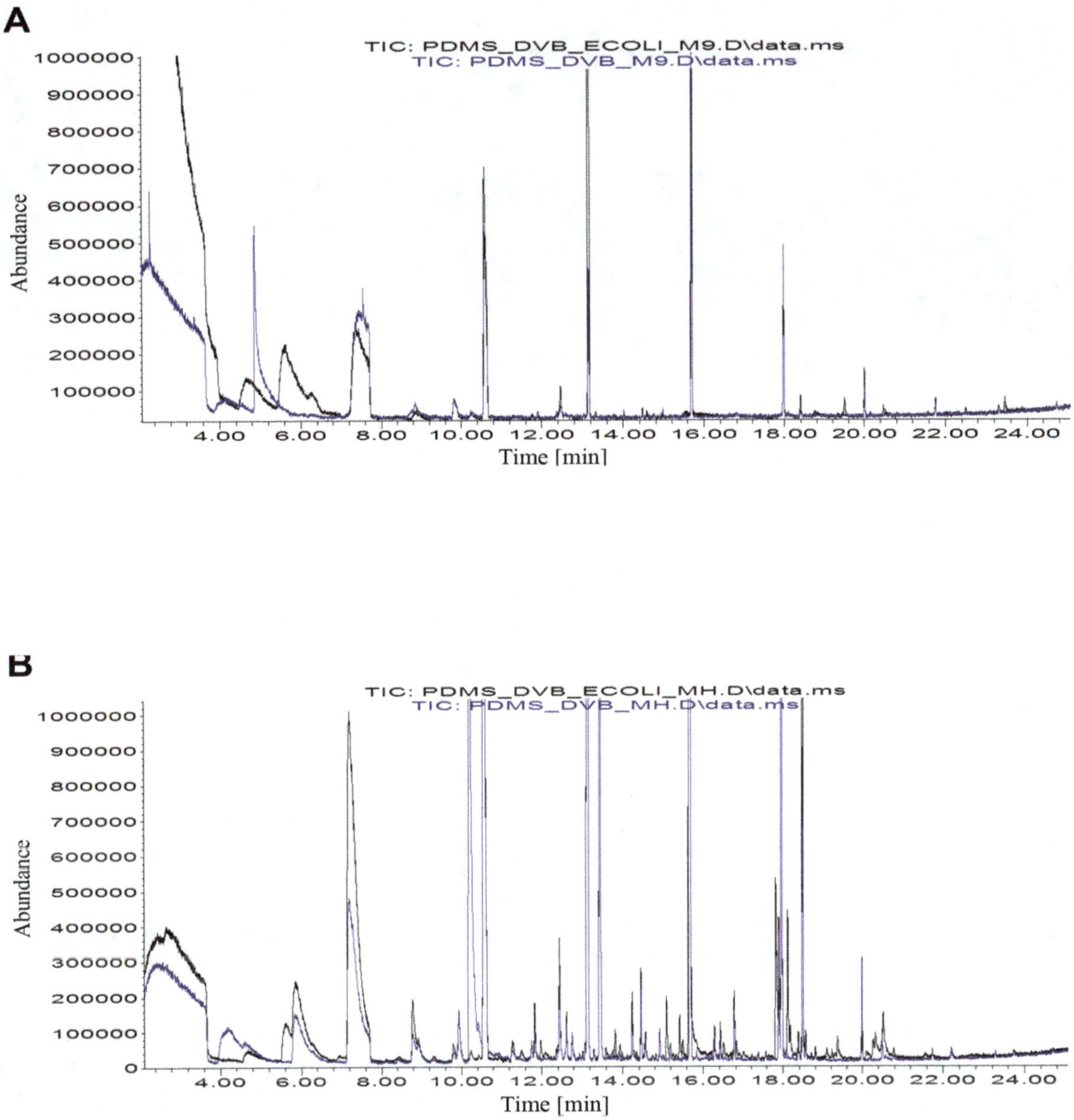

Figure 1. Comparison of overlaid gas chromatography–mass spectrometry (GC-MS) chromatograms obtained for (**A**) *E.coli* bacterium + M9 medium (black) versus pure M9 medium (blue) and (**B**) *E.coli* bacterium + Mueller Hinton (MH) medium (black) versus pure MH medium (blue).

Figure 2 shows a comparison between the two applied sample preparation techniques with the example of E. coli.

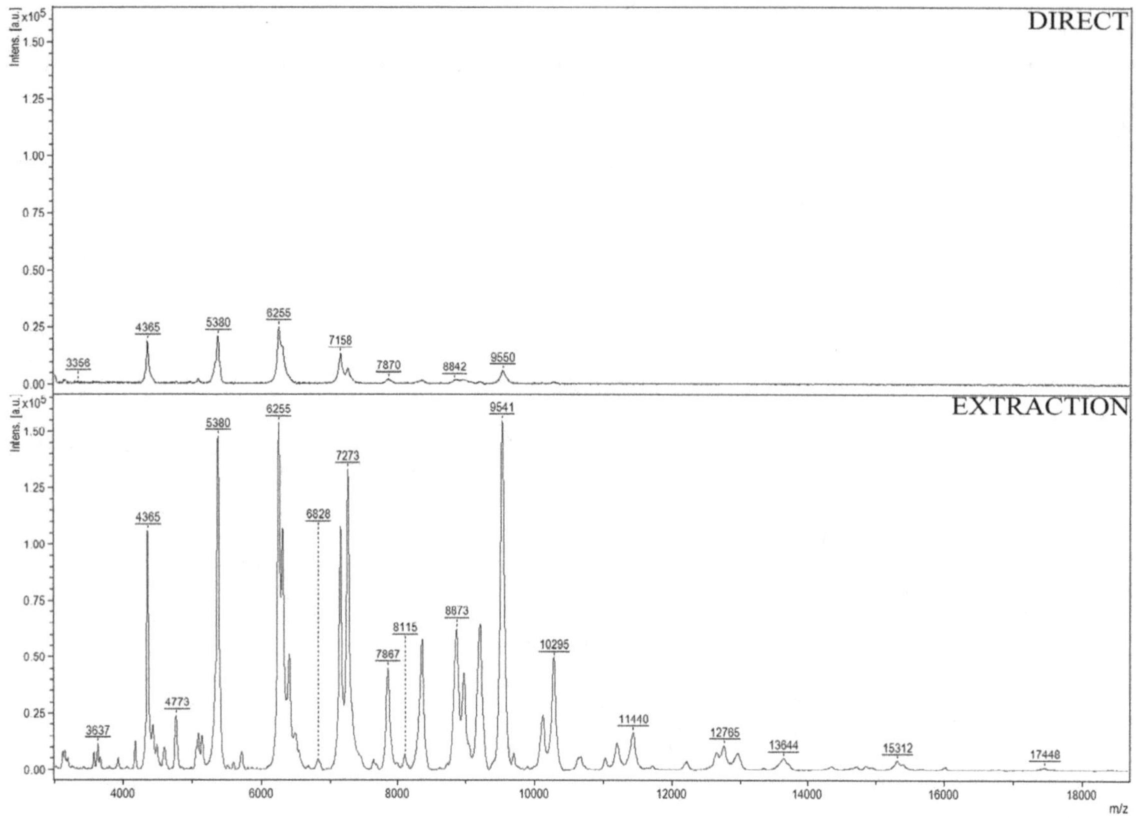

Figure 2. Representative (from triplicate experiment) matrix-assisted laser desorption/ionization–time-of-flight mass spectrometry (MALDI-TOF MS) spectra of *E. coli* in MH medium obtained using the "DIRECT" and "EXTRACTION" procedure.

The differences between MALDI-TOF MS spectra include both the number of detected peaks and their intensity. For E. coli, in the "EXTRACTION" method, we recorded 54 signals with S/N greater than or equal 10. On contrary, for the "DIRECT" procedure, we found only 33 peaks fulfilling this requirement. Moreover, signals obtained for the "EXTRACTION" procedure were several times more intense than the values for the "DIRECT" technique. Similar observations were extended to the other studied bacteria. It indicates that sample treatment using ethanol and formic acid is far more efficient than the method consisting in direct smearing of a sample onto a MALDI target.

3.3. Influence of Silver Nanoparticles on MALDI-TOF MS Spectra and HS-SPME-GC-MS Chromatograms of the Selected Bacteria

To investigate the influence of AgNPs on MALDI-TOF MS spectra of the three model bacteria, the following tests were conducted. In this part of the study, the "EXTRACTION" technique was applied for sample preparation of each bacterial strain, as it was found to be superior to the "DIRECT" procedure in the previous experiment.

Regarding MALDI-TOF MS experiments, the prepared database displayed 1928 most relevant ions, ranging from 3013 to 17,449 *m*/*z*. In GC-MS data, ions addressed as belonging to medium, GC column material, or fiber coating were subtracted from the database, resulting in a total number of 281 computed ions, ranging from 32 to 298 *m*/*z*.

Figure 3 presents the PCA score plot obtained for different protein ions profiles acquired under the mentioned experimental conditions, for each bacterial strain. Profiles belonging to an individual bacterial strain were clearly separated from others, highlighting the discriminative power of ribosomal profiles in bacteria identity. However, still being possible to observe that the performed assays were capable of significantly altering such profiles, in this case, the distinction between the 3 strains was explained by only 14% of the variance.

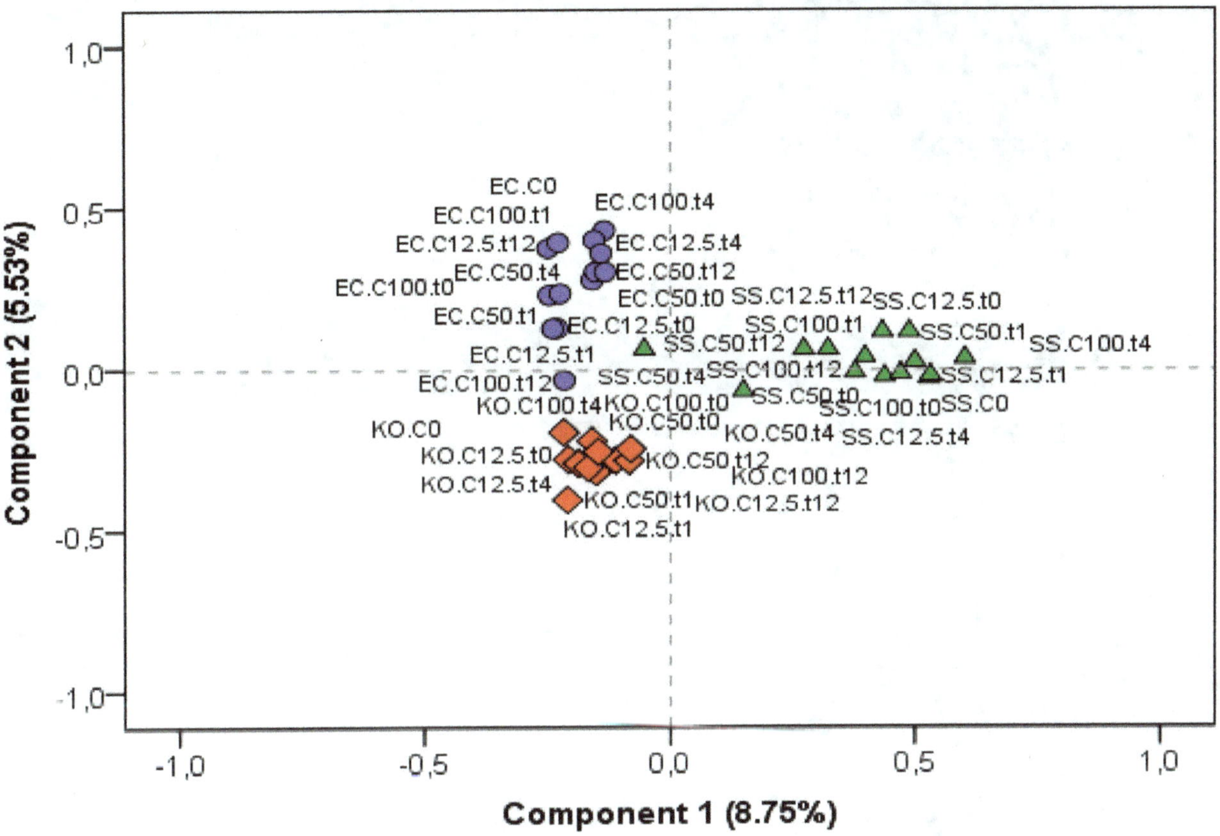

Figure 3. Principal component analysis (PCA) plot of protein ions profiles acquired by MALDI-TOF MS experiments, where diamonds, triangles, and circles represent *K. oxytoca* (KO), *S. saccharolyticus* (SS), and *E. coli* (EC), respectively.

Heatmaps referring to protein ions profiles (Figure 4A) and VOC profiles (Figure 4B) allow inspection of the distribution of ions detected in each experiment. Hierarchical cluster analysis evidencing the similarity between these individual profiles and segregation according to bacterial strain were observed in data extracted both by MALDI-TOF MS and GC-MS results. The ions constituting the profiles were grouped in clusters, which correspond to the main distribution behaviors identified along the samples.

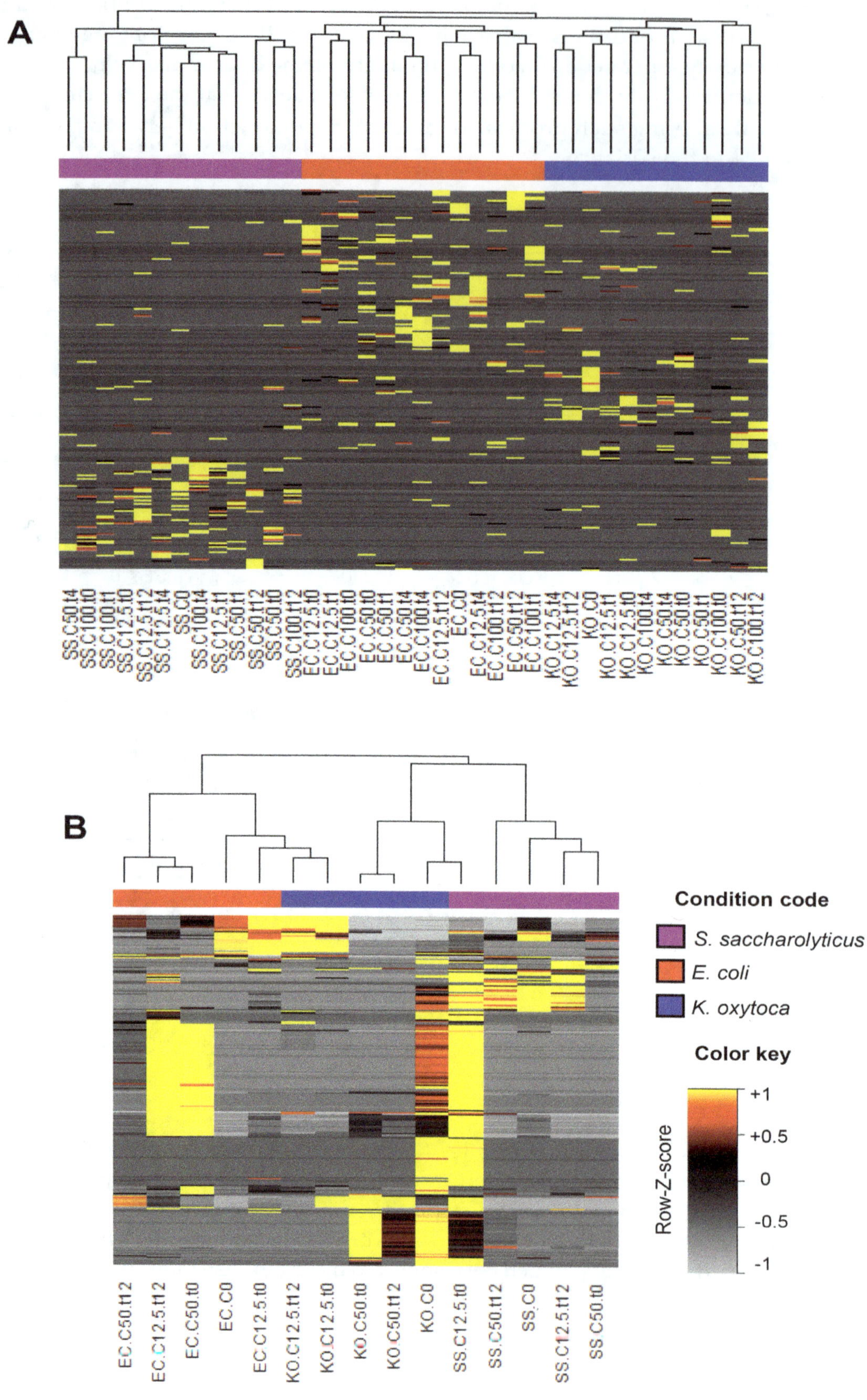

Figure 4. Heatmaps and hierarchical cluster analysis of protein ions (**A**) and volatile organic compound (VOC) profiles (**B**), based on ion areas extracted from MALDI-TOF MS spectra and GC-MS chromatograms, respectively; Horizontal axis = conducted assays, using different bacterial strains, vertical axis = ions organized in clusters.

In order to objectively quantify the overall changes in MALDI-TOF MS spectra after the addition of nanoparticles, the SSS parameter was assessed. The average SSSs calculated for each experiment are displayed in Figure 5. This parameter mathematically represents the average level of similarity between spectra acquired for unstressed strain and the same strain after supplementation with AgNPs. The clusters on the right side of the matrix are based on Euclidian distance and represent more similar behaviors during assay with nanoparticles.

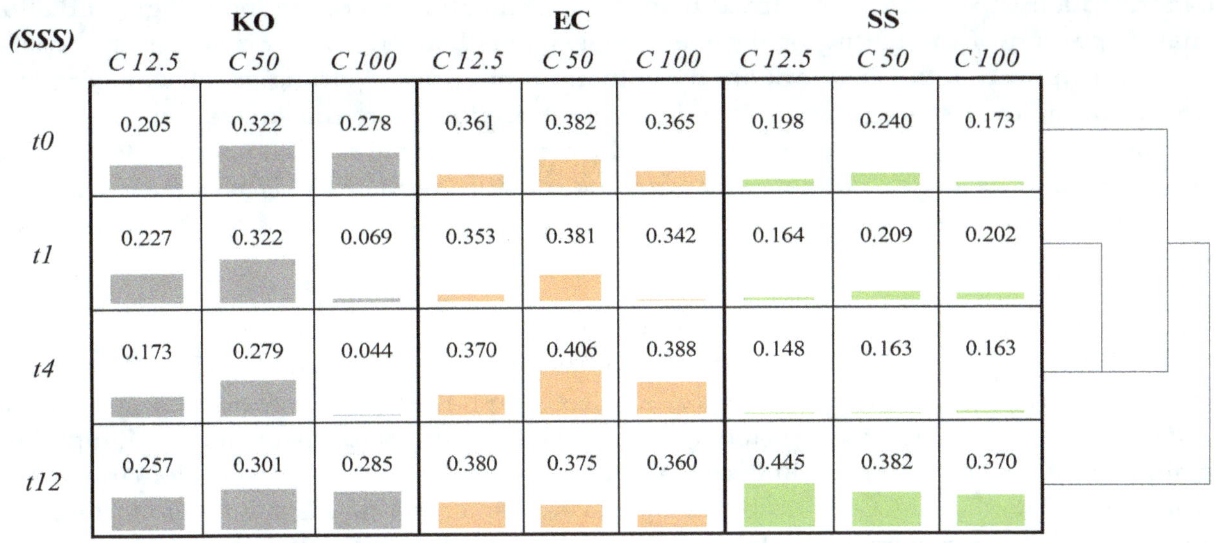

Figure 5. Matrix presenting average values of spectra similarity score (SSS), concerning comparison between unstressed spectrum and assays using silver nanoparticles (AgNPs) at 12.5, 50, and 100 μg mL^{-1}, for periods of time 0, 1, 4, and 12 h. Gray, orange, and green bars refer to *K. oxytoca* (KO), *S. saccharolyticus* (SS), and *E. coli* (EC), respectively; C—concentration (μg mL^{-1}); t—time (h).

For *K. oxytoca*, it can be seen that for concentration 100 μg mL^{-1}, the biggest changes in profiles were obtained for 1 and 4 h after supplementation with AgNPs. After 12 h, an adaptation to the stressing agent is observable resulting in an increased spectrum similarity score to the original native strain. For lower concentrations (12.5 and 50 μg mL^{-1}), *K. oxytoca* manifested stronger resistance to applied silver nanoparticles. *E. coli* was the most resistant for concentration 50 μg mL^{-1}, bigger alternations were noticed for the remaining concentrations. On the other hand, *S. saccharolyticus* appeared to be the most susceptible to added AgNPs. This strain reacted the most in the first hours after supplementation of silver nanoparticles. The strain showed tolerance to stressing agent only after 12 h of influence, regardless of the used concentration. In a general view, the apex of interaction of AgNPs with intercellular portion can be addressed as the higher studied concentration (100 μg mL^{-1}), associated to the incubation time of 4 h for *K. oxytoca* and *S. saccharolyticus* and 1 h for *E. coli*. Once 12 h of incubation was reached, an overall tendency to return to the untreated-like profile is observed for all strains.

With the aim to investigate how the alterations produced in profiles of bacterial proteins are reflected in the VOCs distribution, canonical correlation analysis (CCA) and direct correlation analysis using the Pearson method were conducted. The results are showed in Figure 6. The CCA plot (Figure 6A), along its CCA1 and CCA2 axes, was able to explain 37.71% of the variance of a matrix combining MALDI-TOF MS and GC-MS data. This observation points out the possible relation between VOCs emitted by bacteria and their pattern of small proteins. Although it can be understood that this fraction of proteins is not the only factor governing VOCs production, some particular ions seemed to be closely related to the detected volatiles, regardless of the studied strain. In this plot, length and angle of arrows are related to the contribution of a certain variable to the axes. Variables not accompanied by arrows displayed much weaker influence score than others, not being depicted in the automatically scaled graph. The compounds that presented to be the most affected by bacterial ribosomes were dimethyl disulfide, 2-heptanone, 2-undecanol, dimethyl trisulfide, 3-methyl-1-butanol, 1-nonanol, and 2-tetradecanol. While dimethyl disulfide, 2-heptanone, and 1-nonanol can be interpreted as having correlated behavior between them in the three studied bacteria, hexanal and 2-tetradecanol, for example, demonstrated a much more diverse trend than the aforementioned compounds. Figure 6B allows a visual inspection of the nature of the main connections between the two classes of variables. Variables not showed in this network are those that did not present strong or relevant correlation and, in contrast to the last approach, only individual interactions were considered. Interdependency relationships can be also examined: according to the network analysis, the compounds 2-heptanone, 3-methyl-1-butanol, 3-methylbutanoic acid, and dodecanal have their levels associated with many different related proteins—from this, it can be concluded that their expression is associated with intricate factors.

With basis on what was demonstrated concerning the strong correlations between emitted VOCs and protein ions, it was assumed that the levels of such VOCs could provide indirect information about effectiveness of interaction of the bactericidal agent and colonizing bacteria. This approach has potential usefulness in the monitoring of therapeutic response to antimicrobial treatment. Multiple linear regression analysis was conducted in order to create a model based on VOCs as biomarkers of the extension of AgNPs interaction with bacteria. Level of interaction was used as criterion, using 100-SSS*100 as parameter, since it is related to the percentage of modification of unstressed bacterial spectra. VOCs' responses common to all strains were employed as predictors. As a result, Equation (1) was obtained, with R (coefficient of correlation between observed and predicted values) = 0.89, adjusted R square = 0.79, and standard error of estimate = ±4.10. Such parameters indicate good precision of the generated model:

$$\begin{aligned} \%\text{ of agent effectiveness} &= 42.9 + 1.6 \times 10^{-5} \times A_{\text{dimethyl disulfide}} \\ &- 2.8 \times 10^{-7} \times A_{\text{dimethyl trisulfide}} + 5.3 \times 10^{-6} \times A_{\text{2-heptanone}} - 2.9 \times 10^{-8} \times A_{\text{dodecanal}}. \end{aligned} \quad (1)$$

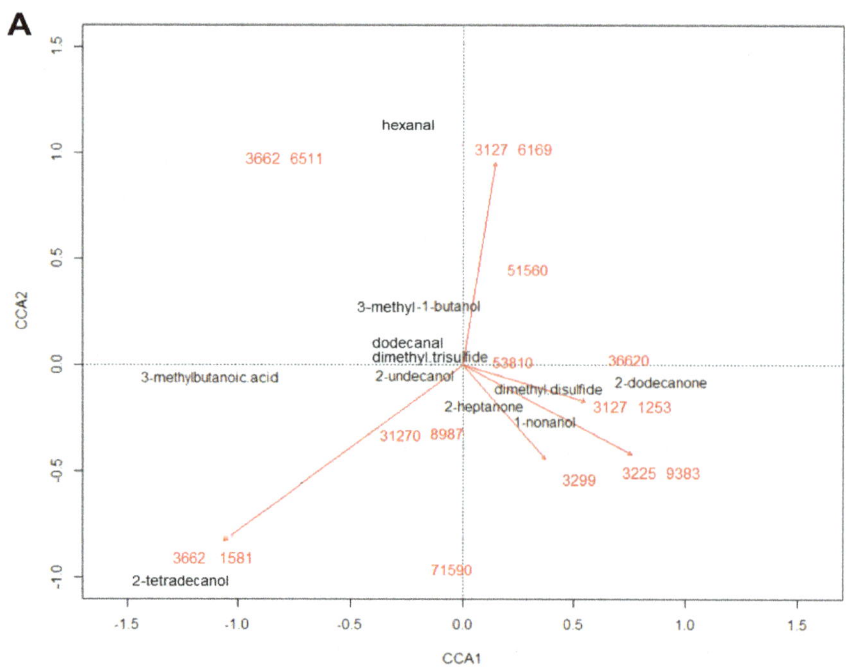

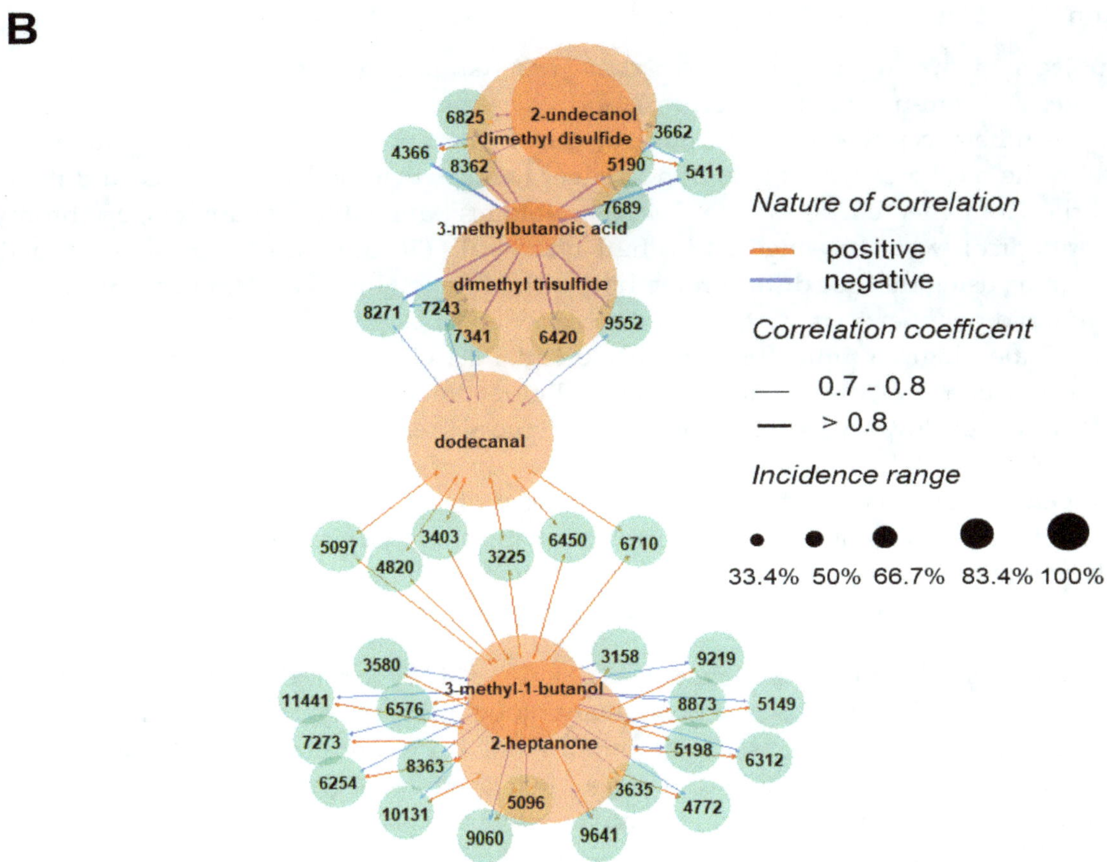

Figure 6. (**A**) Canonical correlation analysis (CCA) biplot showing the correspondence of the main protein ions (red) with emitted VOCs (black), where CCA1 = 22.43% and CCA2 = 15.28%; (**B**) Correlation network depicting main relevant connections (rho ≥ [0.7]) between MALDI-TOF MS ions and identified volatiles.

4. Discussion

The subjects of our work were: *Escherichia coli* (Gram-negative bacterium) and salivary *Klebsiella oxytoca* (Gram-negative bacterium) and *Staphylococcus saccharolyticus* (Gram-positive bacterium). The differences between cell wall structure of Gram-positive and Gram-negative bacteria are essential in the mechanism of interaction of silver nanoparticles with the surface and the inner part of bacteria. Combined effects of AgNPs and antibiotics (ampicillin, kanamycin, erythromycin, and chloramphenicol) were investigated in the Fayaz et al. (2010) study for bactericidal activity against test strains using the disc diffusion method with Mueller Hinton agar plates [36]. In another work, silver colloid nanoparticles synthesized by reduction of $[Ag(NH_3)_2]^+$ complex cation by four saccharides revealed high antimicrobial and bactericidal activity against both Gram-positive and Gram-negative bacteria, including *E. coli* and methicillin-resistant *S. aureus*. Authors claimed that the size of particles and very low concentration of silver are crucial to exhibit bactericidal properties of these nanoparticles [37]. In Krishna et al. (2015), antibacterial activity of silver nanoparticles was tested against the two pathogenic strains *Salmonella typhi* and *Salmonella paratyphi* by well-diffusion method. Complex of AgNPs-ofloxacin demonstrated the augmented effect in comparison to separated components [38]. The example of work showing superiority of Gram-positive bacteria over Gram-negative ones in the meaning of resistance against AgNPs is described by Fayaz et al. (2010).

The tested bacteria from this study were two Gram-positive cocci and two Gram-negative rods, including *E. coli*. The antibacterial activity for all antibiotics (especially ampicillin) increased in the presence of AgNPs against test strains. The minimum inhibitory concentration (MIC) evaluated for synergistic effect of AgNPs and antibiotics showed increased less significant influence on growth of Gram-positive bacteria than on Gram-negative species. Cell wall of Gram-positive bacteria is characterized by a thick peptidoglycan layer (~20–80 nm), whereas in Gram-negative bacteria, the peptidoglycan layer is thinner (~7–8 nm) and sandwiched between two layers of periplasmic space and covered by an outer membrane composed by liposaccharides (LPSs) portion. The Gram-negative wall is considered as more susceptible than the Gram-positive one, because the negative charges liposaccharides are attracted toward the positive relative charge available on silver nanoparticles. Moreover, Fayaz et al. (2010) described also negatively charged AgNPs which can attack this type of bacteria by metal depletion [36]. It was found that *E. coli* cells are more prone to increased permeability after ethylenediaminetetraacetate disodium (EDTA) treatment. Liberation of LPS molecules from outer cell membrane are caused by higher metal depletion which weakens maintaining the assembly of the LPSs in membrane [39]. On the contrary, Gram-positive bacteria with thicker layer of peptidoglycan are more resistant to AgNPs because of hindered penetration of nanoparticles and fewer anchoring points for the AgNPs. The layer is highly composed of rigid structure of linear polysaccharide cross-linked by short peptides [36]. The AgNPs-ampicillin complex prevents unwinding of cellular DNA by preferential binding of silver atoms with cells' DNA [40].

Our work showed that Gram-positive *S. saccharolyticus* was the most resistant strain at all tested AgNPs levels against the remaining Gram-negative ones, when the highest incubation time (12 h) is considered (Figure 5). However, at shorter incubation times *E. coli* and *K. oxytoca* appeared to be more insusceptible for AgNPs influence as reflected in protein profiles acquired by MALDI-TOF MS. After 12 h, bacterial strains exhibited behavior more similar to unstressed ones, deprived of the effect of nanoparticles. Another observation was the fact that both Gram-negative bacteria were more resistant at medium concentration (50 $\mu g\ mL^{-1}$) of AgNPs. Such remark was not noticed for *S. saccharolyticus* strain, making this bacterium more distinctive. In recent work of Al-Sharqi et al. (2019), authors investigated antibacterial efficiencies of photoactivated and not-enhanced AgNPs against *E. coli* and *S. aureus*. Cells not treated with silver nanoparticles served as controls. The results for unmodified *E. coli* show that after 24 h of treatment with 12.5 $\mu g\ mL^{-1}$ AgNPs, bacterial growth was observed to be 93.33% ± 2.88%. Along with increasing concentration of AgNPs, the microbial number decreased significantly reaching the lowest value of survival viability in the level of 76% ± 1.73% for 100 μg mL^{-1} [41]. Our work confirms that with long time of incubation, *E. coli* is more susceptible for AgNPs influence with increasing level of added stressing agent, from 12.5 to 100 μg mL^{-1}.

Protein patterns were processed to obtain heatmap and hierarchical cluster analysis (Figure 4A) that allowed to distinguish three separate clusters belonging to each bacterial strain. It proves effectiveness and appropriateness of the conducted research and shows potential applicability in differentiation purposes. Using lysozyme-stabilized silver nanoparticles, Ashraf et al. (2014) were able to differentiate some of the strains (two *Salmonella enterica*, two *Klebsiella pneumoniae*, four *P. aeruginosa*, two *E. coli*) within the same bacterial species based upon the difference of their antimicrobial activity [42].

The bactericidal effect of silver nanoparticles consists in several mechanisms; (1) AgNPs can adhere onto the surface of cell wall, resulting in membrane damage and altered transport activity [43]. Penetration of cell membrane causes the increased permeability and death of the cell [44]. The damage to membranes is the result of the formation of irregular-shaped pits in the cell surface due to release of LPS molecules [39,45]. (2) Anchoring of silver to cell membrane also inhibits cell wall formation [44,46]. (3) AgNPs modulate cellular signal system and induce oxidative stress caused by generation of reactive oxygen species (ROS) and free radicals [46]. These free radicals can increase porosity of the cell membrane, leading to damage and cell death [44]. (4) AgNPs can be the source of silver ions released by themselves. These Ag^{+} are able to react with thiol groups of enzymes and proteins causing inactivation of them [44,45]. (5) Silver nanoparticles tend to react also with phosphorus-containing compounds such as DNA and prevent its replication as well as cell division and respiratory chain processes [44,45,47]. (6) AgNPs modulate cellular signaling by dephosphorylation of protein substrates in bacteria, resulting in inhibition of cell growth [48]. Finally, changes in nucleoid of bacteria are leading to DNA fragmentation, cell cycle arrest, apoptosis, and inflammatory response [49]. Silver nanoparticles are characterized by many physico-chemical parameters affecting their antimicrobial effectiveness, such as shape, size, concentration, particle dispersion state, and surface charge [43,49].

MALDI-TOF MS technique is often used to identify bacterial strains in timesaving manner and pure culture isolation, such as model organism *E. coli* [50] and other Gram-positive, Gram-negative, anaerobic bacteria and mycobacteria [51,52]. In our work, we applied MALDI-TOF MS technique to obtain protein profiles of bacteria after treatment with silver nanoparticles. In the work of Lok et al. (2006), proteomic analyzes using two-dimensional gel electrophoresis (2-DE) and MS identification revealed that short exposure of *E. coli* cells to AgNPs resulted in alterations in the expressions of a panel of envelope proteins and heat shock proteins (like 30S ribosomal subunit S6) [50]. Twenty protein patterns were identified by MALDI-TOF MS technique from the set of recombinant, human cDNA expression products, together with native proteins isolated from crude mouse brain extracts [53]. Peptide mass fingerprint (PMF) searching of databases appeared to be a cost-effective solution for protein identification purposes. Sixty-two proteins in unsequenced parasitic nematodes were identified by MALDI-TOF MS after evaluation of expressed sequence tag (EST) datasets [54]. This technique was also used, for example, to characterize proteomic patterns in serum from ovarian cancer and healthy control group [55].

MALDI-TOF MS was a suitable technique to investigate binding bare and carbonate-coated AgNPs to the purified tryptophanase (TNase) fragments from *E. coli* to characterize the effect of surface modifications on the binding. It was showed that binding of the protein to AgNPs may sterically block access to the active site caused by lost enzymatic activity of TNase [56]. Using MALDI mass spectra, authors could evaluate the TNase' enhanced affinity for AgNPs, similarly to our present experiments with protein patterns. Metabolic alterations in bacteria after supplementation with nanoparticles were the subject of interest in the study of Gopal et al. (2013) [57]. They examined the interaction of five types of nanoparticles (Ag, NiO, Pt, TiO_2, and ZnO) with *P. aeruginosa* and *S. aureus* and postulated two mechanisms of interaction of the above-mentioned NPs with these two pathogenic bacterial strains. The approach consisting in addition of AgNPs at 0 h of bacterial growth, and incubation with bacteria when they grow in the medium, enabled effective interaction of *P. aeruginosa* with unmodified NPs. For *S. aureus*, NPs were added to fully grown bacterial cultures and incubated—a method similar to the one used in our work. In this case, in MALDI-MS spectra, many bacterial peaks were observed. The changes of proteomic profiles were also the object of the researcher interest in the work of He et al. [58]. They carried out the proteomic analysis of graphene-based silver nanoparticles (AgNPs–GE) together with silver nitrate on *P. aeruginosa*. MALDI–TOF/TOF MS was used to identify proteins from bacteria as outcome of 2-DE experiments with silver agents. Authors discovered seven proteins being induced and nine proteins being suppressed by AgNPs–GE.

The effect of the addition of silver nanoparticles on the *S. aureus* strain was again studied in the work of Chudobova et al. (2013) [59]. These researchers conducted a basic characterization of this strain and found out that AgNPs caused considerable inhibition of the growth of *S. aureus*. The authors proposed two methods for determination of silver nanoparticles inhibition effect: using the growth curves and measurements of inhibition zones. Protein fingerprints for the identification of untreated and silver-supplemented *S. aureus* were obtained by MALDI/TOF mass spectra. The usage of the MALDI-TOF MS technique was extended in the more recent work of Chudobova et al. (2015), dedicated to *S. aureus* strain [60]. They focused on examination of the influence of selected heavy metal ions (Ag^+, Cu^{2+}, Cd^{2+}, Zn^{2+}, and Pb^{2+}) at several concentration levels using biochemical methods and mass spectrometry. Additional peaks in silver-fortified bacteria were found in the obtained MALDI-TOF MS spectra demonstrating modifications at the protein level.

The above-mentioned studies are clear examples of how silver ions or nanoparticles may affect the metabolic and proteomic profiles of bacteria, changes in which are visible using the MALDI MS technique. In the present work, a new approach was introduced: MALDI MS and GC-MS data were processed and correlated using statistical methods that allowed to characterize patterns of small proteins and volatile metabolites associated with the interaction of nanoparticles with bacteria.

Once it was demonstrated that VOC profiles are able to reflect metabolic alterations in bacterial cells, the effective changes in the response of detected volatiles were evaluated. Figure 7 shows VOCs presenting statistically relevant ($p < 0.05$) difference in their distribution when varying amounts of AgNPs were added to the bacterial culture. It is reasonable to assume that the consequences of the presence of nanoparticles in the medium can vary depending on the examined microorganism. For example, after AgNPs addition, dimethyl disulfide levels increased for *K. oxytoca*, and decreased for the other two bacteria; for dimethyl trisulfide, the other sulfur containing metabolite, an opposite trend is observed.

Bacterial strain		**KO**		**EC**		**SS**	
Main related pathways	**VOC**	**C 12.5**	**C 50**	**C 12.5**	**C 50**	**C 12.5**	**C 50**
Pyruvate metabolism, Glycolysis or Gluconeogenesis	acetic acid	**pr**	**pr**	**ab**	**ab**	*ns*	*ns*
Ehrlich pathway (aminoacid metabolism)	3-methylbutanoic acid	-1.1	**ab**	*ns*	*ns*	*ns*	*ns*
	3-methyl-1-butanol	+0.8	+1.8	-0.5	-1.1	**ab**	**ab**
Metabolism of sulfur containing aminoacids	dimethyl disulfide	+3.8	+4.0	-1.2	-1.2	-1.2	-0.9
	dimethyl trisulfide	-4.1	-0.9	+0.2	+4.2	+2.8	+3.3
Fatty alcohols formation (fatty acids biosynthesis)	1-nonanol	+1.3	+4.0	*ns*	*ns*	-1.4	-3.0
Sencodary alcohols formation (fatty acids biosynthesis)	2-undecanol	-4.7	-5.7	+1.0	+1.8	-1.4	**ab**
	2-tetradecanol	**ab**	-1.6	*ns*	*ns*	*ns*	*ns*
Methyl ketones formation (fatty acids biosynthesis)	2-heptanone	-4.1	-3.9	-0.4	+2.0	-4.8	-5.0
	2-octanone	**ab**	**ab**	*ns*	*ns*	*ns*	*ns*
	2-dodecanone	**ab**	*ns*	+1.2	-3.1	-5.2	*ns*
Fatty aldehydes formation (fatty acids biosynthesis), Lipid peroxidation	hexanal	-5.7	**ab**	-7.1	**ab**	*ns*	*ns*
	dodecanal	+0.5	+4.4	+1.0	**ab**	*ns*	+4.4

Figure 7. Combination of charts showing altered VOCs and addressed bacterial metabolic pathways, where numbers inside boxes display the base 2 logarithm of fold-change calculated with respect to the response in untreated strain; pr = produced only after AgNPs addition, ab = absent after AgNPs addition, ns = not significant alteration ($p > 0.05$), KO—*K. oxytoca*, EC—*E. coli*, SS—*S. saccharolyticus*, C—concentration (μg mL^{-1}), VOC—volatile organic compound [61].

The origin of volatiles released by three investigated bacteria is mainly a modification of products of the fatty acid biosynthetic pathway, like hydrocarbons, alcohols, and ketones (Figure 8) [61].

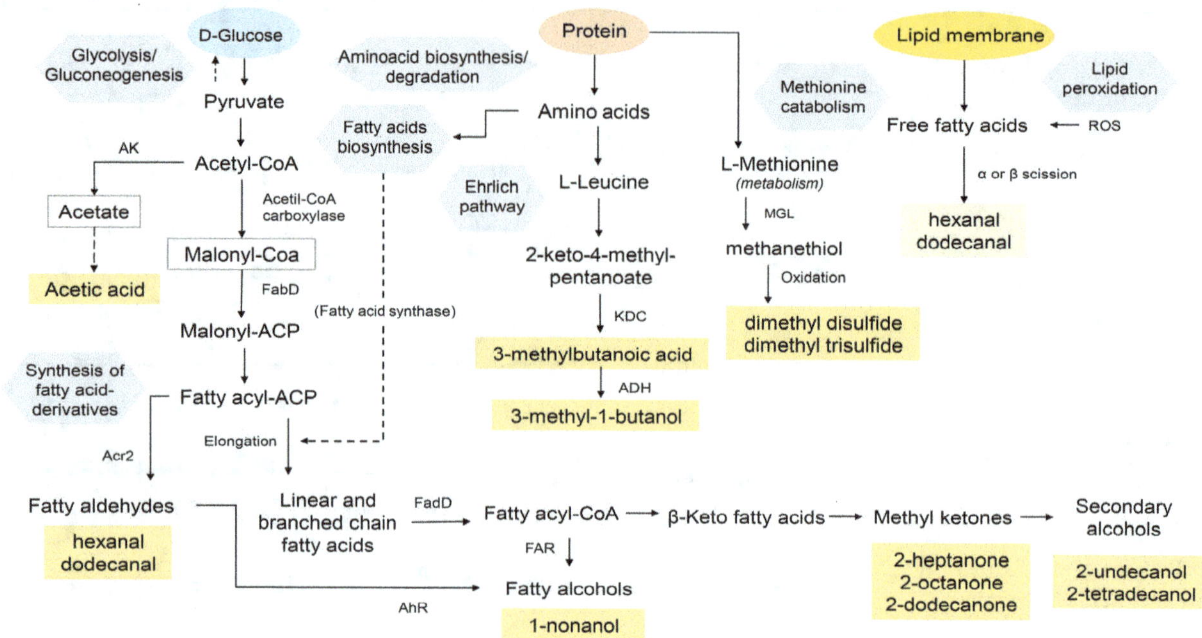

Figure 8. Scheme showing main pathways related to volatile organic metabolites which presented relevant alterations in their responses due to nanoparticles supplementation (AK—acetate kinase; KDC—2-keto acid decarboxylase; ADH—alcohol dehydrogenase; FAR—fatty acid reductase; FabD—malonyl-CoA:ACP transacylase; FadD—fatty acyl-CoA synthase; AhR—aryl hydrocarbon receptor; Acr2—acyl-CoA reductase; MGL—methionine-γ-lyase; ROS—reactive oxygen species).

Volatile organic compounds secreted from *E. coli* were the object of interest of several researchers who used multiple techniques to investigate the headspace of bacteria. Tait et al. (2014) [62] performed optimization of conditions of HS-SPME-GC-MS analysis of *E. coli* VOCs and evaluated the effect of a culture medium type, SPME fiber type, and the employed GC column on the obtained results. Furthermore, volatile profiles of *E. coli* were investigated in the work of Umber et al. (2013) [63] who found elevated levels of such compounds as: dimethyl disulfide, dimethyl trisulfide, and 1-propanol in the headspace of bacteria in LB broth. These volatiles were not observed in chromatograms obtained from *E. coli*/blood mixture. In our research, we detected these three compounds both in the untreated and AgNPs-supplemented strain of *E. coli*.

VOCs from *K. oxytoca* and other species were studied using ion-molecule reaction–mass spectrometry (IMR-MS) by Dolch et al. (2012) [64]. This method allowed to conduct a short analysis time of 3 min per vial and showed the possibility of process automation. For identification of human pathogenic bacteria (like *E. coli* and *K. oxytoca*), Jünger et al. 2012 used multi-capillary column–ion mobility spectrometry (MCC-IMS). Comparisons of volatilomes were confirmed by thermal desorption–gas chromatography–mass spectrometry (TD-GC-MS). VOC patterns from bacteria enabled fast and cost-effective discrimination of investigated pathogens [65]. Another technique employed for volatile extraction from *E. coli*, *K. oxytoca*, and *P. aeruginosa* was a static head-space-sampler (SHS) coupled to a sensory perception system (SPS). Carrillo and Durán 2019 used this method for distinguish polluted water samples after statistical approaches such as pattern recognition techniques [66].

S. saccharolyticus is a bacterial strain responsible for, inter alia, the production of volatile compounds in spoilt mango fruits. GC-MS analyzes revealed the presence of eleven and sixteen volatile organic constituents in healthy and spoilt ripe mango fruits, respectively [67]. There are no other studies concerning volatile profiling of *S. saccharolyticus*. In recent work of Brüggemann et al. (2019),

S. saccharolyticus isolates from blood cultures and prosthetic joint infection specimens were detected and their genomes were sequenced and analyzed. They found that the closest relative of *S. saccharolyticus* is *Staphylococcus capitis* with an average nucleotide identity of 80%. Moreover, *S. saccharolyticus* manifests host tissue-invasive potential and is associated with prosthetic joint infections [68].

5. Conclusions

The reported results confirm that the MALDI-TOF MS technique is an appropriate tool for investigating the influence of silver nanoparticles on metabolism of selected bacterial strains. The comparison between spectra acquired from untreated and silver-enhanced bacteria revealed that addition of AgNPs led to significant changes in their metabolic profiles. Such metabolic alterations were attested by distinguished variations in the emitted bacterial metabolites assessed using GC-MS.

It was demonstrated that interaction between AgNPs and bacteria is deeply associated to the concentration of nanoparticles, incubation time, and strain nature, considerations to be evaluated for the employment of such species as bactericidal agent in medical practice.

Statistical approaches performed in this work reinforced the relation between ribosomal profiles and strain identity, besides that, combination between the variation in protein ion data and VOC patterns allowed the observation of alterations in bacterial inner part closely related with produced volatile metabolites.

Moreover, it can be concluded that the usage of molecular profiles is a promising tool in monitoring of bactericidal performance during infection treatment and to investigate the associated biochemical mechanisms.

Author Contributions: Conceptualization, F.M. and P.P.; Methodology, F.M. and P.P.; Software, F.M. and M.M.; Validation, F.M., P.P. and M.M.; Formal analysis, F.M., P.P. and M.M.; Investigation, F.M. and P.P.; Resources, F.M. and P.P.; Data curation, F.M.; Writing—Original draft preparation, F.M., P.P. and M.M.; Writing—Review and editing, T.L. and B.B.; Visualization, F.M. and M.M.; Supervision, T.L. and B.B.; Project administration, B.B.; Funding acquisition, P.P.

References

1. Ahamed, M.; AlSalhi, M.S.; Siddiqui, M.K.J. Silver nanoparticle applications and human health. *Clin. Chim. Acta* **2010**, *411*, 1841–1848. [CrossRef] [PubMed]
2. León-Silva, S.; Fernández-Luqueño, F.; López-Valdez, F. Silver Nanoparticles (AgNP) in the Environment: A Review of Potential Risks on Human and Environmental Health. *Water Air Soil Pollut.* **2016**, *227*, 306. [CrossRef]
3. Quinteros, M.A.; Cano Aristizábal, V.; Dalmasso, P.R.; Paraje, M.G.; Páez, P.L. Oxidative stress generation of silver nanoparticles in three bacterial genera and its relationship with the antimicrobial activity. *Toxicol. Vitr.* **2016**, *36*, 216–223. [CrossRef] [PubMed]
4. Durán, N.; Durán, M.; de Jesus, M.B.; Seabra, A.B.; Fávaro, W.J.; Nakazato, G. Silver nanoparticles: A new view on mechanistic aspects on antimicrobial activity. *Nanomed. Nanotechnol. Biol. Med.* **2016**, *12*, 789–799. [CrossRef] [PubMed]
5. Saxena, J.; Sharma, P.K.; Sharma, M.M.; Singh, A. Process optimization for green synthesis of silver nanoparticles by Sclerotinia sclerotiorum MTCC 8785 and evaluation of its antibacterial properties. *Springerplus* **2016**, *5*, 861. [CrossRef]
6. Krishnaraj, C.; Ji, B.J.; Harper, S.L.; Yun, S. Il Plant extract-mediated biogenic synthesis of silver, manganese dioxide, silver-doped manganese dioxide nanoparticles and their antibacterial activity against food- and water-borne pathogens. *Bioprocess Biosyst. Eng.* **2016**, *39*, 759–772. [CrossRef]
7. Aazam, E.S.; Zaheer, Z. Growth of Ag-nanoparticles in an aqueous solution and their antimicrobial activities against Gram positive, Gram negative bacterial strains and Candida fungus. *Bioprocess Biosyst. Eng.* **2016**, *39*, 575–584. [CrossRef]
8. Hong, W.; Li, L.; Liang, J.; Wang, J.; Wang, X.; Xu, S.; Wu, L.; Zhao, G.; Xu, A.; Chen, S. Investigating the

environmental factors affecting the toxicity of silver nanoparticles in Escherichia coli with dual fluorescence analysis. *Chemosphere* **2016**, *155*, 329–335. [CrossRef]

9. Railean-Plugaru, V.; Pomastowski, P.; Rafinska, K.; Wypij, M.; Kupczyk, W.; Dahm, H.; Jackowski, M.; Buszewski, B. Antimicrobial properties of biosynthesized silver nanoparticles studied by flow cytometry and related techniques. *Electrophoresis* **2016**, *37*, 752–761. [CrossRef]
10. Singhal, N.; Kumar, M.; Kanaujia, P.K.; Virdi, J.S. MALDI-TOF mass spectrometry: An emerging technology for microbial identification and diagnosis. *Front. Microbiol.* **2015**, *6*, 791. [CrossRef]
11. Rahi, P.; Prakash, O.; Shouche, Y.S. Matrix-assisted laser desorption/ionization time-of-flight mass-spectrometry (MALDI-TOF MS) based microbial identifications: Challenges and scopes for microbial ecologists. *Front. Microbiol.* **2016**, *7*, 1359. [CrossRef] [PubMed]
12. Yari, S.; Tasbiti, A.H.; Ghanei, M.; Shokrgozar, M.A.; Vaziri, B.; Mahdian, R.; Yari, F.; Bahrmand, A. Proteomic analysis of sensitive and multi drug resistant Mycobacterium tuberculosis strains. *Microbiology* **2016**, *85*, 350–358. [CrossRef]
13. Gopal, J.; Wu, H.F.; Lee, C.H. The bifunctional role of Ag nanoparticles on bacteria—A MALDI-MS perspective. *Analyst* **2011**, *136*, 5077–5083. [CrossRef] [PubMed]
14. Lima, D.P.; Diniz, D.G.; Moimaz, S.A.S.; Sumida, D.H.; Okamoto, A.C. Saliva: Reflection of the body. *Int. J. Infect. Dis.* **2010**, *14*, 184–188. [CrossRef] [PubMed]
15. Lee, Y.H.; Wong, D.T. Saliva: An emerging biofluid for early detection of diseases. *Am. J. Dent.* **2009**, *22*, 241–248. [PubMed]
16. Chiappin, S.; Antonelli, G.; Gatti, R.; De Palo, E.F. Saliva specimen: A new laboratory tool for diagnostic and basic investigation. *Clin. Chim. Acta* **2007**, *383*, 30–40. [CrossRef]
17. Milanowski, M.; Pomastowski, P.; Ligor, T.; Buszewski, B. Saliva–Volatile Biomarkers and Profiles. *Crit. Rev. Anal. Chem.* **2017**, *47*, 251–266. [CrossRef]
18. Buszewski, B.; Ulanowska, A.; Ligor, T.; Jackowski, M.; Kłodzińska, E.; Szeliga, J. Identification of volatile organic compounds secreted from cancer tissues and bacterial cultures. *J. Chromatogr. B Anal. Technol. Biomed. Life Sci.* **2008**, *868*, 88–94. [CrossRef]
19. Soini, H.A.; Klouckova, I.; Wiesler, D.; Oberzaucher, E.; Grammer, K.; Dixon, S.J.; Xu, Y.; Brereton, R.G.; Penn, D.J.; Novotny, M.V. Analysis of Volatile Organic Compounds in Human Saliva by a Static Sorptive Extraction Method and Gas Chromatography-Mass Spectrometry. *J. Chem. Ecol.* **2010**, *36*, 1035–1042. [CrossRef]
20. Boots, A.W.; Smolinska, A.; van Berkel, J.J.B.N.; Fijten, R.R.R.; Stobberingh, E.E.; Boumans, M.L.L.; Moonen, E.J.; Wouters, E.F.M.; Dallinga, J.W.; Van Schooten, F.J. Identification of microorganisms based on headspace analysis of volatile organic compounds by gas chromatography–mass spectrometry. *J. Breath Res.* **2014**, *8*, 027106. [CrossRef]
21. Neerincx, A.H.; Geurts, B.P.; Van Loon, J.; Tiemes, V.; Jansen, J.J.; Harren, F.J.M.; Kluijtmans, L.A.J.; Merkus, P.J.F.M.; Cristescu, S.M.; Buydens, L.M.C.; et al. Detection of Staphylococcus aureus in cystic fibrosis patients using breath VOC profiles. *J. Breath Res.* **2016**, *10*, 046014. [CrossRef] [PubMed]
22. Amann, A.; Miekisch, W.; Schubert, J.; Buszewski, B.; Ligor, T.; Jezierski, T.; Pleil, J.; Risby, T. Analysis of Exhaled Breath for Disease Detection. *Ann. Rev. Anal. Chem.* **2014**, *7*, 455–482. [CrossRef] [PubMed]
23. Buszewski, B.; Kęsy, M.; Ligor, T.; Amann, A. Human exhaled air analytics: Biomarkers of diseases. *Biomed. Chromatogr.* **2007**, *21*, 553–566. [CrossRef] [PubMed]
24. Kusano, M.; Mendez, E.; Furton, K.G. Development of headspace SPME method for analysis of volatile organic compounds present in human biological specimens. *Anal. Bioanal. Chem.* **2011**, *400*, 1817–1826. [CrossRef]
25. Kusano, M.; Mendez, E.; Furton, K.G. Comparison of the Volatile Organic Compounds from Different Biological Specimens for Profiling Potential. *J. Forensic Sci.* **2013**, *58*, 29–39. [CrossRef]
26. Brown, J.S.; Prada, P.A.; Curran, A.M.; Furton, K.G. Applicability of emanating volatile organic compounds from various forensic specimens for individual differentiation. *Forensic Sci. Int.* **2013**, *226*, 173–182. [CrossRef]
27. Ratiu, I.A.; Ligor, T.; Bocos-Bintintan, V.; Al-Suod, H.; Kowalkowski, T.; Rafińska, K.; Buszewski, B. The effect of growth medium on an Escherichia coli pathway mirrored into GC/MS profiles. *J. Breath Res.* **2017**, *11*, 036012. [CrossRef]
28. Filipiak, W.; Sponring, A.; Baur, M.M.; Ager, C.; Filipiak, A.; Wiesenhofer, H.; Nagl, M.; Troppmair, J.;

Amann, A. Characterization of volatile metabolites taken up by or released from Streptococcus pneumoniae and Haemophilus influenzae by using GC-MS. *Microbiol (U.K.)* **2012**, *158*, 3044–3053. [CrossRef]

29. Filipiak, W.; Sponring, A.; Baur, M.; Filipiak, A.; Ager, C.; Wiesenhofer, H.; Nagl, M.; Troppmair, J.; Amann, A. Molecular analysis of volatile metabolites released specifically by staphylococcus aureus and pseudomonas aeruginosa. *BMC Microbiol.* **2012**, *12*, 113. [CrossRef]
30. Jo Zimbro, M.; Power, D.A.; Sharon Miller, M.; Wilson, G.E.; Johnson, J.A. *Difco TM & BBL TM Manual of Microbiological Culture*, 2nd ed.; Becton, Dickinson and Company: Sparks, MD, USA, 2009.
31. Railean-Plugaru, V.; Pomastowski, P.; Wypij, M.; Szultka-Mlynska, M.; Rafinska, K.; Golinska, P.; Dahm, H.; Buszewski, B. Study of silver nanoparticles synthesized by acidophilic strain of Actinobacteria isolated from the of Picea sitchensis forest soil. *J. Appl. Microbiol.* **2016**, *120*, 1250–1263. [CrossRef]
32. Buszewski, B.; Milanowski, M.; Ligor, T.; Pomastowski, P. Investigation of bacterial viability from incubated saliva by application of flow cytometry and hyphenated separation techniques. *Electrophoresis* **2017**, *38*, 2081–2088. [CrossRef] [PubMed]
33. Burian, A.; Erdogan, Z.; Jandrisits, C.; Zeitlinger, M. Impact of pH on Activity of Trimethoprim, Fosfomycin, Amikacin, Colistin and Ertapenem in Human Urine. *Pharmacology* **2012**, *90*, 281–287. [CrossRef] [PubMed]
34. Freney, J.; Kloos, W.E.; Hajek, V.; Webster, J.A.; Bes, M.; Brun, Y.; Vernozy-Rozand, C. Recommended minimal standards for description of new staphylococcal species. *Int. J. Syst. Bacteriol.* **1999**, *49*, 489–502. [CrossRef] [PubMed]
35. Knöppel, A.; Knopp, M.; Albrecht, L.M.; Lundin, E.; Lustig, U.; Näsvall, J.; Andersson, D.I. Genetic adaptation to growth under laboratory conditions in Escherichia coli and Salmonella enterica. *Front. Microbiol.* **2018**, *9*, 756. [CrossRef]
36. Fayaz, A.M.; Balaji, K.; Girilal, M.; Yadav, R.; Kalaichelvan, P.T.; Venketesan, R. Biogenic synthesis of silver nanoparticles and their synergistic effect with antibiotics: A study against gram-positive and gram-negative bacteria. *Nanomed. Nanotechnol. Biol. Med.* **2010**, *6*, 103–109. [CrossRef]
37. Panáček, A.; Kvítek, L.; Prucek, R.; Kolář, M.; Večeřová, R.; Pizúrová, N.; Sharma, V.K.; Nevěčná, T.; Zbořil, R. Silver Colloid Nanoparticles: Synthesis, Characterization, and Their Antibacterial Activity. *J. Phys. Chem. B* **2006**, *110*, 16248–16253. [CrossRef]
38. Krishna, G.; Kumar, S.S.; Pranitha, V.; Alha, M.; Charaya, S. Biogenic synthesis of silver nanoparticles and their synergistic effect with antibiotics: A study against Salmonella SP. *Int. J. Pharm. Pharm. Sci.* **2015**, *7*, 84–88.
39. Amro, N.A.; Kotra, L.P.; Wadu-Mesthrige, K.; Bulychev, A.; Mobashery, S.; Liu, G.Y. High-resolution atomic force microscopy studies of the Escherichia coli outer membrane: Structural basis for permeability. *Langmuir* **2000**, *16*, 2789–2796. [CrossRef]
40. Batarseh, K.I. Anomaly and correlation of killing in the therapeutic properties of siliver (I) chelation with glutamic and tartaric acids. *J. Antimicrob. Chemother.* **2004**, *54*, 546–548. [CrossRef]
41. Al-Sharqi, A.; Apun, K.; Vincent, M.; Kanakaraju, D.; Bilung, L.M. Enhancement of the Antibacterial Efficiency of Silver Nanoparticles against Gram-Positive and Gram-Negative Bacteria Using Blue Laser Light. *Int. J. Photoenergy* **2019**, *2019*, 2528490. [CrossRef]
42. Ashraf, S.; Chatha, M.; Ejaz, W.; Janjua, H.; Hussain, I. Lysozyme-coated silver nanoparticles for differentiating bacterial strains on the basis of antibacterial activity. *Nanoscale Res. Lett.* **2014**, *9*, 565. [CrossRef] [PubMed]
43. Dakal, T.C.; Kumar, A.; Majumdar, R.S.; Yadav, V. Mechanistic basis of antimicrobial actions of silver nanoparticles. *Front. Microbiol.* **2016**, *7*, 1831. [CrossRef] [PubMed]
44. Prabhu, S.; Poulose, E.K. Silver nanoparticles: Mechanism of antimicrobial action, synthesis, medical applications, and toxicity effects. *Int. Nano Lett.* **2012**, *2*, 32. [CrossRef]
45. Sondi, I.; Salopek-Sondi, B. Silver nanoparticles as antimicrobial agent: A case study on E. coli as a model for Gram-negative bacteria. *J. Colloid Interface Sci.* **2004**, *275*, 177–182. [CrossRef]
46. Gumel, A.M.; Surayya, M.M.; Yaro, M.N.; Waziri, I.Z.; Amina, A.A. Biogenic synthesis of silver nanoparticles and its synergistic antimicrobial potency: An overview. *J. Appl. Biotechnol. Bioeng.* **2019**, *6*, 22–28.
47. Morones, J.R.; Elechiguerra, J.L.; Camacho, A.; Holt, K.; Kouri, J.B.; Ramírez, J.T.; Yacaman, M.J. The bactericidal effect of silver nanoparticles. *Nanotechnology* **2005**, *16*, 2346–2353. [CrossRef]
48. Shrivastava, S.; Bera, T.; Roy, A.; Singh, G.; Ramachandrarao, P.; Dash, D. Characterization of enhanced antibacterial effects of novel silver nanoparticles. *Nanotechnology* **2007**, *18*, 225103. [CrossRef]

49. Liao, C.; Li, Y.; Tjong, S. Bactericidal and Cytotoxic Properties of Silver Nanoparticles. *Int. J. Mol. Sci.* **2019**, *20*, 449. [CrossRef]
50. Lok, C.N.; Ho, C.M.; Chen, R.; He, Q.Y.; Yu, W.Y.; Sun, H.; Tam, P.K.H.; Chiu, J.F.; Che, C.M. Proteomic analysis of the mode of antibacterial action of silver nanoparticles. *J. Proteome Res.* **2006**, *5*, 916–924. [CrossRef]
51. Siller-Ruiz, M.; Hernández-Egido, S.; Sánchez-Juanes, F.; González-Buitrago, J.M.; Muñoz-Bellido, J.L. Fast methods of fungal and bacterial identification. MALDI-TOF mass spectrometry, chromogenic media. *Enferm. Infecc. Microbiol. Clin. (Engl. Ed.)* **2017**, *35*, 303–313. [CrossRef]
52. Yang, Y.; Lin, Y.; Qiao, L. Direct MALDI-TOF MS Identification of Bacterial Mixtures. *Anal. Chem.* **2018**, *90*, 10400–10408. [CrossRef] [PubMed]
53. Egelhofer, V.; Büssow, K.; Luebbert, C.; Lehrach, H.; Nordhoff, E. Improvements in protein identification by MALDI-TOF-MS peptide mapping. *Anal. Chem.* **2000**, *72*, 2741–2750. [CrossRef] [PubMed]
54. Millares, P.; LaCourse, E.J.; Perally, S.; Ward, D.A.; Prescott, M.C.; Hodgkinson, J.E.; Brophy, P.M.; Rees, H.H. Proteomic profiling and protein identification by MALDI-TOF mass spectrometry in unsequenced parasitic nematodes. *PLoS ONE* **2012**, *7*, e33590. [CrossRef] [PubMed]
55. Swiatly, A.; Horala, A.; Hajduk, J.; Matysiak, J.; Nowak-Markwitz, E.; Kokot, Z.J. MALDI-TOF-MS analysis in discovery and identification of serum proteomic patterns of ovarian cancer. *BMC Cancer* **2017**, *17*, 1–9. [CrossRef] [PubMed]
56. Wigginton, N.S.; De Titta, A.; Piccapietra, F.; Dobias, J.A.N.; Nesatyy, V.J.; Suter, M.J.F.; Bernier-Latmani, R. Binding of silver nanoparticles to bacterial proteins depends on surface modifications and inhibits enzymatic activity. *Environ. Sci. Technol.* **2010**, *44*, 2163–2168. [CrossRef] [PubMed]
57. Gopal, J.; Manikandan, M.; Hasan, N.; Lee, C.-H.; Wu, H.-F. A comparative study on the mode of interaction of different nanoparticles during MALDI-MS of bacterial cells. *J. Mass Spectrom.* **2013**, *48*, 119–127. [CrossRef]
58. He, T.; Liu, H.; Zhou, Y.; Yang, J.; Cheng, X.; Shi, H. Antibacterial effect and proteomic analysis of graphene-based silver nanoparticles on a pathogenic bacterium Pseudomonas aeruginosa. *BioMetals* **2014**, *27*, 673–682. [CrossRef]
59. Chudobova, D.; Maskova, D.; Nejdl, L.; Kopel, P.; Rodrigo, M.A.M.; Adam, V.; Kizek, R. The effect of silver ions and silver nanoparticles on Staphylococcus aureus. *Microb. Pathog. Strateg. Combat. Sci. Technol. Educ.* **2013**, *1*, 728–735.
60. Chudobova, D.; Dostalova, S.; Ruttkay-Nedecky, B.; Guran, R.; Rodrigo, M.A.M.; Tmejova, K.; Krizkova, S.; Zitka, O.; Adam, V.; Kizek, R. The effect of metal ions on Staphylococcus aureus revealed by biochemical and mass spectrometric analyses. *Microbiol. Res.* **2015**, *170*, 147–156. [CrossRef]
61. Schulz, S.; Dickschat, J.S. Bacterial volatiles: The smell of small organisms. *Nat. Prod. Rep.* **2007**, *24*, 814–842. [CrossRef]
62. Tait, E.; Perry, J.D.; Stanforth, S.P.; Dean, J.R. Identification of volatile organic compounds produced by bacteria using HS-SPME-GC-MS. *J. Chromatogr. Sci.* **2014**, *52*, 363–373. [CrossRef] [PubMed]
63. Umber, B.J.; Shin, H.-W.; Meinardi, S.; Leu, S.-Y.; Zaldivar, F.; Cooper, D.M.; Blake, D.R. Gas signatures from Escherichia coli and Escherichia coli-inoculated human whole blood. *Clin. Transl. Med.* **2013**, *2*, 13. [CrossRef] [PubMed]
64. Dolch, M.E.; Hornuss, C.; Klocke, C.; Praun, S.; Villinger, J.; Denzer, W.; Schelling, G.; Schubert, S. Volatile compound profiling for the identification of Gram-negative bacteria by ion-molecule reaction-mass spectrometry. *J. Appl. Microbiol.* **2012**, *113*, 1097–1105. [CrossRef] [PubMed]
65. Jünger, M.; Vautz, W.; Kuhns, M.; Hofmann, L.; Ulbricht, S.; Baumbach, J.I.; Quintel, M.; Perl, T. Ion mobility spectrometry for microbial volatile organic compounds: A new identification tool for human pathogenic bacteria. *Appl. Microbiol. Biotechnol.* **2012**, *93*, 2603–2614. [CrossRef] [PubMed]
66. Carrillo, J.; Durán, C. Fast identification of bacteria for quality control of drinking water through a static headspace sampler coupled to a sensory perception system. *Biosensors* **2019**, *9*, 23. [CrossRef] [PubMed]
67. Ibrahim, A.D.; Oyeleke, B.S.; Muhammad, U.K.; Aliero, A.; Yakubu, S.E.; Safiyanu, H.M. Microorganisms Associated with Volatile Organic Compound Production in Spoilt Mango Fruits. *Indones. J. Biotechnol.* **2011**, *16*, 11–16.
68. Brüggemann, H.; Poehlein, A.; Brzuszkiewicz, E.; Scavenius, C.; Enghild, J.J.; Al-Zeer, M.A.; Brinkmann, V.; Jensen, A.; Söderquist, B. Staphylococcus saccharolyticus Isolated from Blood Cultures and Prosthetic Joint Infections Exhibits Excessive Genome Decay. *Front. Microbiol.* **2019**, *10*, 478. [CrossRef]

3

The Efficacy of Retention Appliances after Fixed Orthodontic Treatment

Antonino Lo Giudice [1], Gaetano Isola [2,*], Lorenzo Rustico [3], Vincenzo Ronsivalle [1], Marco Portelli [3] and Riccardo Nucera [3,*]

1 Department of Medical-Surgical Specialties—Section of Orthodontics, School of Dentistry, University of Catania, Policlinico Universitario "G. Rodolico" Via Santa Sofia 78, 95123 Catania, Italy; nino.logiudice@gmail.com (A.L.G.); vincenzo.ronsivalle@hotmail.it (V.R.)

2 Department of Medical-Surgical Specialties, School of Dentistry, University of Catania, Policlinico Universitario "G. Rodolico" Via Santa Sofia 78, 95123 Catania, Italy

3 Department of Biomedical and Dental Sciences and Morphofunctional Imaging, Section of Orthodontics, School of Dentistry, University of Messina, Policlinico Universitario "G. Martino," 98100 Messina, Italy; lorenzo.rustico@gmail.com (L.R.); mportelli@unime.it (M.P.)

* Correspondence: gaetano.isola@unict.it (G.I.); riccardo.nucera@gmail.com (R.N.)

Abstract: The purpose of this article is to evaluate the amount of the relapse of anterior crowding and the efficacy of retention appliances by reviewing the best available scientific evidence. A survey of articles published up to November 2019 about the stability of dental alignment and retention after fixed orthodontic treatment was performed using seven electronic databases. Study Selection: Only randomized clinical trials investigating patients previously treated with multi-bracket appliances with a follow-up period longer than 6 months were included. Data Extraction: Two authors independently performed the study selection, data extraction, and risk of bias assessment. All pooled data analyses were performed using a random-effects model. Statistical heterogeneity was evaluated. In total, eight randomized clinical trials (RCTs) were included, grouping data from 987 patients. The ages of the patients varied across the studies, ranging between 13 and 17 years. The observation period ranged between 6 and 24 months. The data showed no significant intercanine width modifications during the retention period with both fixed and removable retainers. A significant modification of Little's Index was found for the mandibular removable retainers with a mean difference of 0.72 mm (95% Cl, 0.47 to 0.98) and for the maxillary removable retainers with a mean difference of 0.48 mm (95% Cl, 0.27 to 0.68). No significant changes were found by evaluating Little's Index modification for the mandibular fixed retainers. The results of this meta-analysis showed that all the considered retainers were effective in maintaining dental alignment after fixed orthodontic treatment. However, fixed retainers showed greater efficacy compared to removable retainers.

Keywords: relapse; orthodontic retainers; stability; systematic review; meta-analysis

---

1. Introduction

Stable tooth position after orthodontic treatment is considered a treatment goal. However, evidence shows that the majority of orthodontic treatments move teeth from a stable to an unstable position [1]. In this way, the use of a retainer is considered the only method able to maintain occlusal results [2]. Post-treatment tooth stability can be affected by several different factors, including bone and soft tissue development [3], primary crowding [4–6], dental eruption [7], modification of arch form [8], post-treatment occlusion [9], and the characteristics of pre-treatment malocclusion [10]. Retention can be performed by placing removable or fixed retainers. A recent Cochrane review reported a lack of evidence concerning the effectiveness different retention methods [11]. The efficacy of different retention appliances is of great interest for clinicians to support clinical retention protocols [12–14]. The literature does not provide meta-analytic data reporting and comparing the amount of relapse that occurs when using different retention appliances. The aim of this systematic review and meta-analysis was to evaluate the amount of relapse of anterior crowding and consequently to evaluate the efficacy of retention appliances used after fixed orthodontic treatment according to the best scientific evidence available [15].

2. Materials and Methods

The present systematic review with meta-analysis was performed according to the guidelines provided by the Cochrane Handbook for Systematic Reviews of Interventions (version 5.1.0) and was reported according to the PRISMA statement [16–19]. The protocol of this meta-analysis was preliminary registered on PROSPERO (https://www.crd.york.ac.uk/prospero/). Two authors independently carried out the selection of the studies, data collection, and the assessment of the risk of bias. Any disagreement was resolved by discussion with a third author. The level of agreement between the 2 reviewers was assessed by Cohen kappa statistics, for which a threshold value of 0.90 was preset.

2.1. Information Sources and Search

A survey of articles published up to November 2019 on stability and retention after orthodontic treatment was performed using several electronic databases (Table 1).

Table 1. Performed electronic searches.

Database of Published Trials	Search Strategy Used	Hits
MEDLINE searched via PubMed searched on November 18, 2019 via www.ncbi.nlm.nih.gov/sites/entrez/	((((incisor stability [tiab]) OR post treatment stability [tiab]) OR relapse [mesh])) AND (((orthodontic treatment [tiab] or Orthodontic fixed appliance [tiab]) Or orthodontic retainer [tiab])	254
OvidSP searched on November 18, 2019 via https://ovidsp.tx.ovid.com	(incisor stability OR post treatment stability OR relapse) AND (orthodontic treatment OR orthodontic fixed appliance OR orthodontic retainers)	1135
EMBASE searched via ScienceDirect searched on November 18, 2019 via www.embase.com	(incisor stability or post treatment stability or relapse) AND (orthodontic treatment or orthodontic fixed appliance or orthodontic retainers)	1174
Cochrane Database of Systematic Reviews searched via The Cochrane Library searched on November 18, 2019 via www.thecochranelibrary.com	(incisor stability OR post treatment stability OR relapse) AND (orthodontic treatment OR orthodontic fixed appliance OR orthodontic retainers)	2
Cochrane Central Register of Controlled Trials searched via The Cochrane Library searched on January 18, 2018 via www.thecochranelibrary.com	(incisor stability OR post treatment stability OR relapse) AND (orthodontic treatment OR orthodontic fixed appliance OR orthodontic retainers)	94
Scopus searched on November 18, 2019 via www.scopus.com	(incisor stability OR post treatment stability OR relapse) AND (orthodontic treatment OR orthodontic fixed appliance OR orthodontic retainers)	191
Web of Science searched on November 18, 2019 via http: //scientific.thomson.com/products/wos	(incisor stability or post treatment stability or relapse) AND (orthodontic treatment or orthodontic fixed appliance or orthodontic retainers)	745
Total		3595

Previous systematic reviews and meta-analyses on this topic were also identified, and their reference lists were scanned to find additional trials. No restriction was applied to language, publication year, or status.

2.2. Selection of Studies

Duplicated reports were preliminary excluded. All retrieved records were screened on the basis of their titles and abstracts, and the full texts of the remaining articles were assessed for eligibility in the final analysis.

Studies were considered eligible if they met the following criteria (reported according to the PICO format): clinical trials on human subjects, orthodontic patients treated with multi-bracket appliances with no craniofacial deformity (population), orthodontic retention performed with fixed or removable retainers (intervention), a comparable control group (control group), results analyzed at the beginning of retention and after a follow-up period longer than 6 months (outcomes measured), and analyzed treatment effects that were not influenced by concomitant and/or additional therapeutic procedures.

2.3. Data Extraction and Management

A data extraction form was developed to collect the characteristics (study design, type of retention appliance, sample size, age, sex, orthodontic treatment characteristics, setting, observation time, type of measurements, and follow-up) and outcomes from the included studies. Relapse after orthodontic treatment was investigated by using two parameters: Little's Irregularity Index (LII) for assessment of the degree of crowding and intercanine width for assessment of the transversal anterior dental arch width.

2.4. Assessment of Risk of Bias

The risk of bias assessment was performed using the Cochrane Collaboration's risk of bias tool (Review Manager version 5.2; Nordic Cochrane Centre, Cochrane Collaboration, Copenhagen, Denmark, 2012). Each randomized clinical trial (RCT) was assigned an overall risk of bias rating: low risk (low for all key domains), high risk (high for ≥1 key domain), or unclear risk (unclear for ≥1 key domain).

2.5. Summary Measures and Data Analysis

Two outcomes were considered for the meta-analytic analysis: Little's Irregularity Index and Intercanine width. The published clinical trials evaluating retention protocols do not have a control group with un-retained patients for ethical reasons. As a consequence, all the published trials compare two or more treatment protocols. In order to obtain a quantitative estimation of occlusal changes occurred with different retention protocols, we considered the single-arm data of clinical trials as the data obtained from case-series studies, and we performed a meta-analysis extrapolating and combining these data. In terms of data characteristics, the single-arm data from the RCTs and case series studies data are equivalent, as both studies report data with a mean value and standard deviation. However, the data extrapolated from the single-arm RCTs present less bias compared to the data from the case series studies. Finally, our strategy was supported by the literature. Indeed, when clinical trials with untreated control groups are not available, case-series studies without a control group can be used to perform a meta-analysis [20–22].

The considered effects size used for the meta-analysis was the difference between the outcome values at the end of treatment with fixed appliances and the outcome values after the retention period. Some studies reported the interquartile range rather than standard deviation, and the data extracted from those studies were properly adjusted [23]. The mean differences (MDs) and their corresponding 95% confidence intervals (95% CIs) were used to summarize and combine the data. A random-effects model was applied to estimate all the pooled data. This analysis was performed by means of the OpenMeta [Analyst] computer program (http://www.cebm.brown.edu/openmeta/) [24]. A third outcome (i.e., the fixed retainer failure rate) was considered only for qualitative evaluation.

2.6. *Assessment of Heterogeneity*

Clinical heterogeneity was evaluated by examining the types of participants and the interventions for the outcome in each included study. For all analyses, heterogeneity was assessed with the I^2 index, which is an indicator of true heterogeneity in percentages [14–19].

2.7. *Assessment of Quality of Evidence*

The quality of evidence was assessed using the Grades of Recommendation, Assessment, Development, and Evaluation Pro software (GRADEPro) [25]. The strength of the recommendation for each outcome investigated was assessed using the Strength of Recommendation Taxonomy (SORT) Grading system [26], which addresses the issue of patient-oriented (effectiveness) versus disease-oriented evidence (efficacy). POEMs (patient oriented evidence that matters) allows clinicians to filter information from the medical literature and focus only on what is in fact important for the patient [26].

2.8. *Sensitivity Analysis*

A sensitivity analysis was conducted to evaluate the LII modification in the lower arch with the mandibular removable retention appliances, excluding the RCT with the highest risk of bias (Figure S1).

3. Results

3.1. *This Study Selection*

Figure 1 shows the flow diagram for the selection of studies. Supplementary Table S1 reports the number of excluded studies and the reasons for exclusion. Eleven studies [21–31] were selected for the qualitative analysis and eight studies for the final quantitative synthesis [21–28] (Table 1). The inter-reviewer agreements for study selection were suitable, with a kappa value of 0.987.

3.2. *Study Characteristics*

The characteristics of the 11 RCTs included for the qualitative synthesis are summarized in Table 2. All eight RCTs selected for the meta-analysis evaluated the efficacy of different type of retention appliances (both removable and fixed) after orthodontic treatment with a multi-bracket appliance; the majority of trials took place in university settings. The total number of pooled observed patients was 987. Six studies [27,30–34] included both male and female participants, while in two studies [28,31], the authors did not specify the numbers of male and female participants. Five studies [27,29,30,33,34] reported the patients' ages, with an age range between 13 and 17 years. The appliance features were heterogeneous among the selected studies: Six trials evaluated the effects of vacuum-formed retainers [27,30–34], four trials evaluated the effects of bonded fixed retainers [27–31], two trials evaluated the effects of a Hawley retainer [33,34], one trial evaluated the effects of a Begg retainer [31], and one trial evaluated the effects of a positioner [27].

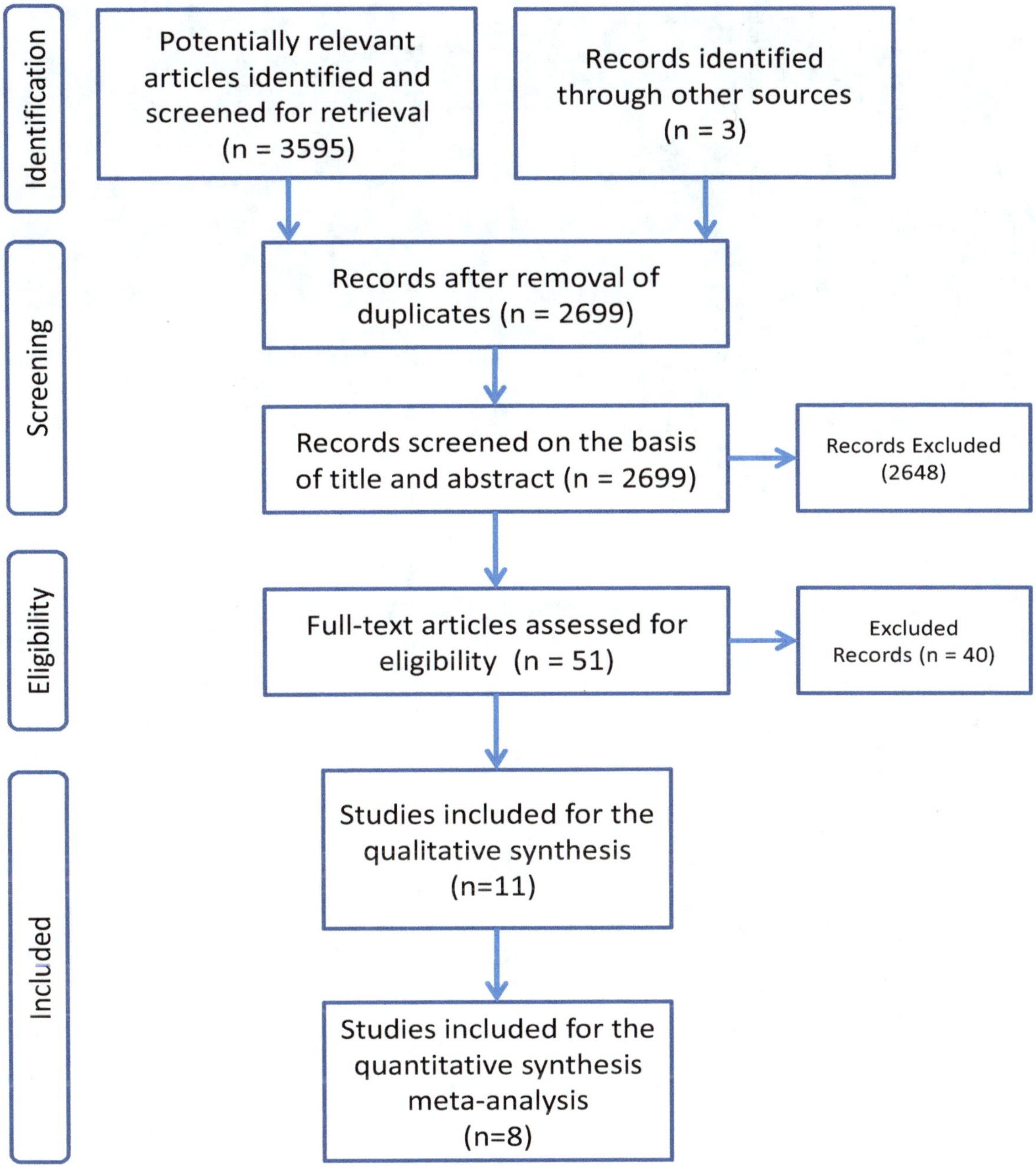

Figure 1. Flow Chart.

Seven studies [27,29,30,32–34] reported the percentage of patients treated with or without extraction, as shown in Table 2. The times of daily wear for the removable appliances (vacuum-formed retainers, Hawley retainers, Begg retainers, and positioners) varied between full-time and night-time among the RCTs, and the observation time varied from 6 to 24 months. The inter-reviewer agreements for study selection were suitable, with a kappa value of 0.968.

Table 2. Study characteristics.

Selected References	Maxillary Retention	Mandibular Retention	Sample	Sex	Age (y)	Orthodontic Treatment Characteristics	Setting	Observation Time	Methods of Measurement
Bolla et al. (2012)	Fixed Retainer (GFR) Fixed Retainer (MST)	Fixed Retainer (GFR) Fixed Retainer (MST)	GFR = 40 MST = 45	F = 28 M = 12 F = 28 M = 17	F = 20.2 M = 23.4 F = 22.6 M = 24.1	No Extraction: 100% Extraction: 0%	Italy	6 years	Failure rate.
Edman Tynelius et al. (2013)	Vacum-Formed Retainer Positioner	Fixed Retainer Positioner	VFR = 47 Positioner = 22 FR = 24	F = 45 M = 30	14,4	No Extraction: 0% Extraction: 100%	National Health Service (NHS) Ystad, Sweden	24 months	Little's irregularity index (LII), intercanine width.
Egli et al. (2017)	//	Fixed Retainer (DB) Fixed Retainer (IB)	FR (DB) = 30 FR (IB) = 30	//	//	//	Postgraduate orthodontic clinic University of Geneva, Switzerland.	24 months	Intercanine width, failure rate.
Forde et al. (2017)	Bonded Retainer Vacum-Formed Retainer	Bonded Retainer Vacum-Formed Retainer	BR = 30 VFR = 26	F = 15 M = 15 F = 18 F = 12	BR = 16 VFR = 17	No Extraction: 31,6% Extraction: 68,4%	St Luke's Hospital, Bradford and York Hospital and Leeds Dental Institute; UK.	12 months	Little's irregularity index (LII), intercanine width.
Gill et al. (2007)	Vacum-Former Retainer	Vacum-Former Retainer	Full-Time = 28 Part-Time = 29	F = 16 M = 12 F = 16 M = 13	FT = 13,7 (2,5) PT = 13,3 (1,4)	No Extraction: 35 Extraction: 65%	Hospital department, London, UK.	6 months	Little's irregularity index (LII), intercanine width.
Kumar et al. (2011)	Vacum-Formed Retainer Begg Retainer	Vacum-Formed Retainer Begg Retainer	VFR = 112 BR = 112	//	//	//	College of Dental Sciences, Davangere, India.	6 months	Little's irregularity index (LII).
O'Rourke et al. (2016)	//	Vacum-Former Retainer Fixed Retainer	VFR = 21 FR = 27	F = 59 M = 23	//	No Extraction: 53,6% Extraction: 46,4%	Hospital, London, UK.	18 months	Little's irregularity index (LII), intercanine width.
Rowland et al. (2006)	Vacum-Former Retainer Hawley Retainer	Vacum-Former Retainer Hawley Retainer	VFR = 201 HR = 196	F = 118 M = 83 F = 123 M = 73	VFR = 14 HR = 15	No Extraction: 66,2% Extraction: 33,8%	Taunton, Bristol, London, and Nottingham, UK.	6 months	Little's irregularity index (LII), intercanine width.
Salehi et al. (2013)	Fixed Retainer (PWR) Fixed Retainer (Multi-Stranded)	Fixed Retainer (PWR) Fixed Retainer (Multi-Stranded)	PWR = 68 Multi-stranded = 74	F = 39 M = 29 F = 44 M = 30	PWR = 18.1 (5,2) PT = 18,2 (4,8)	//	School of Dentistry, Shiraz University of Medical Sciences, Iran	18 months	Failure rate.
Shawesh et al. (2009)	Hawley Retainer	Hawley Retainer	Full-Time = 28 Part-Time = 24	F = 58,8% M = 41,2% F = 75,8% M = 24,2%	FT = 15,6 (1,6) PT = 15,8 (1,2)	No Extraction: 17,9% Extraction: 82,1%	Heaton Mersey, Manchester, UK.	12 months	Little's irregularity index (LII).
Störman et al. (2002)	//	Fixed Retainer (0.0195 Respond®) Fixed Retainer (0.0215 Respond®) Fixed Retainer (Prefabricated 3 to 3)	0.0195 Respond®= 31 0.0215 Respond®= 38 Prefabricated 3 to 3 = 34	//	13 to 17	//	Department of Orthodontics, University of Münster, Germany	24 months	Failure rate.

3.3. *Risk of Bias Assessment*

Although we took only single arm data from the selected studies to perform the meta-analysis, all the pooled data come from RCTs. Therefore, in order to assess the risk of bias, we had to assess the methodological quality of the RCTs; we used the Cochrane Collaboration tool, which is considered the gold standard for this purpose (Table S1). Among the eight studies included for the quantitative synthesis and meta-analysis, only 1 RCT was evaluated to have a high risk of bias [34]. In two RCTs, the risk of bias was unclear [31,33], and five RCTs had a low risk of bias [26–30,32] (Table 3). Consequently, the summary assessments of risk of bias across the studies were considered to be low. The inter-reviewer agreements for risk of bias assessment were suitable, with kappa values of 0.925. Publication bias was not assessed as there were inadequate numbers of included trials to properly develop a funnel plot or more advanced regression-based assessments.

Table 3. Risk of bias assessment.

	Risk of Bias						
STUDIES	**Sequence Generation**	**Allocation Concealment**	**Blinding of Participants, Personnel and Outcomes**	**Incomplete Outcome Data**	**Selective Outcome Reporting**	**Other Risk of Bias**	**Overall Risk of Bias**
Bolla et al. (2012)	Unclear	Unclear	Unclear	High Risk	Unclear	High Risk	High Risk
Edman et al. (2013)	Low Risk	Low Risk	Low Risk	Low Risk	Low Risk	Low Risk	Low Risk
Egli et al. (2017)	Low Risk	Low Risk	Low Risk	Low Risk	Low Risk	Low Risk	Low Risk
Forde et al. (2017)	Low Risk	Low Risk	Low Risk	Low Risk	Low Risk	Low Risk	Low Risk
Gill et al. (2007)	Low Risk	Low Risk	Low Risk	Low Risk	Low Risk	Low Risk	Low Risk
Kumar et al. (2011)	Unclear	Unclear	Low Risk	Low Risk	Unclear	Unclear	Unclear
O'Rourke et al. (2016)	Low Risk	Low Risk	Low Risk	Low Risk	Low Risk	Low Risk	Low Risk
Rowland et al. (2006)	Low Risk	Low Risk	Low Risk	Low Risk	Unclear	Low Risk	Unclear
Salehi et al. (2013)	Low Risk	Unclear	Low Risk	Low Risk	Low Risk	Low Risk	Unclear
Shawesh et al. (2009)	Low Risk	Low Risk	Low Risk	Low Risk	Low Risk	High Risk	High Risk
Störmann et al. (2002)	Unclear	Unclear	Low Risk	Low Risk	Low Risk	Unclear	Unclear

3.4. *Quantitative Data Synthesis*

The data showed that the mean difference of intercanine width during the retention period was 0.05 mm (95% Cl, −0.41 to 0.51; $P = 0.84$; $I^2 = 99\%$) for the mandibular fixed retainers (Figure 2a), 0.01 mm (95% Cl, −0.26 to 0.28; $P = 0.95$; $I^2 = 100\%$) for the mandibular removable retainers (Figure 2b), and −0.13 mm (95% Cl, −0.52 to 0.27; $P = 0.53$; $I^2 = 99\%$) for the maxillary removable retainers (Figure 2c). The mean difference of Little's Index during the retention period was 0.48 mm (95% Cl, −0.04 to 1.01; $P = 0.07$; $I^2 = 98\%$) for the mandibular fixed retainers (Figure 2d), 0.73 mm (95% Cl, 0.47 to 0.98; $P = 0.00001$; $I^2 = 100\%$) for the mandibular removable retainers (Figure 2e), and 0.48 mm (95% Cl, 0.27 to 0.68; $\mathrm{P} = 0.00001$; $I^2 = 91\%$) for the maxillary removable retainers (Figure 2f).

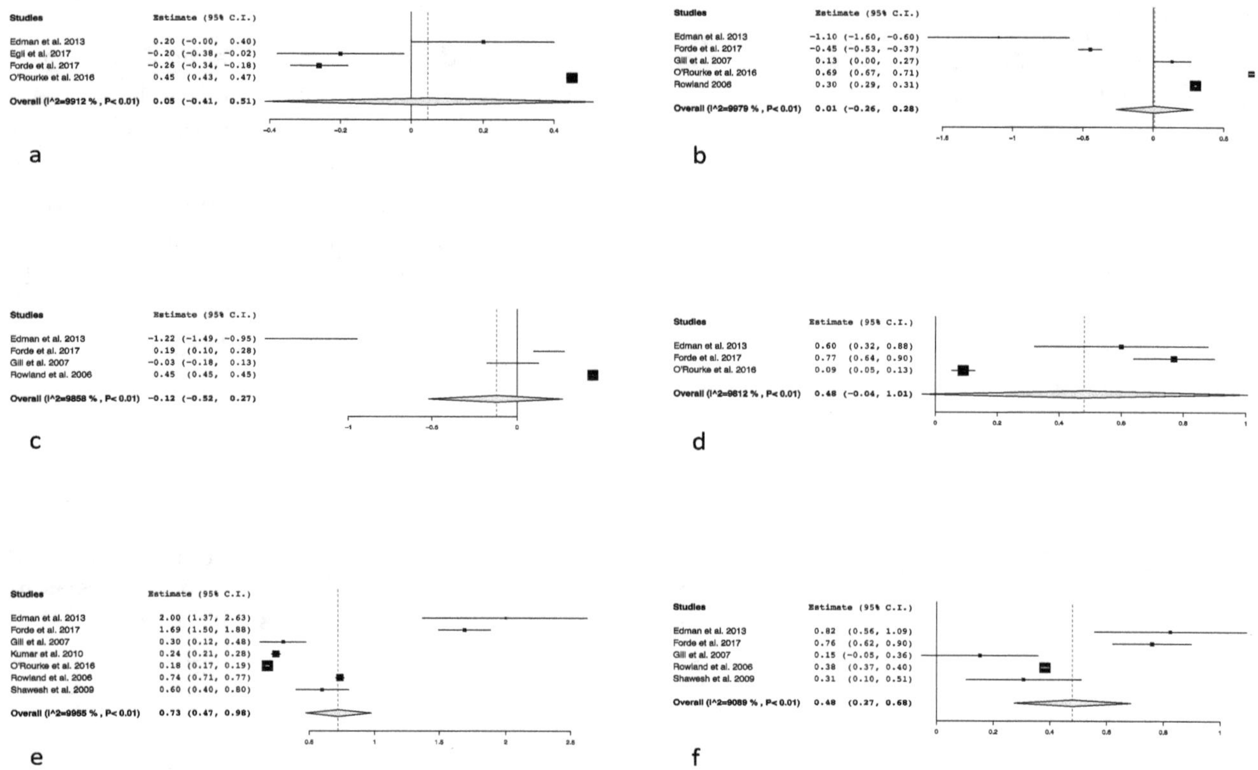

Figure 2. (**a**) Forest plot of the intercanine width modification: mandibular fixed retainers; (**b**) mandibular removable retainers; (**c**) maxillary removable retainers; (**d**) forest plot of the Little's Index modification: mandibular fixed retainers; (**e**) mandibular removable retainers; (**f**) maxillary removable retainers.

3.5. Fixed Retainer Failure Rate

Among the 11 studies included for qualitative synthesis, four RCTs [28,35–37] reported the failure rate of the fixed retainers during the observation period. The summarized failure rate was 41.3% (72/174) for the maxillary arch and 36.7% (115/313) for the mandibular arch (Table 4). Among the four studies, only one RCT had a high risk of bias [35]. For two RCTs, the risk of bias was unclear [36,37], and one RCT had a low risk of bias [28] (Table 3).

Table 4. Fixed retainer failure rate.

	Retainer Characteristics	Maxillary Arch	Mandibular Arch
Bolla et al. (2012)	Glass-Fiber reinforced	4/14 (28.5%)	7/34 (20.5%)
	Multistranded	7/18 (38.8%)	10/32 (31.2%)
Egli et al. (2017)	Direct Bonding	//	11/30 (37%)
	Indirect Bonding	//	13/30 (43%)
Salehi et al. (2013)	Polyethylene Woven Ribbon	27/74 (36.5%)	14/37 (37.8%)
	0.0175 in flexible spiral wire	34/68 (50%)	29/68 (42.6%)
Störmann et al. (2002)	0.0195 Respond®	//	10/30 (33.3%)
	0.0215 Respond®	//	18/36 (50%)
	Prefabricated 3 to 3	//	3/16 (18.7%)
Total		**72/174 (41.3%)**	**115/313 (36.7%)**

3.6. Assessment of Quality of Evidence

According to the GRADE [25], there was low level of evidence for all the LII outcomes (Table 5) and for the mandibular and maxillary intercanine width outcomes with both fixed and removable retainers (Table 6). According to the SORT approach [26], the strength of the recommendations was classified as A for LII and C for intercanine width (Table 7).

Table 5. Should fixed retainers or removable retainers be used for maintaining the alignment of anterior teeth?

Certainty Assessment							№ of Patients		Effect		Certainty	Importance
№ of Studies	**Study Design**	**Risk of Bias**	**Inconsistency**	**Indirectness**	**Imprecision**	**Other Considerations**	**Fixed Retainers**	**Removable Retainers**	**Relative (95% CI)**	**Absolute (95% CI)**		
Mandibular Fixed												
3	randomised trials	not serious	very serious [a]	not serious	not serious	none	96	96	-	MD 0.48 higher (0.04 lower to 1 higher)	⊕⊕○○ LOW	CRITICAL
Mandibular Removable												
7	randomised trials	very serious [b]	very serious [a]	not serious	not serious	none	818	818	-	MD 0.72 higher (0.47 higher to 0.98 higher)	⊕○○○ VERY LOW	CRITICAL
Maxillary Removable												
5	randomised trials	very serious [c]	very serious [a]	not serious	not serious	none	605	605	-	MD 0.8 higher (0.35 higher to 1.24 higher)	⊕○○○ VERY LOW	CRITICAL
Acrylic Removable Retainers (mandibular)												
3	randomised trials	very serious [b]	very serious [a]	not serious	not serious	none	360	360	-	MD 1.08 higher (0.53 higher to 1.63 higher)	⊕○○○ VERY LOW	CRITICAL
Vacum-Formed Removable Retainers (mandibular)												
5	randomised trials	serious [d]	very serious [a]	not serious	not serious	none	436	436	-	MD 0.51 higher (0.33 higher to 0.69 higher)	⊕○○○ VERY LOW	CRITICAL

CI: Confidence interval; **MD:** Mean difference. (**a**) Heterogeneity > 75%; (**b**) in one study, the risk of bias was unclear for "Sequence generation", "Allocation concealment", "Selective Outcome Reporting", and "Other Risk of bias". In one study, the risk of bias was unclear for "Selective Outcome Reporting". In one study, the risk of bias was high for "Other Risk of bias"; (**c**) in one study the risk of bias was unclear for "Selective Outcome Reporting". In one study, the risk of bias was high for "Other Risk of bias"; (**d**) in one study, the risk of bias was unclear for "Sequence generation", "Allocation concealment", "Selective Outcome Reporting", and "Other Risk of bias". In one study, the risk of bias was unclear for "Selective Outcome Reporting".

Table 6. Should fixed retainers or removable retainers be used for maintaining intercanine width?

Certainty Assessment							№ of Patients		Effect		Certainty	Importance
№ of Studies	Study Design	Risk of Bias	Inconsistency	Indirectness	Imprecision	Other Considerations	Fixed Retainers	Removable Retainers	Relative (95% CI)	Absolute (95% CI)		
Mandibular Fixed												
4	randomised trials	not serious	very serious [a]	not serious	not serious	none	126	126	-	MD 0.05 higher (0.41 lower to 0.51 higher)	⨁⨁◯◯ LOW	CRITICAL
Mandibular Removable												
5	randomised trials	not serious	very serious [a]	not serious	not serious	none	542	542	-	MD 0.01 higher (0.27 lower to 0.28 higher)	⨁⨁◯◯ LOW	CRITICAL
Maxillary Removable												
4	randomised trials	not serious	very serious [a]	not serious	not serious	none	553	553	-	MD 0.13 lower (0.52 lower to 0.27 higher)	⨁⨁◯◯ LOW	CRITICAL

CI: Confidence interval; **MD:** Mean difference. (**a**) Heterogeneity > 75%.

Table 7. Strength of recommendations for each outcome investigated in the present study.

Outcomes	Study Quality *	Consistency *	Strength of Recommendation *	Explanation
Intercanine width				
Mandibular fixed retainer	Level 3	Yes	C	Disease-oriented outcome Meta-analysis including 4 RCTs
Mandibular removable retainer	Level 3	Yes	C	Disease-oriented outcome Meta-analysis including 5 RCTs
Maxillary removable retainer	Level 3	Yes	C	Disease-oriented outcome Meta-analysis including 4 RCTs
Irregularity Index				
Mandibular fixed retainer	Level 1	Yes	A	Patient-oriented outcome Meta-analysis including 3 RCTs
Mandibular removable retainer	Level 1	Yes	A	Patient-oriented outcome Meta-analysis including 7 RCTs
Maxillary removable retainer	Level 1	Yes	A	Patient-oriented outcome Meta-analysis including 5 RCTs
Acrylic removable retainer	Level 1	Yes	A	Disease-oriented outcome Meta-analysis including 3 RCTs
Vacuum-Formed Removable retainer	Level 1	Yes	A	Disease-oriented outcome Meta-analysis including 5 RCTs

* Reports of the levels of study quality, consistency of measured outcomes, and strength of recommendations according to the Strength of Recommendation Taxonomy (SORT) system.

4. Discussion

To the best of our knowledge, this is the first review with meta-analysis that investigates the current literature with the best evidence (RCTs) on the efficacy of orthodontic retainers to maintain the occlusal results after fixed orthodontic treatment. The results of this meta-analysis will provide clinicians a quantitative evaluation of the efficacy of fixed and removable retainers and consequently a quantitative evaluation of orthodontic relapse during the retention period.

The pooled data show that the intercanine width does not change significantly during retention with all evaluated retention appliances [37–44].

The data show that the fixed retainers are also able to avoid significant modifications of LII ($p = 0.07$). However, this datum should be interpreted with caution because of the fewer number of considered trials. Conversely, the use of removable retainers showed a significant increase of LII. This datum was obtained by pooling the data from five trials for the maxillary arch (Figure 2f) and from seven trials for the mandibular arch (Figure 2e); it can be considered a consistent meta-analytic datum. The amount of variation for LII is 0.48 and 0.72 mm, respectively, for the maxillary and mandibular arch. This result clearly shows that, despite the use of a removable retainer appliance, the teeth of both arches present a small statistically significant (but clinically insignificant) alignment alteration. These results, especially for intercanine width, must be interpreted with caution due to the young age of the sample participants, as this type of alteration can influence the outcome due to residual growth and patient compliance.

Interestingly, our data show a significant alteration of LII in the absence of modification of the intercanine width. These results could be explained by interpreting the alteration of LII as a consequence of a single tooth rotational relapse, rather than a transversal inter-canine diameter relapse. The reported modifications of LII could be related to specific factors associated with the use of removable retainers, such as patient compliance and the limitations of using retainers nocturnally. This last hypothesis, however, does not seem to be supported by the evidence. Indeed, one of the considered RCTs compared removable retainers used full time and removable retainers used part-time [45–55]. The authors did not find significant differences in terms of relapse after 12 months of retention.

Compliance is certainly an issue related to removable retainers. However, the results of this review clearly show that fixed retainers are not free of issues. In fact, the failure rate of fixed retainers (caused by wire breakage or bonding failure) is, on average, 41% and 36% for maxillary and mandibular retainers, respectively (Table 4). These data are in accordance with previously published data [14,56–61].

One limitation of this meta-analysis is the small number of included trials; this aspect affected the I2 index, undervaluing the extent of between-study heterogeneity [62,63]. The I2 values reported a high total variation across the studies, with a mean value and a standard deviation equal to 97.8% and 2.2%, respectively. This variation was assumed to be due to the clinical heterogeneity of the different appliances used in the considered RCTs. Moreover, the source of heterogeneity could be related to other factors such as patient compliance, final occlusal results, orthodontist expertise, type of malocclusion, and type of treatment (with or without extractions) [13,64–77].

The I2 values potentially affected the level of evidence of our findings, which ranged from very low to low, according to the GRADE approach. Although we selected only published trials offering the highest level of evidence (RCTs), the GRADE score showed that the included studies provided, in most cases, a very low quality of evidence (Tables 5 and 6). This result should be assessed while considering the difficulties in conducting RCTs for orthodontics [46].

All these aspects increased the heterogeneity of the different clinical trials and, consequently, contributed to limiting the methodological GRADE score of the orthodontic trials.

The SORT approach (Table 7) revealed a high strength of recommendations for the LII outcome and a poor strength of recommendations for the intercanine width outcome, likely because the LII represents a clinical outcome that directly affect smile aesthetics and appearance (i.e., a patient-oriented outcome).

The sensitivity analysis showed a similar outcome compared with the results of this meta-analysis for the same parameter (0.74) (95% Cl, 0.47 to 1.01; $P = 0.00001$; $I^2 = 100\%$), confirming the validity of the performed meta-analysis.

5. Conclusions

The results of this meta-analysis show that all the considered retainers are effective in maintaining dental alignment after fixed orthodontic treatment. However, the fixed retainers showed greater efficacy than the removable retainers.

The most important issues for fixed and removable retainers are, respectively, the risk of failure and patient compliance. Further RCT studies with longer observation periods are needed in order to assess the long-term efficacy of orthodontic retainers.

Author Contributions: Conceptualization, A.L.G. and L.R.; methodology, M.P., G.I.; software, V.R.; writing—original draft preparation, writing—review and editing R.N. and G.I. All authors have read and agreed to the published version of the manuscript.

References

1. Little, R.M.; Wallen, T.R.; Riedel, R.A. Stability and relapse of mandibular anterior alignment—First premolar extraction cases treated by traditional edgewise orthodontics. *Am. J. Orthod.* **1981**, *80*, 349–365. [CrossRef]
2. Blake, M.; Bibby, K. Retention and stability: A review of the literature. *Am. J. Orthod. Dentofac. Orthop.* **1998**, *114*, 299–306. [CrossRef]
3. Nucera, R.; Lo Giudice, A.; Bellocchio, M.; Spinuzza, P.; Caprioglio, A.; Cordasco, G. Diagnostic concordance between skeletal cephalometrics, radiographbased soft-tissue cephalometrics, and photograph-based soft-tissue cephalometrics. *Eur. J. Orthod.* **2017**, *39*, 352–357. [PubMed]
4. Lo Giudice, A.; Nucera, R.; Leonardi, R.; Paiusco, A.; Baldoni, M.; Caccianiga, G. A Comparative Assessment of the Efficiency of Orthodontic Treatment with and without Photobiomodulation during Mandibular Decrowding in Young Subjects: A Single-Center, Single-Blind Randomized Controlled Trial. *Photobiomodul Photomed. Laser Surg.* **2020**. [CrossRef] [PubMed]

5. Richardson, M.E. Late lower arch crowding in relation to primary crowding. *Angle Orthod.* **1982**, *44*, 56–61.
6. Lo Giudice, A.; Nucera, R.; Perillo, L.; Paiusco, A.; Caccianiga, G. Is low-level laser therapy an effective method to alleviate pain induced by active orthodontic alignment archwire? A randomized clinical trial. *J. Evid. Based Dent. Prac.* **2019**, *19*, 71–78. [CrossRef]
7. Richardson, M.E. Late lower arch crowding in relation to the direction of eruption. *Eur. J. Orthod.* **1996**, *18*, 341–347. [CrossRef]
8. Bondemark, L.; Holm, A.K.; Hansen, K.; Axelsson, S.; Mohlin, B.; Brattstrom, V.; Paulin, G.; Pietila, T. Long term stability of orthodontic treatment and patient satisfaction: A systematic review. *Angle Orthod.* **2007**, *77*, 181–191. [CrossRef]
9. Weiland, F. The role of occlusal discrepancies in the long-term stability of the mandibular arch. *Eur. J. Orthod.* **1994**, *16*, 521–529. [CrossRef]
10. Little, R.M.; Riedel, R.A. Postretention evaluation of stability and relapse—Mandibular arches with generalized spacing. *Am. J. Orthod. Dentofac. Orthop.* **1989**, *95*, 37–41. [CrossRef]
11. Littlewood, S.J.; Millett, D.T.; Doubleday, B.; Bearn, D.R.; Worthington, H.V. Retention procedures for stabilising tooth position after treatment with orthodontic braces. *Cochrane Database Syst. Rev.* **2016**. [CrossRef]
12. Al-Moghrabi, D.; Pandis, N.; Fleming, P.S. The effects of fixed and removable orthodontic retainers: A systematic review. *Prog. Orthod.* **2016**, *17*, 24. [CrossRef] [PubMed]
13. Nucera, R.; Gatto, E.; Borsellino, C.; Aceto, P.; Fabiano, F.; Matarese, G.; Perillo, L.; Cordasco, G. Influence of bracket-slot design on the forces released by superelastic nickel-titanium alignment wires in different deflection configurations. *Angle Orthod.* **2014**, *84*, 541–547. [CrossRef] [PubMed]
14. Lo Giudice, G.; Lo Giudice, A.; Isola, G.; Fabiano, F.; Artemisia, A.; Fabiano, V.; Nucera, R.; Matarese, G. Evaluation of bond strength and detachment interface distribution of different bracket base designs. *Acta Med. Mediterr.* **2015**, *31*, 585–590.
15. Papadopoulos, M.A. Meta-analysis in evidence-based orthodontics. *Orthod. Craniofac. Res* **2003**, *6*, 112–126. [CrossRef]
16. Nucera, R.; Militi, A.; Lo Giudice, A.; Longo, V.; Fastuca, R.; Caprioglio, A.; Cordasco, G.; Papadopoulos, M.A. Skeletal and Dental Effectiveness of Treatment of Class II Malocclusion with Headgear: A Systematic Review and Meta-analysis. *J. Evid. Based Dent. Prac.* **2018**, *18*, 41–58. [CrossRef]
17. Higgins, J.P.T.; Green, S. (Eds.) *Cochrane Handbook for Systematic Reviews of Interventions*, (version 5.1.0, updated March 2016); The Cochrane Collaboration: London, UK, 2016.
18. Nucera, R.; Lo Giudice, A.; Rustico, L.; Matarese, G.; Papadopoulos, M.A.; Cordasco, G. Effectiveness of orthodontic treatment with functional appliances on maxillary growth in the short term: A systematic review and meta-analysis. *Am. J. Orthod. Dentofac. Orthop.* **2016**, *149*, 600–611.e3. [CrossRef]
19. Liberati, A.; Altman, D.G.; Tetzlaff, J.; Mulrow, C.; Gotzsche, P.C.; Ioannidis, J.P.A.; Clarke, M.; Devereaux, P.J.; Kleijnen, J.; Moher, D. The PRISMA statement for reporting systematic reviews and meta-analyses of studies that evaluate health care interventions: Explanation and elaboration. *J. Clin. Epidemiol.* **2009**, *62*, e1–e34. [CrossRef]
20. Fitzpatrick-Lewis, D.; Ciliska, D.; Thomas, H. *The Methods for the Synthesis of Studies without Control Groups*; National Collaborating Centre for Methods and Tools: Hamilton, ON, Canada, 2009.
21. Chambers, D.; Rodgers, M.; Woolacott, N. Not only randomized controlled trials, but also case series should be considered in systematic reviews of rapidly developing technologies. *J. Clin. Epidemiol.* **2009**, *62*, 1253–1260.e4. [CrossRef]
22. Dalziel, K.; Round, A.; Stein, K.; Garside, R.; Castelnuovo, E.; Payne, L. Do the findings of case series studies vary significantly according to methodological characteristics? *Health Technol Assess.* **2005**, *9*, 1–148. [CrossRef]
23. Hozo, S.L.; Djulbegovic, B.; Hozo, I. Estimating the mean and variance from the median, range, and the size of a sample. *BMC Med. Res. Methodol.* **2005**, *5*, 13. [CrossRef] [PubMed]
24. Wallace, B.C.; Dahabreh, I.J.; Trikalinos, T.A.; Lau, J.; Trow, P.; Schmid, C.H. Closing the Gap between Methodologists and End-Users: R as a Computational Back-End. *J. Stat. Softw.* **2012**, *49*, 1–15. [CrossRef]
25. Falck-Ytter, Y.; Guyatt, G.H.; Vist, G.; Kunz, R. Rating quality of evidence and strength of recommendations GRADE: An emerging consensus on rating quality of evidence and strength of recommendations. *BMJ* **2008**, *336*, 924–926.

26. Newman, M.G.; Weyant, R.; Hujoel, P. JEBDP improves grading system and adopts strength of recommendation taxonomy grading (SORT) for guidelines and systematic reviews. *J. Evid. Based Dent. Prac.* **2007**, *7*, 147–150. [CrossRef] [PubMed]
27. Edman Tynelius, G.; Bondemark, L.; Lilja-Karlander, E. A randomized controlled trial of three orthodontic retention methods in Class I four premolar extraction cases—Stability after 2 years in retention. *Orthod. Craniofac. Res.* **2013**, *16*, 105–115. [CrossRef] [PubMed]
28. Egli, F.; Bovali, E.; Kiliaridis, S.; Cornelis, M.A. Indirect vs direct bonding of mandibular fixed retainers in orthodontic patients: Comparison of retainer failures and posttreatment stability. A 2-year follow-up of a single-center randomized controlled trial. *Am. J. Orthod. Dentofac. Orthop.* **2017**, *151*, 15–27. [CrossRef]
29. Forde, K.; Storey, M.; Littlewood, S.J.; Paul Scott, P.; Luther, F.; Kang, J. Bonded versus vacuum-formed retainers: A randomized controlled trial. Part 1: Stability, retainer survival, and patient satisfaction outcomes after 12 months. *Eur. J. Orthod.* **2018**, *40*, 387–398. [CrossRef]
30. Gill, D.S.; Naini, F.B.; Jones, A.; Tredwin, C.J. Part-time versus full-time retainer wear following fixed appliance therapy: A randomized prospective controlled trial. *World J. Orthod.* **2007**, *8*, 300–306.
31. Kumar, A.G.; Bansal, A. Effectiveness and acceptability of Essix and Begg retainers: A prospective study. *Aust. Orthod. J.* **2011**, *27*, 52–56.
32. O'Rourke, N.; Albeedh, H.; Sharma, P.; Johal, A. Effectiveness of bonded and vacuum-formed retainers: A prospective randomized controlled clinical trial. *Am. J. Orthod. Dentofac. Orthop.* **2016**, *150*, 406–415. [CrossRef]
33. Rowland, H.; Hichens, L.; Williams, A.; Hills, D.; Killingback, N. The effectiveness of Hawley and vacuum-formed retainers: A single-center randomized controlled trial. *Am. J. Orthod. Dentofac. Orthop.* **2007**, *132*, 730–737. [CrossRef]
34. Shawesh, M.; Bhatti, B.; Usmani, T.; Mandall, N. Hawley retainers full- or part-time? A randomized clinical trial. *Eur. J. Orthod.* **2010**, *32*, 165–170. [CrossRef]
35. Bolla, E.; Cozzani, M.; Doldo, T.; Fontana, M. Failure evaluation after a 6-year retention period: A comparison between glass fiber-reinforced (GFR) and multistranded bonded retainers. *Int. Orthod.* **2012**, *10*, 16–28. [CrossRef] [PubMed]
36. Salehi, P.; Zarif Najafi, H.; Roeinpeikar, S.M. Comparison of survival time between two types of orthodontic fixed retainer: A prospective randomized clinical trial. *Prog. Orthod.* **2013**, *14*, 25. [CrossRef] [PubMed]
37. Störmann, I.; Ehmer, U. A prospective randomized study of different retainer types. *J. Orofac. Orthop.* **2002**, *63*, 42–50. [CrossRef] [PubMed]
38. Isola, G.; Anastasi, G.P.; Matarese, G.; Williams, R.C.; Cutroneo, G.; Bracco, P.; Piancino, M.G. Functional and molecular outcomes of the human masticatory muscles. *Oral Dis.* **2018**, *24*, 1428–1441. [CrossRef]
39. Isola, G.; Polizzi, A.; Santonocito, S.; Alibrandi, A.; Ferlito, S. Expression of Salivary and Serum Malondialdehyde and Lipid Profile of Patients with Periodontitis and Coronary Heart Disease. *Int. J. Mol. Sci.* **2019**, *20*, 6061. [CrossRef]
40. Isola, G.; Perillo, L.; Migliorati, M.; Matarese, M.; Dalessandri, D.; Grassia, V.; Alibrandi, A.; Matarese, G. The impact of temporomandibular joint arthritis on functional disability and global health in patients with juvenile idiopathic arthritis. *Eur. J. Orthod.* **2019**, *41*, 117–124. [CrossRef]
41. Mev, J. Are random controlled trials appropriate for orthodontics? *Evid. Based Dent.* **2002**, *3*, 35–36.
42. Leonardi, R.; Lo Giudice, A.; Rugeri, M.; Muraglie, S.; Cordasco, G.; Barbato, E. Three-dimensional evaluation on digital casts of maxillary palatal size and morphology in patients with functional posterior crossbite. *Eur. J. Orthod.* **2018**, *40*, 556–562. [CrossRef]
43. Leonardi, R. Cone-beam computed tomography and three-dimensional orthodontics. Where we are and future perspectives. *J. Orthod.* **2019**, *46* (Suppl. 1), 45–48. [CrossRef] [PubMed]
44. Caccianiga, G.; Crestale, C.; Cozzani, M.; Piras, A.; Mutinelli, S.; Lo Giudice, A.; Cordasco, G. Low-level laser therapy and invisible removal aligners. *J. Biol. Regul. Homeost. Agents* **2016**, *30* (Suppl. 1), 107–113. [PubMed]
45. Isola, G.; Alibrandi, A.; Rapisarda, E.; Matarese, G.; Williams, R.C.; Leonardi, R. Association of vitamin d in patients with periodontal and cardiovascular disease: A cross-sectional study. *J. Periodontal. Res.* **2020**. [CrossRef]
46. Isola, G.; Alibrandi, A.; Currò, M.; Matarese, M.; Ricca, S.; Matarese, G.; Ientile, R.; Kocher, T. Evaluation of

salivary and serum ADMA levels in patients with periodontal and cardiovascular disease as subclinical marker of cardiovascular risk. *J. Periodontol.* **2020**. [CrossRef]

47. Isola, G.; Polizzi, A.; Alibrandi, A.; Indelicato, F.; Ferlito, S. Analysis of Endothelin-1 concentrations in individuals with periodontitis. *Sci. Rep.* **2020**. [CrossRef] [PubMed]
48. Isola, G.; Matarese, G.; Ramaglia, L.; Pedullà, E.; Rapisarda, E.; Iorio-Siciliano, V. Association between periodontitis and glycosylated haemoglobin before diabetes onset: A cross-sectional study. *Clin. Oral Investig.* 2019. [CrossRef]
49. Cutroneo, G.; Piancino, M.G.; Ramieri, G.; Bracco, P.; Vita, G.; Isola, G.; Vermiglio, G.; Favaloro, A.; Anastasi, G.; Trimarchi, F. Expression of muscle-specific integrins in masseter muscle fibers during malocclusion disease. *Int. J. Mol. Med.* **2012**, *30*, 235–242. [CrossRef]
50. Isola, G.; Matarese, M.; Ramaglia, L.; Cicciù, M.; Matarese, G. Evaluation of the efficacy of celecoxib and ibuprofen on postoperative pain, swelling, and mouth opening after surgical removal of impacted third molars: A randomized, controlled clinical trial. *Int. J. Oral Maxillofac. Surg.* **2019**, *48*, 1348–1354. [CrossRef]
51. Isola, G.; Alibrandi, A.; Pedullà, E.; Grassia, V.; Ferlito, S.; Perillo, L.; Rapisarda, E. Analysis of the Effectiveness of Lornoxicam and Flurbiprofen on Management of Pain and Sequelae Following Third Molar Surgery: A Randomized, Controlled, Clinical Trial. *J. Clin. Med.* **2019**, *8*, 325. [CrossRef]
52. Isola, G.; Matarese, G.; Alibrandi, A.; Dalessandri, D.; Migliorati, M.; Pedullà, E.; Rapisarda, E. Comparison of Effectiveness of Etoricoxib and Diclofenac on Pain and Perioperative Sequelae After Surgical Avulsion of Mandibular Third Molars: A Randomized, Controlled, Clinical Trial. *Clin. J. Pain* **2019**, *35*, 908–915. [CrossRef]
53. Lo Giudice, A.; Brewer, I.; Leonardi, R.; Roberts, N.; Bagnato, G.5. Pain threshold and temporomandibular function in systemic sclerosis: Comparison with psoriatic arthritis. *Clin. Rheumatol.* **2018**, *37*, 1861–1867. [CrossRef] [PubMed]
54. Lo Giudice, A.; Nucera, R.; Matarese, G.; Portelli, M.; Cervino, G.; Lo Giudice, G.; Militi, A.; Caccianiga, G.; Cicciù, M.; Cordasco, G. Analysis of resistance to sliding expressed during first order correction with conventional and self-ligating brackets: An in-vitro study. *Int. J. Clin. Exp. Med.* **2016**, *9*, 15575–15581.
55. Piancino, M.G.; Isola, G.; Cannavale, R.; Cutroneo, G.; Vermiglio, G.; Bracco, P.; Anastasi, G.P. From periodontal mechanoreceptors to chewing motor control: A systematic review. *Arch. Oral Biol.* **2017**, *78*, 109–121. [CrossRef] [PubMed]
56. Perillo, L.; Padricelli, G.; Isola, G.; Femiano, F.; Chiodini, P.; Matarese, G. Class II malocclusion division 1:.A new classification method by cephalometric analysis. *Eur. J. Paediatr. Dent.* **2012**, *13*, 192–196.
57. Isola, G.; Giudice, A.L.; Polizzi, A.; Alibrandi, A.; Patini, R.; Ferlito, S. Periodontitis and Tooth Loss Have Negative Systemic Impact on Circulating Progenitor Cell Levels: A Clinical Study. *Genes* **2019**, *10*, 1022. [CrossRef]
58. Isola, G.; Polizzi, A.; Muraglie, S.; Leonardi, R.M.; Lo Giudice, A. Assessment Of vitamin C And Antioxidants Profiles In Saliva And Serum In Patients With Periodontitis And Ischemic Heart Disease. *Nutrients* **2019**, *11*, 2956. [CrossRef]
59. Cannavale, R.; Matarese, G.; Isola, G.; Grassia, V.; Perillo, L. Early treatment of an ectopic premolar to prevent molar-premolar transposition. *Am. J. Orthod. Dentofac. Orthop.* **2013**, *143*, 559–569. [CrossRef]
60. Lo Giudice, A.; Barbato, E.; Cosentino, L.; Ferraro, C.M.; Leonardi, R. Alveolar bone changes after rapid maxillary expansion with tooth-born appliances: A systematic review. *Eur J Orthod.* **2018**, *40*, 296–303. [CrossRef]
61. Isola, G.; Matarese, M.; Briguglio, F.; Grassia, V.; Picciolo, G.; Fiorillo, L.; Matarese, G. Effectiveness of Low-Level Laser Therapy during Tooth Movement: A Randomized Clinical Trial. *Materials* **2019**, *12*, 2187. [CrossRef]
62. Lo Giudice, A.; Rustico, L.; Caprioglio, A.; Migliorati, M.; Nucera, R. Evaluation of condylar cortical bone thickness in patient groups with different vertical facial dimensions using cone-beam computed tomography. *Odontology* **2020**, in press. [CrossRef]
63. Lo Giudice, A.; Fastuca, R.; Portelli, M.; Militi, A.; Bellocchio, M.; Spinuzza, P.; Briguglio, F.; Caprioglio, A.; Nucera, R. Effects of rapid vs slow maxillary expansion on nasal cavity dimensions in growing subjects: A methodological and reproducibility study. *Eur. J. Paediatr. Dent.* **2017**, *18*, 299–304. [PubMed]

64. Caccianiga, G.; Paiusco, A.; Perillo, L.; Nucera, R.; Pinsino, A.; Maddalone, M.; Cordasco, G.; Lo Giudice, A. Does Low-Level Laser Therapy Enhance the Efficiency of Orthodontic Dental Alignment? Results from a Randomized Pilot Study. *Photomed Laser Surg.* **2017**, *35*, 421–426. [CrossRef] [PubMed]
65. Matarese, G.; Portelli, M.; Mazza, M.; Militi, A.; Nucera, R.; Gatto, E.; Cordasco, G. Evaluation of skin dose in a low dose spiral CT protocol. *Eur. J. Paediatr. Dent.* **2006**, *7*, 77–80.
66. Caprioglio, A.; Bergamini, C.; Franchi, L.; Vercellini, N.; Zecca, P.A. ; Nucera R, Fastuca R Prediction of Class II improvement after rapid maxillary expansion in early mixed dentition. *Prog. Orthod.* **2017**, *18*, 9. [CrossRef] [PubMed]
67. Nucera, R.; Lo Giudice, A.; Matarese, G.; Artemisia, A.; Cordasco, G.; Bramanti, E. Analysis of the characteristics of slot design affecting resistance to sliding during active archwire configurations. *Prog Orthod.* **2013**, *14*, 35. [CrossRef] [PubMed]
68. Isola, G.; Matarese, G.; Cordasco, G.; Rotondo, F.; Crupi, A.; Ramaglia, L. Anticoagulant therapy in patients undergoing dental interventions: A critical review of the literature and current perspectives. *Minerva Stomatol.* **2015**, *64*, 21–46.
69. Matarese, G.; Isola, G.; Anastasi, G.P.; Cutroneo, G.; Favaloro, A.; Vita, G.; Cordasco, G.; Milardi, D.; Zizzari, V.L.; Tetè, S.; et al. Transforming Growth Factor Beta 1 and Vascular Endothelial Growth Factor levels in the pathogenesis of periodontal disease. *Eur. J. Inflamm.* **2013**, *11*, 479–488. [CrossRef]
70. Isola, G.; Williams, R.C.; Lo Gullo, A.; Ramaglia, L.; Matarese, M.; Iorio-Siciliano, V.; Cosio, C.; Matarese, G. Risk association between scleroderma disease characteristics, periodontitis, and tooth loss. *Clin. Rheumatol.* **2017**, *36*, 2733–2741. [CrossRef]
71. Matarese, G.; Isola, G.; Alibrandi, A.; Lo Gullo, A.; Bagnato, G.; Cordasco, G.; Perillo, L. Occlusal and MRI characterizations in systemic sclerosis patients: A prospective study from Southern Italian cohort. *Joint. Bone. Spine.* **2016**, *83*, 57–62. [CrossRef]
72. Ametrano, G.; D'Antò, V.; Di Caprio, M.P.; Simeone, M.; Rengo, S.; Spagnuolo, G. Effects of sodium hypochlorite and ethylenediaminetetraacetic acid on rotary nickel-titanium instruments evaluated using atomic force microscopy. *Int. Endod. J.* **2011**, *44*, 203–209. [CrossRef]
73. Spagnuolo, G.; Ametrano, G.; D'Antò, V.; Formisano, A.; Simeone, M.; Riccitiello, F.; Amato, M.; Rengo, S. Microcomputed tomography analysis of mesiobuccal orifices and major apical foramen in first maxillary molars. *Open. Dent. J.* **2012**, *6*, 118–125. [CrossRef] [PubMed]
74. Krifka, S.; Petzel, C.; Bolay, C.; Hiller, K.A.; Spagnuolo, G.; Schmalz, G.; Schweikl, H. Activation of stress-regulated transcription factors by triethylene glycol dimethacrylate monomer. *Biomaterials* **2011**, *32*, 1787–1795. [CrossRef] [PubMed]
75. Pelo, S.; Saponaro, G.; Patini, R.; Staderini, E.; Giordano, A.; Gasparini, G.; Garagiola, U.; Azzuni, C.; Cordaro, M.; Foresta, E.; et al. Risks in surgery-first orthognathic approach: Complications of segmental osteotomies of the jaws. A systematic review. *Eur. Rev. Med. Pharmacol. Sci.* **2017**, *21*, 4–12. [PubMed]
76. Facciolo, M.T.; Riva, F.; Gallenzi, P.; Patini, R.; Gaglioti, D. A rare case of oral multisystem Langerhans cell histiocytosis. *J. Clin. Expd. Dent.* **2017**, *9*, e820–e824. [CrossRef]
77. Cordasco, G.; Lo Giudice, A.; Militi, A.; Nucera, R.; Triolo, G.; Matarese, G. In vitro evaluation of resistance to sliding in self-ligating and conventional bracket systems during dental alignment. *Korean J. Orthod.* **2012**, *42*, 218–224. [CrossRef]

4

Oral Microbiome in Four Female Centenarians

Yoshiaki Nomura [1,*], Erika Kakuta [2], Ayako Okada [1], Ryoko Otsuka [1], Mieko Shimada [3], Yasuko Tomizawa [4], Chieko Taguchi [5], Kazumune Arikawa [5], Hideki Daikoku [6], Tamotsu Sato [6] and Nobuhiro Hanada [1]

1 Department of Translational Research, Tsurumi University School of Dental Medicine, Kanagawa 230-8501, Japan; okada-a@tsurumi-u.ac.jp (A.O.); otsuka-ryoko@tsurumi-u.ac.jp (R.O.); hanada-n@tsurumi-u.ac.jp (N.H.)

2 Department of Oral bacteriology, Tsurumi University School of Dental Medicine, Kanagawa 230-8501, Japan; kakuta-erika@tsurumi-u.ac.jp

3 Chiba Prefecture University of Health Sciences, Chiba 261-0014, Japan; mieko.shimada@cpuhs.ac.jp

4 Department of Cardiovascular Surgery, Tokyo Women's Medical University, Tokyo 162-8666, Japan; tomizawa.yasuko@twmu.ac.jp

5 Department of Preventive and Public Oral Health, Nihon University School of Dentistry at Matsudo, Matsudo 271-8587, Japan; taguchi.chieko@nihon-u.ac.jp (C.T.); arikawa.kazumune@nihon-u.ac.jp (K.A.)

6 Iwate Dental Association, Morioka 470-2101, Japan; dai-koku@nifty.com (H.D.); tamosato-dent@k-2inc.jp (T.S.)

* Correspondence: nomura-y@tsurumi-u.ac.jp

Abstract: The oral microbiome of healthy older adults has valuable information about a healthy microbiome. In this study, we collected and analyzed the oral microbiome of denture plaque and tongue coating samples from four female centenarians. After DNA extraction and purification, pyrosequencing of the V3–V4 hypervariable regions of the 16S rRNA was carried out. The bacterial taxonomy for each lead was assigned based on a search of the EzBioCloud 16S database. We obtained a total of 199,723 valid, quality-controlled reads for denture plaque and 210,750 reads for tongue coating. The reads were assigned 407 operational taxonomic units with a 97% identity cutoff. Twenty-nine species were detected in both denture plaque and tongue coatings from all subjects. *Firmicutes* was the most abundant phylum; the *Streptococcus salivarius* group was the most abundant species in both the denture plaque and tongue coatings; and the *Fusobacterium nucleatum* group was detected in all subjects. In the bacterial profile, species formed clusters composed of bacteria with a wide range of prevalence and abundance, not dependent on phyla; each cluster may have specific species that could be candidates for a core microbiome. *Firmicutes* and *Veillonella* were abundant phyla on both plaque and tongue coatings of centenarians.

Keywords: oral microbiome; core microbiome; centenarian; next-generation sequencing

1. Introduction

The human microbiome changes with age [1] and health affects the composition of the microflora. It has been suggested that aging is accompanied by an underlying inflammatory state [2] that interacts with the microbiota of older adults and makes them more susceptible to age-related diseases [3–5]. Changes in the gut microbiome are explained by diseases, including metabolic changes and inflammatory conditions. Studies of intestinal microbiota in the elderly show that the microbiome affects a variety of clinical problems, including physical weakness, *Clostridium difficile* infection, colitis, vulvar vaginal atrophy, colorectal cancer, and atherosclerosis [6]. Other research has focused on the metabolism of nutrients. The microbiota has been shown to correlate with the declining metabolism of essential amino acids by aging [7].

In addition to the intestinal microbiome, the oral microbiome has been intensively studied. Both are affected by development, aging, and the state of oral disease. The formation of the first oral flora is strongly influenced by the mother [8–10]. Breast milk provides a source of bacteria that act as an inoculum for newborns [11–14]. The production and excretion of metabolites by pioneering colonies, such as *Streptococcus* and *Actinomyces*, alter the anaerobic oral environment. Under such conditions, anaerobic bacteria such as *Veillonella* and fusobacteria colonize [8,15]. With development, the microbial community evolves and microbial diversity increases [16,17]. Current knowledge shows that adult-like stability is reached around age two [15]. The established oral microbiota is disturbed by oral diseases. The development of dental caries has been associated with changes in microbial composition over time [18]. Differences in bacterial communities on the phylogenetic level were observed between healthy people and patients with periodontal disease [19,20]. The oral microbiota includes some pathogenic bacteria for systemic diseases. Therefore, the oral microbiome affects health and varies with health or disease [21]. Oral diseases, especially periodontal disease, can be the main risk factor for several systemic diseases [22–27]. Periodontal bacteria and their surface lipopolysaccharides were the agents of systemic diseases [28]. Recent advances of research on systemic diseases and oral health showed that there exist protective host factors for systemic diseases in relation to periodontal diseases [29–31]. The number of studies on the oral microbiota of community-dwelling older persons is limited [32–37].

In this study, denture plaque and tongue surface samples were obtained from people over 100 years old. The samples were analyzed by high-throughput sequencing of 16S rRNA through a metagenomics approach. We describe the commonly prevalent and highly abundant species of four female centenarians and compare them with the healthy oral microbiome proposed in previous studies. In addition, differences in sampling sites and the co-prevalence of species were analyzed.

2. Materials and Methods

2.1. Subject and Setting

Originally, the aim of the survey was to investigate the relationship between oral health and systemic health in 80-year-old adults. This survey is known as the 8020 Data Bank Survey. A 20-year follow-up study was conducted from 1996 to 2017 with subjects 80 years of age (born in 1917) residing in the 8 districts served by one health center in Iwate Prefecture. The sampling method was cluster sampling, and the sampling frame was a complete count survey for all subjects. For the baseline survey, based on residential registration, public health nurses visited 944 homes where 80-year-olds lived, and 666 subjects participated in these checkups.

The follow-up survey was conducted by the resident register with surviving subjects who participated in the baseline survey. After 20 years, 12 subjects survived. Among them, 5 lived in their own home with their families; the others lived in nursing homes. Four subjects who lived in their own home agreed to participate in the survey. We visited their homes at 10:00 in the morning to minimize the effect of food intake. Details of the survey were described in our previous report [27,28,37,38].

2.2. Oral Examination

Two dentists visited the homes of the subjects. An oral examination was carried out with a penlight and a dental mirror. The definition and diagnosis of dental caries were based on the criteria of the World Health Organization [39].

2.3. Sample Collection

As all subjects wore complete dentures, plaque samples were collected from the denture surface based on a method described in previous reports [40,41]. Briefly, the denture was brushed around the buccal surface with a toothbrush for 2 min, followed by immersion of the toothbrush with the attached plaque in sterilized, phosphate-buffered saline (PBS). Tongue coating samples were collected by using a mucosal brush (ERAC 510Lion, Tokyo, Japan). The tongue surface was brushed one way, from back to front, 5 times. Samples were treated in the same way as denture plaque samples. Samples were kept on ice before being transported to the Iwate Dental Association in an ice box with refrigerant, then were stored at −20 °C for further analysis.

2.4. Microbial DNA Extraction

Denture plaque and tongue surface samples suspended in PBS were collected by a centrifuge at 3000 rpm for 10 min. DNA extraction was performed by a Maxwell 16 LEV Blood DNA Kit (Promega KK, Tokyo, Japan)according to the manufacturer's instructions. DNA concentration was measured by a NanoDrop ND-2000 (Thermo Fisher Scientific KK, Tokyo, Japan). Degradation of DNA was visually checked by electrophoresis on 1% agarose gel. Degradation of DNA and contamination of RNA were checked by a Qubit dsDNA BR Assay Kit (Thermo Fisher Scientific KK, Tokyo, Japan).

Samples meeting the following criteria were used for further sequence analysis: conc > 20 ng/μL, volume ≥ 20 μL, A260/280 ≥ 1.8, and A260/230 > 1.5. In this study, all samples met the criteria.

2.5. Microbial Community Analysis

Extracted DNA was analyzed in a laboratory (Chun Lab, Seoul, Korea). Polymerase chain reaction (PCR) amplification was performed using primers specific to the V3–V4 region pyrosequencing tags of the 16S rRNA gene in the extracted bacterial DNA. Taxonomic classification of each read was assigned based on a search of the EzBioCloud 16S database [42,43], which contains the 16S rRNA genes of type strains that have valid published names and representative species-level phylotypes of both cultured and uncultured entries in the GenBank database, with complete hierarchical taxonomic classification from the phylum to species level [44].

2.6. Bioinformatics Analysis

The number of 16S rRNA gene copies (absolute abundance) of operational taxonomic units (OTUs) was calculated by multiplying their respective relative abundance by the total number of 16S rRNA gene copies. Bioinformatics analysis was performed by the microbiome package on the Bioconductor of R software [45].

3. Results

3.1. Characteristics of Subjects Who Participated in this Study

All four subjects who participated in this study were women, 100 years old, and wore complete dentures. One subject had five residual roots (sample ID 1), with complete dentures designed over the stump root. Blood tests and medical examinations were conducted to confirm the health of the subjects. Blood tests showed values in the normal range. Two subjects had hypertension. According to this continuous study, one subject had high blood pressure at age 85 (sample ID 1) and one had normal blood pressure at age 90 (sample ID 2). Other than that, there were no specific symptoms on examination.

3.2. Sequence Data Details

Out of eight samples from the four subjects, 199,723 reads for denture plaque (min, max: 42,792, 54,898) and 210,750 for tongue coatings (45,193, 57,753) passed quality control. From these reads, sequences clustered into 15 phyla, 31 classes, 49 orders, 71 families, 142 genera, and 406 species. A heatmap of all 407 species detected in this study is shown in Figure S1. All sequence data are provided in the Supplementary Materials.

The ACE, Chao1, jackknife, Shannon, and Simpson alpha diversity indices were calculated to analyze the diversity and richness of all samples. By comparing the samples of denture plaque and tongues, the ACE, Chao1, jackknife, and Shannon indices were not significantly different ($P > 0.05$), proving that bacterial diversity and richness were similar in the samples collected from denture plaque and tongues. The values of these indices are shown in Table S1. Statistics of taxonomic assignment are shown in Table S2. A rarefaction curve is shown in Figure S2.

3.3. Oral Microbiome Profile of Centenarians

Figure 1A shows the relative abundance of detected bacteria at the phylum level. On both denture plaque and the tongue, Firmicutes were abundant. Figure 1B shows the phylum level proportion of bacteria of the four subjects. For three subjects, Firmicutes were abundant in both saliva and the tongue. Proteobacteria were relatively abundant in the saliva and tongue of one subject. Dynamic pie charts are presented in the Supplementary Materials.

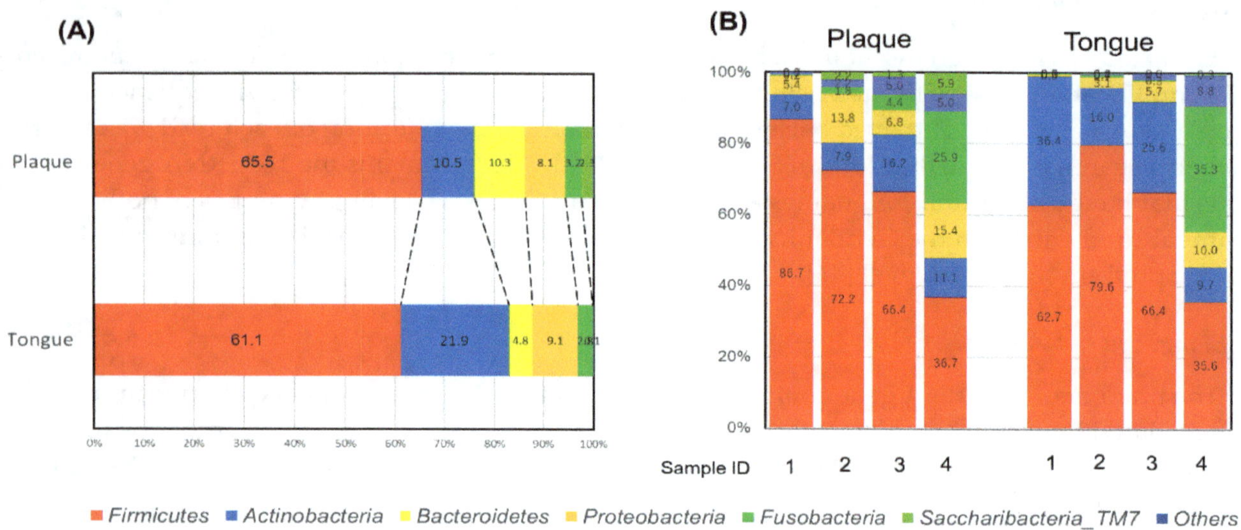

Figure 1. Proportion of phyla in denture plaque and the tongue: (**A**) total, and (**B**) individual subjects.

3.4. Core Microbiome Analysis

Figure 2 shows the prevalence of taxa in terms of abundance. Abundant species belonged to *Firmicutes*, *Proteobacteria*, and *Bacteroides*. In this study, 29 species were detected from all subjects in denture plaque and the tongue. Table 1 shows the species detected from all subjects, and Table S3 shows the 15 species in plaque and 7 species in the tongue. The most abundant bacteria were Firmicutes at the phylum level and the *Streptococcus salivarius* group at the species level in both plaque and the tongue. The *Fusobacterium nucleatum* group was detected from all subjects. A heatmap of the candidates for the core microbiome is shown in Figure S3.

Table 1. Bacteria detected in denture plaque and tongue from all subjects.

Phylum	Genus	Species	Abundance (%)	
			Plaque	Tongue
Firmicutes	*Streptococcus*	*Streptococcus salivarius* group	9.72	25.06
		Streptococcus sinensis group	4.12	13.22
		Streptococcus pneumoniae group	4.46	1.92
		Streptococcus parasanguinis group	2.30	3.83
		Streptococcus gordonii group	4.80	0.62
		Streptococcus peroris group	0.82	1.03
		Streptococcus sanguinis	0.87	0.08
		Streptococcus_uc	0.40	0.32
	Veillonella	*Veillonella dispar*	5.63	4.89
		Veillonella parvula group	7.40	0.51
		Veillonella atypica	1.90	1.95
		Veillonella_uc	0.05	0.09
	Gemella	*Gemella haemolysans* group	0.23	0.54
	Granulicatella	*Granulicatella adiacens* group	0.43	1.67
	Lachnoanaerobaculum	*Lachnoanaerobaculum orale* group	0.13	0.08
	Lactobacillus	*Lactobacillus salivarius*	3.95	0.33
	Megasphaera	*Megasphaera micronuciformis*	0.29	0.07
	Moryella	*Stomatobaculum longum*	0.17	0.22
Actinobacteria	*Actinomyces*	*KE952139_s*	0.71	2.39
		CAGY_s	0.11	0.30
		JRMV_s	0.02	0.37
	Atopobium	*Atopobium parvulum*	0.76	0.27
	Rothia	*Rothia mucilaginosa*	0.65	17.17
		Rothia dentocariosa	4.34	0.52
		Rothia_uc	0.02	0.10
Bacteroidetes	*Prevotella*	*Prevotella histicola*	3.95	0.54
		Prevotella jejuni	0.32	1.06
		Prevotella salivae	0.35	0.08
Fusobacteria	*Fusobacterium*	*Fusobacterium nucleatum* group	0.37	0.04

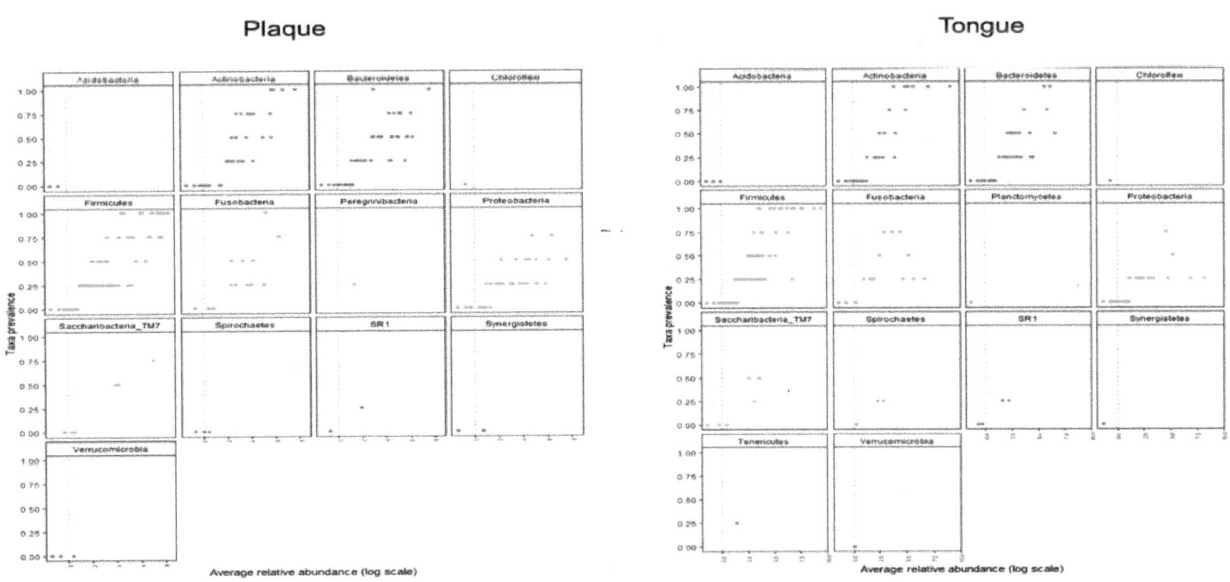

Figure 2. Prevalence of taxa in terms of abundance for 14 different phyla.

3.5. Analysis of Co-prevalent Species

Then, the levels of species co-prevalence were analyzed by t-distributed stochastic neighbor embedding (tSNE). As shown in Figure 3, species were constructed in clusters that were not dependent on the phylum. The list of classified species and detection in 3 of 4 subjects (75%) is shown in Table S2.

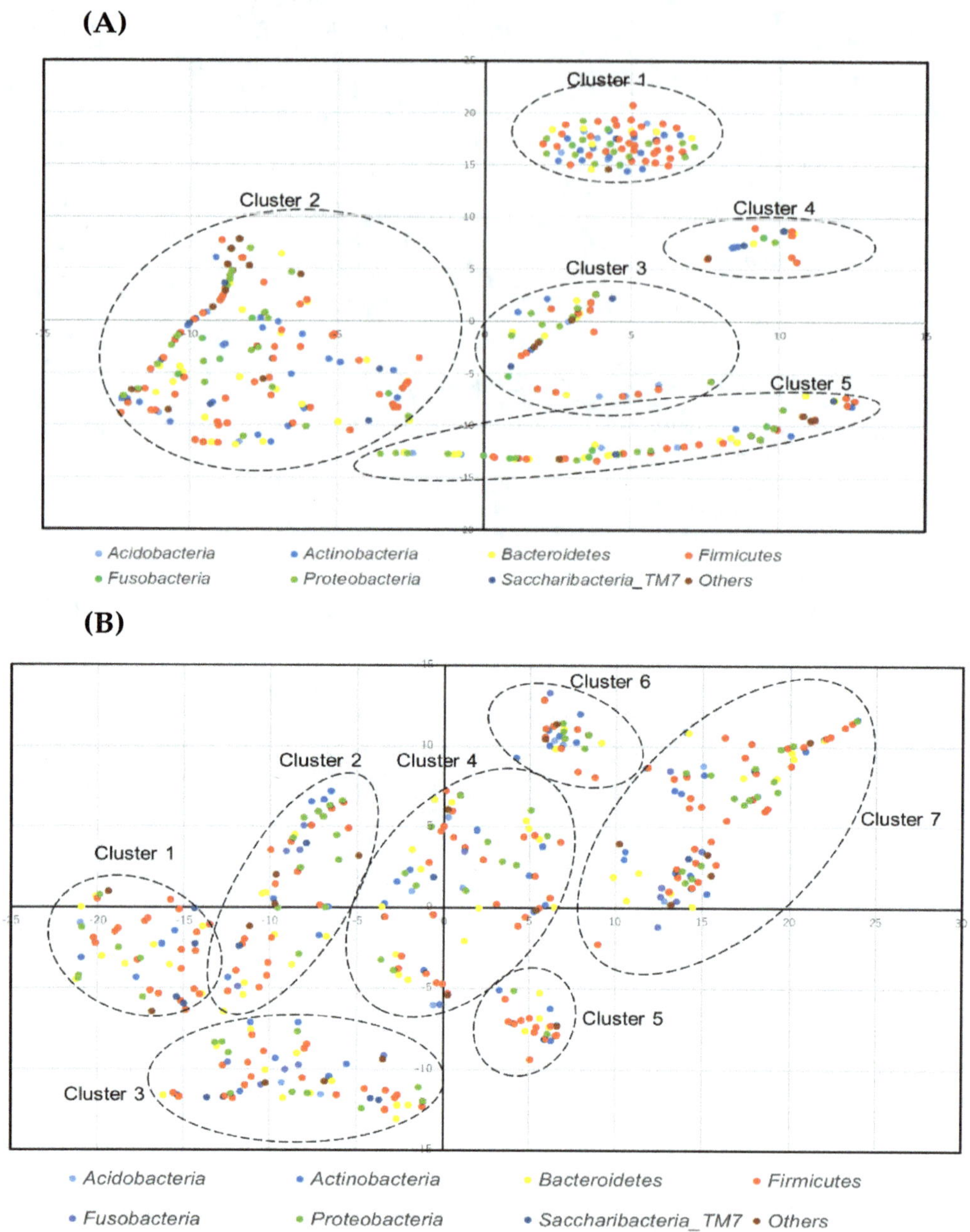

Figure 3. t-distributed stochastic neighbor embedding (tSNE) plot of species: (**A**) denture plaque, and (**B**) the tongue.

4. Discussion

This study describes microbial profiles of the oral cavities of four female centenarians by high throughput sequencing. Highly prevalent and abundant species are described. In addition, differences in sampling sites and co-prevalence of species are presented.

A total of 406 species were detected. Studies indicate that the diversity of bacteria is reduced with the frailty of older adults [3,46]. All participants in this study were female centenarians. Bacterial diversity was not reduced when compared to another study [16].

Firmicutes was the most abundant phylum for both the denture plaque and tongue samples. Several studies have shown that *Firmicutes* is the most abundant phylum in the saliva of infants [16] and young children aged 6–8 years [47], swabs of the oral cavities of youths and adults [48], and dental plaque from older adults [34]. *Firmicutes*, *Streptococcus*, and *Veillonella* were detected in all subjects in both the denture plaque and the tongue. The result that *Firmicutes* was the most abundant, followed by *Veillonella*, is consistent with the proportions of oral microorganisms in the Human Oral Microbiome Database [49]. The abundant genera after *Veillonella* vary between studies. *Streptococcus*, *Veillonella*, and *Neisseria* were the predominant bacterial genera present in infants. Abundant genera that coat the tooth surface first are *Streptococcus* and *Veillonella* [50]. *Streptococcus*, *Veillonella*, and *Neisseria* are the predominant bacterial genera present in infants [16]. *Streptococcus* and *Veillonella* are known as early colonizers. *Neisseria* settles down at the age of 1–2 years [18].

In this study, *Neisseria* was not detected in all subjects. Differences at the species level in previous reports may be due to the sample difference. All subjects surveyed in this study wore complete dentures, so the plaque sample was denture plaque, not dental plaque attached to the tooth surface. Additionally, the small sample size may have affected the difference.

In this study, *Streptococcus salivarius* was the most abundant species in both the denture plaque and the tongue. This result is consistent with another study that investigated the tongues of Japanese older adults [16]. The results of the study show that more than 5% of abundant species were *Streptococcus salivarius*, *Prevotella melaninogenica*, *Rothia mucilaginosa*, *Veillonella atypica*, and *Neisseria flavescens*. Except for *Neisseria flavescens*, the other four species were common to our results. Another study showed that *Streptococcus oralis* was by far the most prevalent species [51]. As described above, Firmicutes and *Veillonella* are abundant phyla. Each study has different bacterial profiles at the genus or species level.

The bacterial profile of the denture plaque was similar to that of oral mucosa. Actinobacteria was abundant in the denture plaque and Bacilli were abundant in the dental plaque [52]. In this study, the proportion of these bacteria varies between samples: 5.4%, 15.5%, 10.8%, and 6.5% for Actinobacteria and 82.45%, 44.4%, 21.5%, and 48.1% for Bacilli. The small sample size may have affected the results.

A previous study had shown that oral microbiome profiles were related to the risk of death by pneumonia for older persons residing in nursing homes [53]. *Neisseria flavescens*, the *Fusobacterium periodonticum* group, and the *Haemophilus parainfluenzae* group were abundant in the risk group. In this study, one subject (Sample ID 4) had higher levels of these bacteria than the mean values of the risk group.

As shown in Figure 3 the bacterial community formed clusters with a low prevalence or abundance of bacteria. The clustering was not phylum dependent.

The clusters were composed of bacteria with a wide range of prevalence and abundance. This indicates that some bacteria were the core of the cluster. There may be an interaction or symbiotic mechanism between core bacteria and low-prevalence or low-abundance bacteria. Therefore, there may be healthy microbiome candidates within the core bacteria of each cluster.

A limitation of this study was the small sample size of four people. The design was a cross-sectional study. The data presented in this study were from Japanese older persons. Even though dietary habits have little effect on the oral microbiome [54], regional or cultural differences could have an effect on the oral microbiome [44]. The health status of the subjects who participated in this study was limited. Subjects with specific diseases were not included. For comparison, healthy and pathogenic conditions should be considered. Longevity is not simply explained by microflora. Further study is needed to evaluate the host factors such as nutraceutical agent [29], serum malondialdehyde [30], and progenitor cell levels [31]. In addition, the subjects investigated in this study were all female and edentulous.

5. Conclusions

The oral microbiome was preserved in Japanese centenarians at the phylum level. At the species level, bacterial profiles were not consistent with other studies. *Firmicutes* and *Veillonella* were abundant phyla in both the plaque and the tongue. In the bacterial profile, bacteria formed clusters. The oral microbiome of the centenarian investigated in this study was similar to that of other age groups from previous studies at phylum level. Further study is needed to define a common bacterial profile at the species level.

Author Contributions: Y.N. planned the study design and management and analysis of the data and wrote the original draft. E.K., A.O., R.O., M.S., Y.T., C.T., and K.A. collected and managed the data. Y.N., H.D., T.S., and N.H. contributed to funding acquisition, planning the study design, and reviewing and editing the manuscript. All authors have read and agreed to the published version of the manuscript.

References

1. Yatsunenko, Y.; Rey, F.E.T.; Manary, M.J.; Trehan, I.; Dominguez-Bello, M.G.; Contreras, M.; Magris, M.; Hidalgo, G.; Baldassano, R.N.; Anokhin, A.P.; et al. Human gut microbiome viewed across age and geography. *Nature* **2012**, *486*, 222–227. [CrossRef]
2. Chung, H.Y.; Lee, E.K.; Choi, Y.J.; Kim, J.M.; Kim, D.H.; Zou, Y.; Kim, C.H.; Lee, J.; Kim, H.S.; Kim, N.D.; et al. Molecular inflammation as an underlying mechanism of the aging process and age-related diseases. *J. Dent. Res.* **2011**, *90*, 830–840. [CrossRef] [PubMed]
3. Claesson, M.J.; Cusack, S.; O'Sullivan, O.; Greene-Diniz, R.; de Weerd, H.; Flannery, E.; Marchesi, J.R.; Falush, D.; Dinan, T.; Fitzgerald, G.; et al. Composition, variability, and temporal stability of the intestinal microbiota of the elderly. *Proc. Natl. Acad. Sci. USA* **2011**, *108*, 4586–4591. [CrossRef]
4. O'Toole, P.W.; Jeffery, I.B. Gut microbiota and aging. *Science* **2015**, *350*, 1214–1215. [CrossRef]
5. Jackson, M.A.; Jeffery, I.B.; Beaumont, M.; Bell, J.T.; Clark, A.G.; Ley, R.E.; O'Toole, P.W.; Spector, T.D.; Steves, C.J. Signatures of early frailty in the gut microbiota. *Genome Med.* **2016**, *8*, 8. [CrossRef]
6. Zapata, H.J.; Quagliarello, V.J. The microbiota and microbiome in aging: Potential implications in health and age-related diseases. *J. Am. Geriatr. Soc.* **2015**, *63*, 776–781. [CrossRef]
7. Rampelli, S.; Candela, M.; Turroni, S.; Biagi, E.; Collino, S.; Franceschi, C.; O'Toole, P.W.; Brigidi, P. Functional metagenomic profiling of intestinal microbiome in extreme ageing. *Aging* **2013**, *5*, 902–912. [CrossRef]
8. Sampaio-Maia, B.; Monteiro-Silva, F. Acquisition and maturation of oral microbiome throughout childhood: An update. *Dent. Res. J.* **2014**, *11*, 291–301.
9. Flores, G.E.; Caporaso, J.G.; Henley, J.B.; Rideout, J.R.; Domogala, D.; Chase, J.; Leff, J.W.; Vázquez-Baeza, Y.; Gonzalez, A.; Knight, R.; et al. Temporal variability is a personalized feature of the human microbiome. *Genome Biol.* **2014**, *15*, 531. [CrossRef] [PubMed]
10. Teng, F.; Yang, F.; Huang, S.; Bo, C.; Xu, Z.Z.; Amir, A.; Knight, R.; Ling, J.; Xu, J. Prediction of early childhood caries via spatial-temporal variations of oral microbiota. *Cell Host Microbe* **2015**, *18*, 296–306. [CrossRef] [PubMed]
11. Boix-Amorós, A.; Collado, M.C.; Mira, A. Relationship between milk microbiota, bacterial load, macronutrients, and human cells during lactation. *Front Microbiol.* **2016**, *7*, 492. [CrossRef] [PubMed]
12. Fernández, L.; Langa, S.; Martín, V.; Maldonado, A.; Jiménez, E.; Martín, R.; Rodríguez, J.M. The human milk microbiota: Origin and potential roles in health and disease. *Pharmacol. Res.* **2013**, *69*, 1–10. [CrossRef] [PubMed]
13. Fitzstevens, J.L.; Smith, K.C.; Hagadorn, J.I.; Caimano, M.J.; Matson, A.P.; Brownell, E.A. Systematic review of the human milk microbiota. *Nutr. Clin. Pract.* **2016**, *32*, 354–364. [CrossRef] [PubMed]
14. Rodriguez, J.M. The origin of human milk bacteria: Is there a bacterial entero-mammary pathway during late pregnancy and lactation? *Adv. Nutr. Int. Rev. J.* **2014**, *5*, 779–784. [CrossRef]
15. Gomez, A.; Nelson, K.E. The oral microbiome of children: Development, disease, and implications beyond oral health. *Microb. Ecol.* **2017**, *73*, 492–503. [CrossRef]
16. Cephas, K.D.; Kim, J.; Mathai, R.A.; Barry, K.A.; Dowd, S.E.; Meline, B.S.; Swanson, K.S. Comparative analysis of salivary bacterial microbiome diversity in edentulous infants and their mothers or primary care givers using pyrosequencing. *PLoS ONE* **2011**, *6*, e23503. [CrossRef]
17. Lif Holgerson, P.; Öhman, C.; Rönnlund, A.; Johansson, I. Maturation of oral microbiota in children with or without dental caries. *PLoS ONE* **2015**, *10*, e0128534. [CrossRef]

18. Dzidic, M.; Collado, M.C.; Abrahamsson, T.; Artacho, A.; Stensson, M.; Jenmalm, M.C.; Mira, A. Oral microbiome development during childhood: An ecological succession influenced by postnatal factors and associated with tooth decay. *ISME J.* **2018**, *12*, 2292–2306. [CrossRef]
19. Chen, W.P.; Chang, S.H.; Tang, C.Y.; Liou, M.L.; Tsai, S.J.; Lin, Y.L. Composition Analysis and Feature Selection of the Oral Microbiota Associated with Periodontal Disease. *Biomed. Res. Int.* **2018**, *2018*, 3130607. [CrossRef]
20. Minty, M.; Canceil, T.; Serino, M.; Burcelin, R.; Tercé, F.; Blasco-Baque, V. Oral microbiota-induced periodontitis: A new risk factor of metabolic diseases. *Rev. Endocr. Metab. Disord.* **2019**, *20*, 449–459. [CrossRef]
21. Graves, D.T.; Corrêa, J.D.; Silva, T.A. The Oral Microbiota Is Modified by Systemic Diseases. *J. Dent Res.* **2019**, *98*, 148–156. [CrossRef] [PubMed]
22. Jensen, E.; Allen, G.; Bednarz, J.; Couper, J.; Peña, A. Periodontal risk markers in children and adolescents with type 1 diabetes: A systematic review and meta-analysis. *Diabetes Metab. Res. Rev.* **2020**, e3368. [CrossRef] [PubMed]
23. Wang, J.; Yang, X.; Zou, X.; Zhang, Y.; Wang, J.; Wang, Y. Relationship between periodontal disease and lung cancer: A systematic review and meta-analysis. *J. Periodontal Res.* **2020**. [CrossRef]
24. Nadim, R.; Tang, J.; Dilmohamed, A.; Yuan, S.; Wu, C.; Bakre, A.T.; Partridge, M.; Ni, J.; Copeland, J.R.; Anstey, K.J.; et al. Influence of periodontal disease on risk of dementia: A systematic literature review and a meta-analysis. *Eur. J. Epidemiol.* **2020**. [CrossRef] [PubMed]
25. Priyamvara, A.; Dey, A.K.; Bandyopadhyay, D.; Katikineni, V.; Zaghlol, R.; Basyal, B.; Barssoum, K.; Amarin, R.; Bhatt, D.L.; Lavie, C.J. Periodontal Inflammation and the Risk of Cardiovascular Disease. *Curr. Atheroscler. Rep.* **2020**, *22*, 28. [CrossRef] [PubMed]
26. Orlandi, M.; Graziani, F.; D'Aiuto, F. Periodontal therapy and cardiovascular risk. *Periodontol 2000* **2020**. [CrossRef]
27. Jepsen, S.; Suvan, J.; Deschner, J. The association of periodontal diseases with metabolic syndrome and obesity. *Periodontol 2000* **2020**. [CrossRef]
28. Mulhall, H.; Huck, O.; Amar, S. Porphyromonas gingivalis, a Long-Range Pathogen: Systemic Impact and Therapeutic Implications. *Microorganisms* **2020**, *8*, 869. [CrossRef]
29. Isola, G.; Polizzi, A.; Iorio Siciliano, V.; Alibrandi, A.; Ramaglia, L.; Leonardi, R. Effectiveness of a nutraceutical agent in the non-surgical periodontal therapy: A randomized, controlled clinical trial. *Clin. Oral Investig.* **2020**. [CrossRef]
30. Isola, G.; Polizzi, A.; Santonocito, S.; Alibrandi, A.; Ferlito, S. Expression of Salivary and Serum Malondialdehyde and Lipid Profile of Patients with Periodontitis and Coronary Heart Disease. *Int. J. Mol. Sci.* **2019**, *20*, 6061. [CrossRef]
31. Isola, G.; Giudice, A.L.; Polizzi, A.; Alibrandi, A.; Patini, R.; Ferlito, S. Periodontitis and Tooth Loss Have Negative Systemic Impact on Circulating Progenitor Cell Levels: A Clinical Study. *Genes* **2019**, *10*, 1022. [CrossRef]
32. Asakawa, M.; Takeshita, T.; Furuta, M.; Kageyama, S.; Takeuchi, K.; Hata, J.; Ninomiya, T.; Yamashita, Y. Tongue Microbiota and Oral Health Status in Community-Dwelling Elderly Adults. *mSphere* **2018**, *3*. [CrossRef] [PubMed]
33. Feres, M.; Teles, F.; Teles, R.; Figueiredo, L.C.; Faveri, M. The subgingival periodontal microbiota of the aging mouth. *Periodontol 2000* **2016**, *72*, 30–53. [CrossRef] [PubMed]
34. Jiang, Q.; Liu, J.; Chen, L.; Gan, N.; Yang, D. The Oral Microbiome in the Elderly with Dental Caries and Health. *Front. Cell Infect. Microbiol.* **2019**, *8*, 442. [CrossRef] [PubMed]
35. Iwauchi, M.; Horigome, A.; Ishikawa, K.; Mikuni, A.; Nakano, M.; Xiao, J.Z.; Odamaki, T.; Hironaka, S. Relationship between oral and gut microbiota in elderly people. *Immun. Inflamm. Dis.* **2019**, *7*, 229–236. [CrossRef] [PubMed]
36. Ogawa, T.; Hirose, Y.; Honda-Ogawa, M.; Sugimoto, M.; Sasaki, S.; Kibi, M.; Kawabata, S.; Ikebe, K.; Maeda, Y. Composition of salivary microbiota in elderly subjects. *Sci. Rep.* **2018**, *8*, 414. [CrossRef] [PubMed]
37. Zakaria, M.N.; Furuta, M.; Takeshita, T.; Shibata, Y.; Sundari, R.; Eshima, N.; Ninomiya, T.; Yamashita, Y. Oral microbiome in community-dwelling elderly and its relation to oral and general health conditions. *Oral Dis.* **2017**, *23*, 973–982. [CrossRef]

38. Nomura, Y.; Kakuta, E.; Okada, A.; Otsuka, R.; Shimada, M.; Tomizawa, Y.; Taguchi, C.; Arikawa, K.; Daikoku, H.; Sato, T.; et al. Effects of self-assessed chewing ability, tooth loss and serum albumin on mortality in 80-year-old individuals: A 20-year follow-up study. *BMC Oral Health.* **2020**, *20*, 122. [CrossRef]
39. World Health Organization. *Oral Health Surveys: Basic Methods*, 5th ed.; World Health Organization: Geneva, Switzerland, 2013.
40. Okada, M.; Hayashi, F.; Nagasaka, N. PCR detection of 5 Putative periodontal pathogens in dental plaque samples from children 2 to 12 years of age. *J. Clin. Periodontol.* **2001**, *28*, 576–582. [CrossRef]
41. Okada, A.; Sogabe, K.; Takeuchi, H.; Okamoto, M.; Nomura, Y.; Hanada, N. Characterization of specimens obtained by different sampling methods for evaluation of periodontal bacteria. *J. Oral Sci.* **2017**, *59*, 491–498. [CrossRef]
42. Kim, O.S.; Cho, Y.J.; Lee, K.; Yoon, S.H.; Kim, M.; Na, H.; Park, S.C.; Jeon, Y.S.; Lee, J.H.; Yi, H.; et al. Introducing EzTaxon-e: A prokaryotic 16S rRNA gene sequence database with phylotypes that represent uncultured species. *Int. J. Syst. Evol. Microbiol.* **2012**, *62*, 716–721. [CrossRef] [PubMed]
43. Yoon, S.H.; Ha, S.M.; Kwon, S.; Lim, J.; Kim, Y.; Seo, H.; Chun, J. Introducing EzBioCloud: A taxonomically united database of 16S rRNA and whole genome assemblies. *Int. J. Syst. Evol. Microbiol.* **2017**, *67*, 1613–1617. [CrossRef]
44. Nomura, Y.; Otsuka, R.; Hasegawa, R.; Hanada, N. Oral Microbiome of Children Living in an Isolated Area in Myanmar. *Int. J. Environ. Res. Public Health* **2020**, *17*, 4033. [CrossRef] [PubMed]
45. Lahti, L.; Shetty, S. Introduction to the Microbiome R Package, 2020. Available online: https://microbiome.github.io/tutorials/ (accessed on 31 July 2020).
46. Saraswati, S.; Sitaraman, R. Aging and the human gut microbiota-from correlation to causality. *Front. Microbiol.* **2014**, *5*, 764. [CrossRef] [PubMed]
47. Xu, Y.; Jia, Y.H.; Chen, L.; Huang, W.M.; Yang, D.Q. Metagenomic analysis of oral microbiome in young children aged 6–8 years living in a rural isolated Chinese province. *Oral Dis.* **2018**, *24*, 1115–1125. [CrossRef]
48. Burcham, Z.M.; Garneau, N.L.; Comstock, S.S.; Tucker, R.M.; Knight, R.; Metcalf, J.L. Patterns of Oral Microbiota Diversity in Adults and Children: A Crowdsourced Population Study. *Sci. Rep.* **2020**, *10*, 2133. [CrossRef]
49. Forsyth Institutes. eHOMED Expanded Human Oral Microbiome Database. Available online: http://www.homd.org/ (accessed on 31 July 2020).
50. Kolenbrander, P.E.; Palmer, R.J.; Periasamy, S.; Jakubovics, N.S. Oral multispecies biofilm development and the key role of cell-cell distance. *Nat. Rev. Microbiol.* **2010**, *8*, 471–480. [CrossRef]
51. Aas, J.A.; Paster, B.J.; Stokes, L.N.; Olsen, I.; Dewhirst, F.E. Defining the normal bacterial flora of the oral cavity. *J. Clin. Microbiol.* **2005**, *43*, 5721–5732. [CrossRef]
52. O'Donnell, L.E.; Robertson, D.; Nile, C.J.; Cross, L.J.; Riggio, M.; Sherriff, A.; Bradshaw, D.; Lambert, M.; Malcolm, J.; Buijs, M.J.; et al. The Oral Microbiome of Denture wearers is influenced by levels of natural dentition. *PLoS ONE* **2015**, *10*, e0137717. [CrossRef]
53. Kageyama, S.; Takeshita, T.; Furuta, M.; Tomioka, M.; Asakawa, M.; Suma, S.; Takeuchi, K.; Shibata, Y.; Iwasa, Y.; Yamashita, Y. Relationships of Variations in the Tongue Microbiota and Pneumonia Mortality in Nursing Home Residents. *J. Gerontol. A Biol. Sci. Med. Sci.* **2018**, *73*, 1097–1102. [CrossRef]
54. De Filippis, F.; Vannini, L.; LaStoria, A.; Laghi, L.; Piombino, P.; Stellato, G.; Serrazanetti, D.I.; Gozzi, G.; Turroni, S.; Ferrocino, I.; et al. The same microbiota and a potentially discriminant metabolome in the saliva of omnivore, ovo-lacto-vegetarian and Vegan individuals. *PLoS ONE* **2014**, *9*, e112373. [CrossRef] [PubMed]

5

Association of Salivary Human Papillomavirus Infection and Oral and Oropharyngeal Cancer

Óscar Rapado-González [1,2,3], Cristina Martínez-Reglero [4], Ángel Salgado-Barreira [4], Almudena Rodríguez-Fernández [5], Santiago Aguín-Losada [6], Luis León-Mateos [6], Laura Muinelo-Romay [2,3], Rafael López-López [3,6,*] and María Mercedes Suarez-Cunqueiro [1,3,7,*]

1 Department of Surgery and Medical-Surgical Specialties, Medicine and Dentistry School, Universidade de Santiago de Compostela (USC), 15782 Santiago de Compostela, Spain; oscar.rapado@rai.usc.es
2 Liquid Biopsy Analysis Unit, Translational Medical Oncology (Oncomet), Health Research Institute of Santiago (IDIS), 15706 Santiago de Compostela, Spain; lmuirom@gmail.com
3 Centro de Investigación Biomédica en Red en Cáncer (CIBERONC), Instituto de Salud Carlos III, 28029 Madrid, Spain
4 Methodology and Statistics Unit, Galicia Sur Health Research Institute (IISGS), 36312 Vigo, Spain; cristina.martinez@iisgaliciasur.es (C.M.-R.); angel.salgado.barreira@sergas.es (Á.S.-B.)
5 Department of Preventive and Public Health, Universidade de Santiago de Compostela (USC), 15782 Santiago de Compostela, Spain; almudena.rodríguez@usc.es
6 Translational Medical Oncology (Oncomet), Health Research Institute of Santiago (IDIS), Complexo Hospitalario Universitario de Santiago de Compostela (SERGAS), 15706 Santiago de Compostela, Spain; lanfear22@hotmail.com (S.A.-L.); Luis.Angel.Leon.Mateos@sergas.es (L.L.-M.)
7 Translational Medical Oncology (Oncomet), Health Research Institute of Santiago (IDIS), 15706 Santiago de Compostela, Spain
* Correspondence: rafa.lopez.lopez@gmail.com (R.L.-L.); mariamercedes.suarez@usc.es (M.M.S.-C.)

Abstract: Background. Human papillomavirus (HPV) infection has been recognized as an important risk factor in cancer. The purpose of this systematic review and meta-analysis was to determine the prevalence and effect size of association between salivary HPV DNA and the risk of developing oral and oropharyngeal cancer. Methods. A systematic literature search of PubMed, EMBASE, Web of Science, LILACS, Scopus and the Cochrane Library was performed, without language restrictions or specified start date. Pooled data were analyzed by calculating odds ratios (ORs) and 95% confidence intervals (CIs). Quality assessment was performed using the Newcastle–Ottawa Scale (NOS). Results. A total of 1672 studies were screened and 14 met inclusion criteria for the meta-analysis. The overall prevalence of salivary HPV DNA for oral and oropharyngeal carcinoma was 43.2%, and the prevalence of salivary HPV16 genotype was 27.5%. Pooled results showed a significant association between salivary HPV and oral and oropharyngeal cancer (OR = 4.94; 2.82–8.67), oral cancer (OR = 2.58; 1.67–3.99) and oropharyngeal cancer (OR = 17.71; 6.42–48.84). Significant associations were also found between salivary HPV16 and oral and oropharyngeal cancer (OR = 10.07; 3.65–27.82), oral cancer (OR = 2.95; 1.23–7.08) and oropharyngeal cancer (OR = 38.50; 22.43–66.07). Conclusions. Our meta-analysis demonstrated the association between salivary HPV infection and the incidence of oral and oropharyngeal cancer indicating its value as a predictive indicator.

Keywords: human papillomavirus; oral cancer; oropharyngeal cancer; saliva; meta-analysis

1. Introduction

Human papillomavirus (HPV) infection has been recognized as an important risk factor in a subset of head and neck squamous cell carcinomas, independently of traditional risk factors such as tobacco or alcohol use [1,2]. Globally, around 38,000 cases of head and neck cancer are attributed to the HPV infection. Of these, around 76% are cases of oropharynx cancer, 12% of oral cavity cancer and 10% of larynx cancer [3]. Currently, it is well known that HPV-status determines the molecular landscape of these tumors and their clinical evolution, with a better prognosis and response to therapy being found in HPV-positive patients [4,5].

HPVs are small, non-enveloped, close-circular, double-stranded DNA viruses of approximately 8000 base-pairs which present a specific tissue tropism infecting epithelial cells of the skin and mucosae of the anogenital and upper aero-digestive tract [6]. More than 200 different HPV types have been identified and classified into low-risk and high-risk according to their oncogenic potential. In this sense, high-risk HPV (HR-HPV) can promote the malignant transformation of HPV-infected cells through E6 and E7 viral oncoproteins, responsible for inactivating the *TP53* and *Rb* (retinoblastoma tumor suppressor gene) [7]. A subset of 12 alpha HR-HPV (16, 18, 31, 33, 35, 39, 45, 51, 52, 56, 58, and 59) has been classified as carcinogenic to humans according to the International Agency of Research in Cancer [8]. HR-HPV is considered the main cause of cervical cancer, genotypes 16 and 18 being responsible for 70% of cases [9]. In addition, several studies have also demonstrated the pathogenic role of HPV in other anogenital cancers [10–12] as well as in head and neck cancers [13]. Currently, HPV16 is widely recognized as an etiological factor in oropharynx tumors [14], however, not enough evidence exists regarding the HPV relationship and the anatomic subsites of head and neck squamous cell carcinoma [15].

Nowadays, a variety of molecular biological methods have been developed for the detection and genotyping of HPV at DNA, mRNA, and protein levels by polymerase chain reaction (PCR), real-time PCR, in situ hybridization, immunohistochemistry and serum antibody assays [16]. In addition, next-generation HPV sequencing approaches provide accurate information on genotype composition and pathways to better understand functional consequences [17]. Certain collection approaches present difficulties. For example, tumoral tissue biopsy is invasive and tumors may be inaccessible. For its part, the collection of oral exfoliated cells with cotton swabs or cytobrush is restricted to a specific and accessible oral area, making collection difficult for non-visual tumors and early molecular alterations. To overcome these drawbacks, the detection of HPV in oral exfoliated cells from saliva (with or without oral rinses) represents a quick and easy non-invasive alternative for oral and oropharyngeal cancer screening in high-risk populations. In this sense, several researchers have analyzed the prevalence of salivary HPV DNA from head and neck cancer, however, to our knowledge, no previous systematic review has elucidated evidence of this relationship. Therefore, the aim of the present systematic review and meta-analysis was to determine the prevalence and effect size of association between salivary HPV DNA and the risk of developing oral and oropharyngeal cancer.

2. Materials and Methods

2.1. Protocol and Registration

This study was conducted according to Preferred Reporting Items for Systematic Reviews and Meta-Analysis (PRISMA) guidelines [18] and the protocol was registered with the International Prospective Register of Systematic Reviews (reference No. CRD42020161345).

2.2. Search Strategy and Study Selection

The systematic literature search was performed in PubMed, EMBASE, Web of Science, LILACS, Scopus and the Cochrane Library through 9 January 2020, without language restrictions or specified start date. The following combinations of keywords and medical subject headings were used: (human papilloma virus OR HPV) AND (saliva OR oral rinses OR mouthwash) AND (oral squamous cell carcinoma OR OSCC OR oropharyngeal squamous cell carcinoma OR OPSCC OR oral cancer OR oropharyngeal cancer). All studies were screened based on the title and abstract, and eligible manuscripts were retrieved for full-text review. Additionally, we manually searched the reference lists in each original and review article in order to avoid missing potential studies. The literature search was performed independently by two researchers (ORG and MMSC), and any disagreements were resolved by consensus. The studies selected through the search strategy and other references were managed using RefWorks software, and duplicated items were removed using the associated tools.

2.3. *Eligibility Criteria*

We included the studies that met the following criteria: (1) case-control studies of patients with oral and/or oropharyngeal cancer and healthy controls, (2) HPV DNA prevalence determined in salivary samples (whole saliva or oral rinses), and (3) sufficient data to calculate odds ratios (ORs) with 95% confidence intervals (CIs). The exclusion criteria were as follows: (1) in vitro or animal study, (2) reviews, letters, personal opinions, book chapters, case reports, and conference abstracts, and (3) duplicate articles or suspicion of data overlap.

2.4. *Protocol and Registration*

Two researchers (ORG and MMSC) independently assessed each eligible manuscript, extracted data using a pre-established form, and collated the data into a Microsoft Excel spreadsheet (Microsoft Corp. Redmond, WA, USA). Any disagreement among reviewers was resolved by consensus. The following information was extracted from each study: author, publication year, country, type of sample, method of collection, tumor location, sample size, HPV detection method, number of cases and HPV-positive cases, number of controls and HPV-positive controls, HPV-positive genotypes, overall HPV DNA prevalence (number of subjects testing positive for any HPV type) and type-specific HPV DNA prevalence (number of subjects testing positive for specific HPV types: HPV16 or HPV18, HR-HPV and LR-HPV). If the required data were incomplete, attempts were made to contact the authors to obtain the missing information.

2.5. *Assessment of Risk Bias*

The Newcastle-Ottawa Scale (NOS) [19] was used to evaluate the individual quality of the selected studies by three independent researchers (ORG, ARF, and MMSC), and discrepancies were resolved by consensus. The NOS assesses the quality of non-randomized studies based on design, content and ease of use directed to the task of incorporating the quality assessments in the interpretation of meta-analytic results. This 'star system' consists of 8 items classified into three broad perspectives: the selection of study groups; the comparability of the groups; and the ascertainment of either the exposure or outcome of interest for case-control or cohort studies. The highest quality studies were allotted a maximum of one star for each item, except for, the item related to comparability, which was allowed the assignment of a maximum of two stars. The NOS score ranged from 0 to 9 stars and validity criteria were as follows: 8–9, high quality; 6–7, medium quality; <5 low quality.

2.6. *Statistical Analysis*

Statistical analysis was conducted using the meta package of free R software (v.3.6.2; https://www.r-project.org). Firstly, to evaluate the statistical model applied to the meta analytic database, heterogeneity was assessed using the Cochran's Q statistic test-based Chi-squared test and I2 statistics. Heterogeneity was considered significant when I2 > 50% and/or presence of a $p < 0.10$ for the Cochran's Q test. The prevalence of HPV DNA and HPV genotypes in oral and/or oropharyngeal cancer was calculated using fixed or random effects depending on the heterogeneity. The relationship between saliva HPV DNA infection and oral and/oropharyngeal cancer risk was evaluated by pooled odds ratio (OR) and 95% confidence intervals (CIs) comparing cases to controls. If significant heterogeneity was detected, the DerSimonian and Laird random-effects model was applied to calculate the pooled OR with 95% CIs; otherwise, the Mantel–Haenszel fixed-effects model was used. Then, subgroup analyses were performed to explore the potential sources of heterogeneity among studies according to the anatomic tumor location and HPV genotypes. Additionally, publication bias was checked with Begg's and Egger's tests and by visual inspection in funnel plots demonstrating the relationship between the individual log ORs and their standard errors [20,21]. p-values of <0.05 were considered to indicate statistical significance.

3. Results

3.1. Study Selection

A total of 1669 articles were identified across the six electronic databases and three additional reports from the reference lists. After removing duplicates, a total of 1542 articles were screened based on the title and abstract, and 1494 were excluded for lack of adherence to our inclusion criteria. Therefore, full-text articles were retrieved for the remaining 48 articles. After a full-text review, 34 articles were excluded for the following reasons: non case-control studies (22); controls under risk conditions (2); suspicious of data overlap (3); insufficient data (3); and reviews, letters, and meta-analysis (4). Finally, 14 articles met all the inclusion criteria and were included in the final analysis. A detailed flowchart showing the selection process is shown in Figure 1.

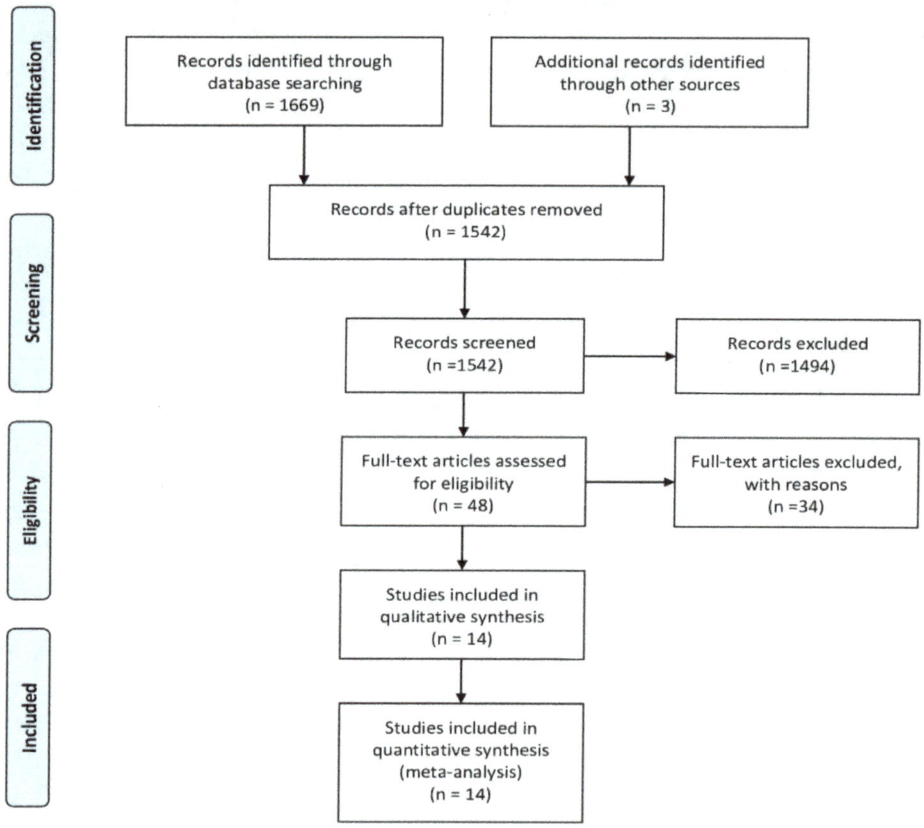

Figure 1. Preferred Reporting Items for Systematic Reviews and Meta-Analysis (PRISMA) flow diagram of the literature selection process, including identification, screening, eligibility and total studies included in qualitative and quantitative synthesis.

3.2. Study Characteristics

Individual characteristics of the included studies are summarized in Table 1. A total of 14 articles evaluating HPV prevalence in oral and/or oropharyngeal cancer were included in this meta-analysis, and these studies were carried out from 2005 to 2019. Study sample sizes ranged from 42 to 677 subjects.

The study units in this meta-analysis comprised a total of 2320 cases (658 from the oral cavity, 1160 from the oral cavity plus oropharynx and 502 from the oropharynx), and 5868 controls (2210 from the oral cavity, 2304 from the oral cavity plus oropharynx and 1354 from the oropharynx). As reported in Table 1, four studies were conducted in India [22–25], three in the USA [26–28], and two in Sweden [29,30], whereas the remaining studies were carried out in the following countries: Canada [31], France [32], Hungary [33], Pakistan [34], and Iran [35]. In terms of sampling, oral rinses and saliva ($n = 7$, 50%, respectively) were analyzed for HPV positivity and genotyping. The methods most used for saliva HPV-DNA determination were conventional PCR, nested PCR and quantitative PCR. However, other analytical strategies such as next generation sequencing or immunoassays were also employed for salivary HPV genotyping (Table 1).

3.3. *Study Quality*

Assessment of risk of bias and quality was performed according to NOS (Table S1). Regarding the selection domain, adequate description about characteristics and selection criteria for cases and controls were provided by all of the included studies. Regarding the comparability domain, six out of the 14 studies matched for age and at least one additional factor. Insofar as the exposure domain, few studies reported the blinding of analyses or non-response rates. The mean NOS score in our meta-analysis was six.

3.4. *Meta-Analysis*

3.4.1. Salivary HPV Association with Oral and Oropharyngeal Cancer

Overall, the prevalence of salivary HPV for oral and oropharyngeal carcinoma was of 43.2% ($n = 1160$) while the infection rate in the healthy control group was of 8.9% ($n = 2304$). Salivary HPV16 was the most common type of HPV DNA positive cases ($n = 1116$), representing 27.5% (Figure 2).

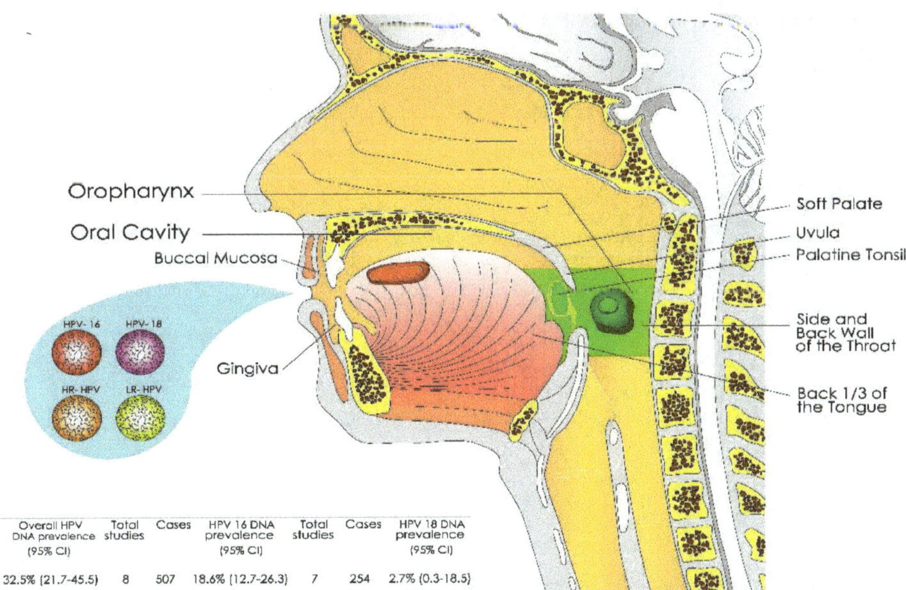

	Total studies	Cases	Overall HPV DNA prevalence (95% CI)	Total studies	Cases	HPV 16 DNA prevalence (95% CI)	Total studies	Cases	HPV 18 DNA prevalence (95% CI)
Oral	12	658	32.5% (21.7-45.5)	8	507	18.6% (12.7-26.3)	7	254	2.7% (0.3-18.5)
Oropharyngeal	8	502	51.9% (41.8-61.9)	7	456	39.6% (24.1-57.5)	5	363	1.4% (0.6-3.3)
Overall	14	1160	43.2% (35.8-50.8)	12	1116	27.5% (20.6-35.7)	10	748	2.3% (0.6-8.5)

Figure 2. Schematic drawing of salivary HPV and prevalence of oral and/or oropharyngeal cancer. Oral tissue sheds pathogen-infected cells containing different HPV DNA genotypes (HPV16, HPV18, HR-HPV, and LR-HPV) into saliva (with or without oral rinses). The prevalence of salivary HPV DNA varied according to anatomic tumor location, showing the highest infection rate in oropharyngeal carcinomas. In addition, the type-specific prevalence in saliva was also different according to the anatomic tumor location.

Table 1. Characteristics of the 14 case-control studies included in this meta-analysis.

	Country	Tumor Location (*n*)	Type of Sample/ Method of Collection	HPV-Positive Cases (n/N)	HPV-Positive Case Types	HPV-Positive Controls (n/N)	HPV-Positive Control Types	HPV Detection Method
Hansson et al.; 2005	Sweden	OC (85) OPC (46)	Oral rinse/7 mL of 0.9% NaCl solution for 30s	39/131	16, 18, 33, 45, 58, 59, 13, 32, 62, 10, 76	14/320	16, 67, 54, 55, 62, 87, 75, 76, RTRX9	Nested PCR (MY09/ MY11 and GP5+/6+ primers) DNA sequencing
SahebJamee et al.; 2009	Iran	OC (22)	Oral rinse/10 mL of normal saline	9/22	16, 18, 6/11	5/20	16, 6/11	PCR (GP5+/ 6+ primers for L1 region)
Kulkarni et al.; 2011	India	OC (34)	Saliva	24/34	16, 18	255/396	16, 18	PCR (16 and 18 specific primers)
Goot-Heah et al.; 2012	India	OC (14)	Saliva	0/14	-	0/30	-	Nested PCR (MY09/11 and GP5+/6+ primers for L1 region)
Chen et al.; 2013	USA	OC (32) OPC (52)	Saliva/Oragene DNA kits (DNA Genotek)	38/84	16	1/19	16	qPCR (specific primers and probe for E6 region of HPV16)
Nordfors et al.; 2014	Sweden	OPC (47)	Oral rinse/15 mL 50% Listerine®(Johnson and Johnson) for 30s	25/47	16, 18, 67, 6, 51	0/37	-	Bead-based multiplex assay on a MagPix instrument (Luminex Corporation), GP5+/6+ primers for the L1 region and specific primers and probe for E6 region of HPV16
Khyani et al.; 2015	Pakistan	OC (35)	Saliva	15/35	16, 18	3/35	16	qPCR using Real-time PCR Kit HPV16/18 Real-TM Quant (Sacace Biotechnologies)
Modak et al.; 2016	India	OC (235)	Saliva	149/235	16	193/409	16	PCR (HPV 16 specific primer)

Table 1. *Cont.*

	Country	Tumor Location (*n*)	Type of Sample/ Method of Collection	HPV-Positive Cases (n/N)	HPV-Positive Case Types	HPV-Positive Controls (n/N)	HPV-Positive Control Types	HPV Detection Method
Rosenthal et al.; 2017	USA	OC (61) OPC (45)	Oral rinse/10 mL of 0.9% NaCl solution for 30s	44/106	16, 18, * HR-HPV other	3/81	16, * HR-HPV other	qPCR from the HPV L1 region (Cobas®HPV Test-Roche Diagnostics)
Auguste et al.; 2017	France	OC (22) OPC (41)	Saliva/Oragene OG-500 kit (DNA Genotek)	21/63	16, 33, 51	80/308	16	PCR (SPF10 primer system for L1 region, INNO-LiPA®HPV Genotyping Extra; Innogenetics)
Laprise et al.; 2017	Canada	OC (72) OPC (183)	Oral rinse/alcohol-based solution for 15–30s	125/255	16, 18, ** HPV α-9 other than HPV16, *** HPV other	61/422	16, 18, ** HPV α-9 other than HPV16, *** HPV other	PCR (MY09/11 primers for HPV) and genotyping by Linear Array assay (Roche Molecular diagnostics)
Hettman et al.; 2018	Hungary	OPC (12)	Unstimulated saliva	4/12	16, 13	2/57	13, 11	PCR (MY09/11 primers for L1 region) Nested PCR (MY09/11 and GP5+/6+ primers for L1 region), sequencing for genotyping
Ramesh et al.; 2018	India	OC (30)	Oral rinse/10mL of 0.9% normal saline	13/30	16, 18	18/60	16, 18	Nested PCR (MY09/ 11 primers for L1 region)
Dang et al.; 2019	USA	OC (16) OPC (76)	Oral rinse/Original Mint Scope®mouthwash or Crest®Alcohol-free mouthwash (Proctor and Gamble) for 30s	37/92	16, NV14.4, NV69.1, NV95	1/110	18	qPCR (HPV16 E7/HPV18 E7 primers and probe) FAP-PCR from the L1 region NGS and Sanger sequencing

Abbreviations: OC, oral cancer; OPC, oropharynx cancer; PCR, polymerase chain reaction; qPCR, quantitative PCR; FAP-PCR, fluorescent arbitrarily primed PCR; NGS, next-generation sequencing; * HR-HPV other: 31, 33, 35, 39, 45, 51, 52, 56, 58, 59, 66, and 68; ** HPV α-9 other than HPV16: 31,33,35,52,58, and 67; *** HPV other: 6, 11, 18, 26, 34, 39, 40, 42, 44, 45, 51, 53, 54, 56, 59, 61, 62, 66, 68, 69, 70, 71, 72, 73, 81, 82, 83, 84, and 89.

Our meta-analysis included a total of 1160 cases and 2304 controls. The pooled analysis showed a significant association between positive salivary HPV DNA status and oral and oropharyngeal cancer with a pooled OR of 4.94 (95% CI = 2.82–8.67; $p < 0.01$) (Figure 3).

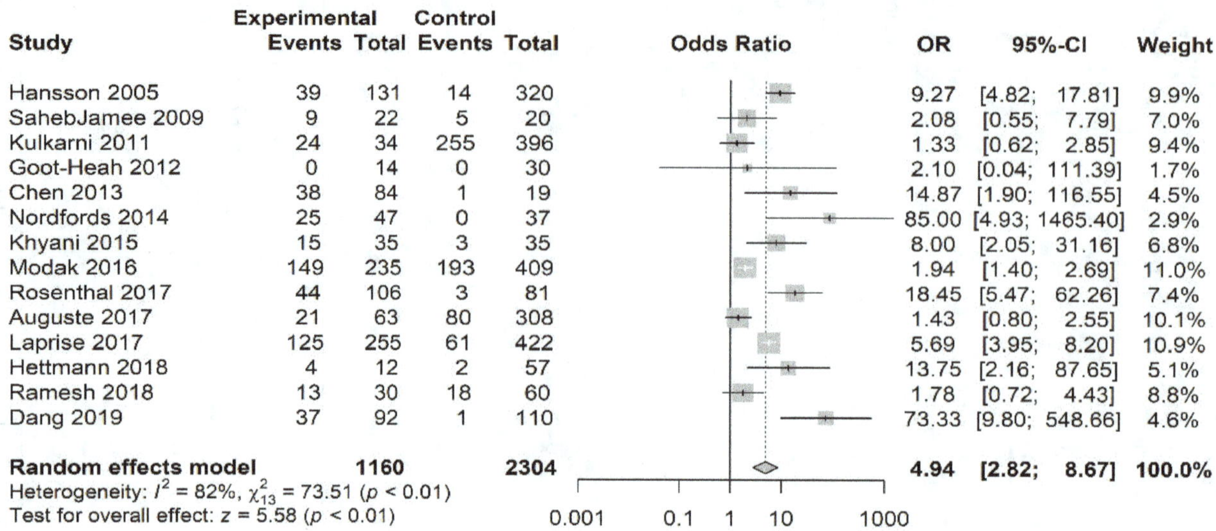

Figure 3. Forest plot for the studies on the association between salivary HPV and oral and oropharyngeal cancer. The squares indicate the ORs (odds ratios) in each study, with square sizes inversely proportional to the standard error of the OR. The diamond shape indicates the pooled ORs. Horizontal lines represent 95% CIs (confidence intervals), I2 > 50% indicates severe heterogeneity.

A random-effects model was used because heterogeneity was identified among the 14 studies (I2 = 82%). Visual inspection of the funnel plot revealed a symmetrical (Egger's test, $p = 0.159$; Begg's test, $p = 0.298$) distribution of the studies, indicating no evidence of publication bias (Figure 4).

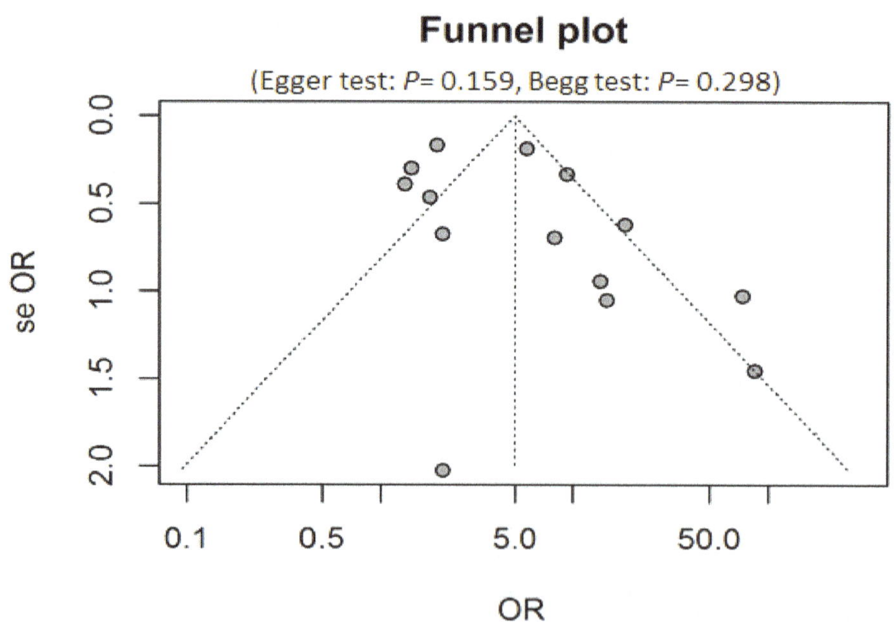

Figure 4. Funnel plot for studies (of 14 studies) on the association between salivary HPV and oral and oropharyngeal cancer. The vertical line represents the pooled OR using random-effect meta-analysis. Two diagonal lines represent (pseudo) 95% confidence limits around the OR for each standard error on the vertical axis. In the absence of heterogeneity, 95% of the studies should lie within the funnel defined by these diagonal lines. Abbreviations: se OR, standard error of odds ratio.

For the type-specific analysis (Figure 5), salivary HPV16 showed a significant association with a pooled OR of 10.07 (95% CI = 3.65–27.82; $p < 0.01$). However, salivary HPV18 did not show any significant increased risk for oral and oropharyngeal cancer with a pooled OR of 1.80 (95% CI = 0.66–4.90). In addition, a significant association was found for salivary HR-HPV with OR of 5.94 (95% CI = 2.78–12.69; $p < 0.01$), whereas salivary LR-HPV did not show any significant increased risk with OR of 1.45 (95% CI = 0.70–2.98). The respective funnel plots are represented in Figures S1–S4.

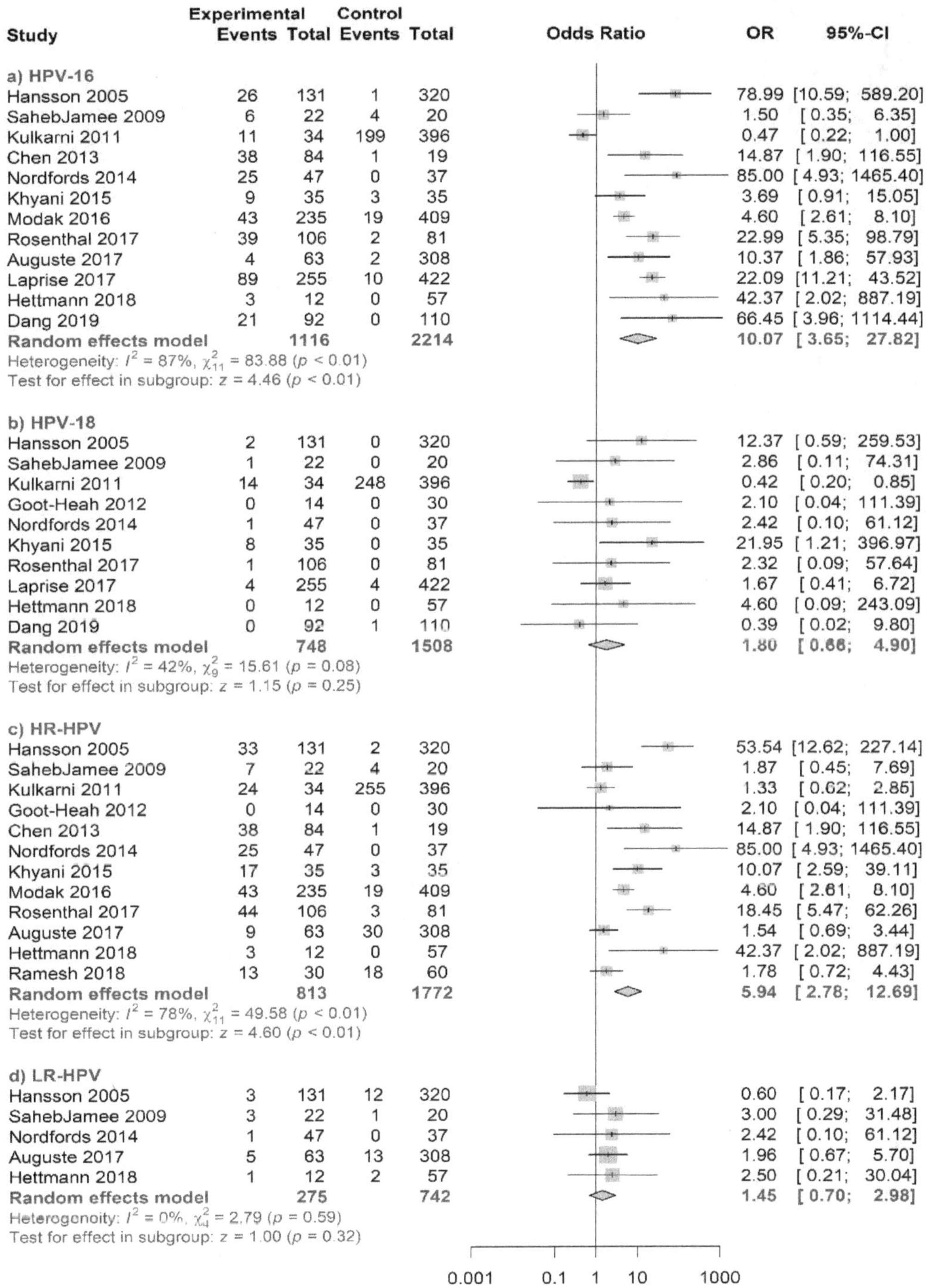

Figure 5. Forest plot for the studies on the association between salivary HPV and oral and oropharyngeal cancer. The squares indicate the ORs in each study, with square sizes inversely proportional to the standard error of the OR. The diamond shape indicates the pooled ORs. Horizontal lines represent 95% CIs. I2 > 50% indicates severe heterogeneity. (**a**) HPV16, (**b**) HPV18, (**c**) HR-HPV, and (**d**) LR-HPV.

3.4.2. Type-Specific Salivary HPV Association with Oropharyngeal Cancer

Our subgroup meta-analysis consisted of eight studies, including 502 cases and 1354 controls. In the pooled analysis, salivary HPV DNA infection and oropharyngeal cancer showed a significant association with a pooled OR of 17.71 (95% CI = 6.42–48.84; $p < 0.01$) (Figure 6).

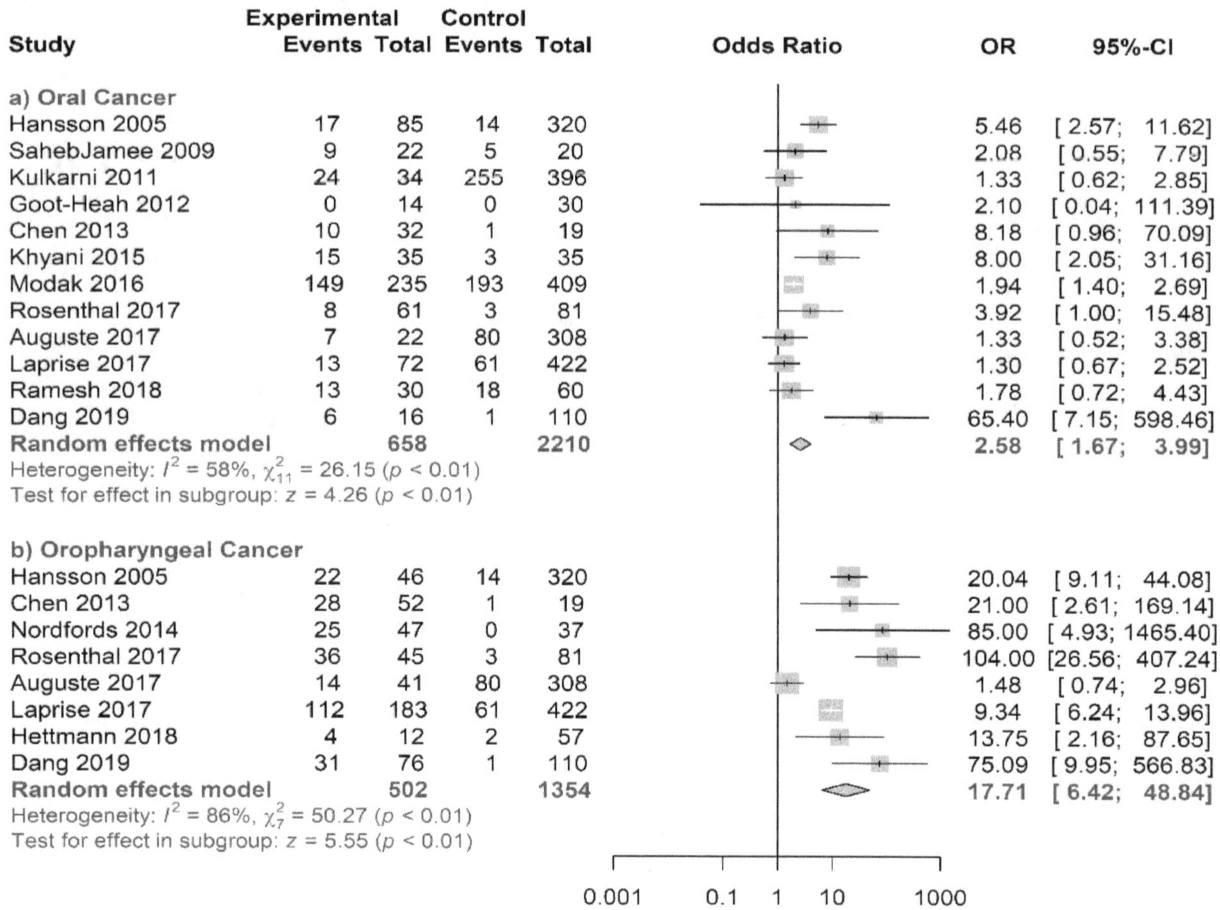

Figure 6. Forest plot for the studies on the association between salivary HPV and anatomic tumor subsites. The squares indicate the ORs in each study, with square sizes inversely proportional to the standard error of the OR. The diamond shape indicates the pooled ORs. Horizontal lines represent 95% CIs. I2 > 50% indicates severe heterogeneity. (**a**) Oral Cancer and (**b**) Oropharyngeal Cancer.

According to type-specific analysis (Figure 7), salivary HPV16 showed a significant association with a pooled OR of 38.50 (95% CI = 22.43–66.07; $p < 0.01$) whereas salivary HPV18 showed no significant association with a pooled OR of 1.92 (95% CI = 0.63–5.91). In addition, a significant association was found for salivary HR-HPV with a pooled OR of 26.69 (95% CI = 3.46–206.17; $p < 0.01$) whereas no significant association was found for salivary LR-HPV with a pooled OR of 2.08 (95% CI = 0.75–5.81). Their respective funnel plots are shown in Figures S5–S9.

Study	Experimental Events	Experimental Total	Control Events	Control Total	OR	95%-CI
a) HPV-16						
Chen 2013	28	52	1	19	21.00	[2.61; 169.14]
Nordfords 2014	25	47	0	37	85.00	[4.93; 1465.40]
Rosenthal 2017	33	45	2	81	108.62	[23.03; 512.34]
Auguste 2017	4	41	2	308	16.54	[2.93; 93.42]
Laprise 2017	84	183	10	422	34.96	[17.51; 69.79]
Hettmann 2018	3	12	0	57	42.37	[2.02; 887.19]
Dang 2019	19	76	0	110	74.95	[4.44; 1263.88]
Random effects model		**456**		**1034**	**38.50**	**[22.43; 66.07]**
Heterogeneity: $I^2 = 0\%$, $\chi^2_6 = 3.63$ ($p = 0.73$)						
Test for effect in subgroup: $z = 13.25$ ($p < 0.01$)						
b) HPV-18						
Nordfords 2014	1	47	0	37	2.42	[0.10; 61.12]
Rosenthal 2017	1	45	0	81	5.49	[0.22; 137.71]
Laprise 2017	3	183	4	422	1.74	[0.39; 7.86]
Hettmann 2018	0	12	0	57	4.60	[0.09; 243.09]
Dang 2019	0	76	1	110	0.48	[0.02; 11.87]
Random effects model		**363**		**707**	**1.92**	**[0.63; 5.91]**
Heterogeneity: $I^2 = 0\%$, $\chi^2_4 = 1.35$ ($p = 0.85$)						
Test for effect in subgroup: $z = 1.14$ ($p = 0.25$)						
c) HR-HPV						
Chen 2013	28	52	1	19	21.00	[2.61; 169.14]
Nordfords 2014	25	47	0	37	85.00	[4.93; 1465.40]
Rosenthal 2017	37	45	3	81	120.25	[30.15; 479.60]
Auguste 2017	9	41	30	308	2.61	[1.14; 5.98]
Hettmann 2018	3	12	0	57	42.37	[2.02; 887.19]
Random effects model		**197**		**502**	**26.69**	**[3.46; 206.17]**
Heterogeneity: $I^2 = 86\%$, $\chi^2_4 = 27.6$ ($p < 0.01$)						
Test for effect in subgroup: $z = 3.15$ ($p < 0.01$)						
d) LR-HPV						
Hansson 2005	1	46	12	320	0.57	[0.07, 4.49]
Nordfords 2014	1	47	0	37	2.42	[0.10; 61.12]
Auguste 2017	5	41	13	308	3.15	[1.06; 9.35]
Random effects model		**134**		**665**	**2.08**	**[0.75; 5.81]**
Heterogeneity: $I^2 = 9\%$, $\chi^2_2 = 2.19$ ($p = 0.33$)						
Test for effect in subgroup: $z = 1.40$ ($p = 0.16$)						

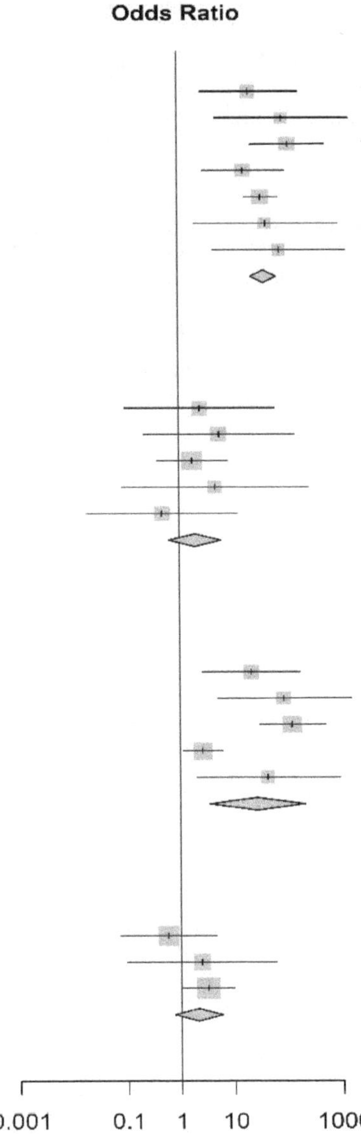

Figure 7. Forest plot for the studies on the association between salivary HPV and oropharyngeal cancer. The squares indicate the ORs in each study, with square sizes inversely proportional to the standard error of the OR. The diamond shape indicates the pooled ORs. Horizontal lines represent 95% CIs. I2 > 50% indicates severe heterogeneity. (**a**) HPV16, (**b**) HPV18, (**c**) HR-HPV, and (**d**) LR-HPV.

3.4.3. Type-Specific Salivary HPV Association with Oral Cancer

Our subgroup meta-analysis consisted of 12 studies, including 658 cases and 2210 controls. In the pooled analysis, salivary HPV DNA infection and oral cancer showed a significant association with a pooled OR of 2.58 (95% CI = 1.67–3.99; $p < 0.01$) (Figure 6). According to type-specific analysis (Figure 8), salivary HPV16 showed a significant association with a pooled OR of 2.95 (95% CI = 1.23–7.08; $p = 0.02$), whereas no significant association was observed for salivary HPV18 with a pooled OR of 1.51 (95% CI = 0.45–5.15). In addition, a significant association was observed for salivary HR-HPV with a pooled OR of 4.44 (95% CI – 2.47–7.98; $p < 0.01$). However, salivary LR-HPV did not show any significantly increased risk for oral cancer with OR of 1.79 (95% CI = 0.67–4.74). Their respective funnel plots are shown in Figures S10–S14.

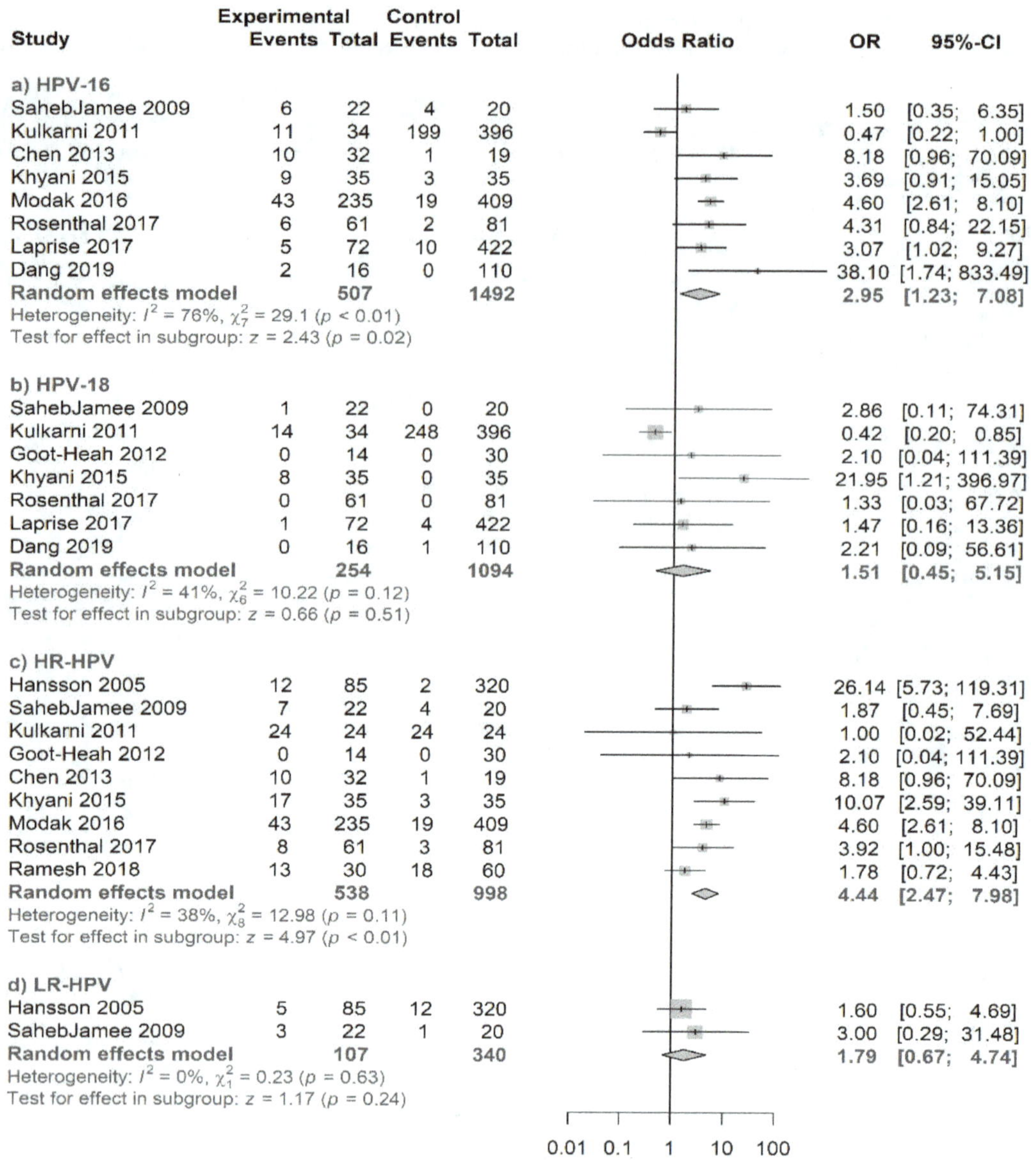

Figure 8. Forest plot for the studies on the association between salivary HPV and oral cancer. The squares indicate the ORs in each study, with square sizes inversely proportional to the standard error of the OR. The diamond shape indicates the pooled ORs. Horizontal lines represent 95% CIs. I2 > 50% indicates severe heterogeneity. (**a**) HPV16, (**b**) HPV18, (**c**) HR-HPV, and (**d**) LR-HPV.

4. Discussion

In the present study the overall pooled prevalence of salivary HPV-related to oral and oropharyngeal cancer was 43.2%. Similarly, a meta-analysis based on 11 case-control studies evaluating the HPV infection in oral and oropharyngeal cancer found an HPV DNA prevalence of 39.27% [36]. In terms of anatomic tumor location, we observed the highest prevalence of salivary HPV in oropharyngeal cancer (51.9%), whereas the overall percentage in the oral cavity was 32.5%. Similarly, a large comprehensive meta-analysis based on data from 148 studies estimated a pooled HPV DNA prevalence of 45.8% in oropharynx tumors and 24.5% in oral cavity tumors [37]. Although our meta-analysis did not evaluate HPV DNA prevalence in different oropharynx subsites, evidence shows that HPV is most prevalent in tonsils and base of tongue cancers compared to tumors located in walls of oropharynx, uvula and soft palate [38].

Overall, in our study, salivary HPV16 was the most commonly detected oncogenic type, accounting for around 28% of cases. As we expected, salivary HPV16 showed a higher prevalence in oropharyngeal cancer (39.6%) than oral cancer (18.6%), in accordance with previous studies [37,39,40]. In particular, the salivary HPV16 prevalence in our study was slightly higher in oral cancer than reported in a meta-analysis by Nydiae et al. [37] (18.6% vs 14.9%), however, other authors have reported higher rates of HPV16 prevalence in oral carcinoma, ranging from 20% to 50% [41–43]. Salivary HPV18 was another oncogenic HPV type commonly evaluated by the included studies. Unlike salivary HPV16, HPV18 positivity was found much less frequently, with an overall prevalence of 2.3%. Salivary HPV18 prevalence was even lower in oropharynx tumors (1.7%) as compared to oral cavity tumors (2.7%). One plausible explanation for the decreased prevalence of salivary HPV18 in both oral and oropharyngeal cancers is its specific tropism for glandular tissue and adenocarcinomas, while most head and neck cancers are predominantly of the squamous cell carcinoma type [44]. In addition, HR-HPV has developed a variety of mechanisms facilitating HPV evasion of recognition and clearance by the host immune system [45], which probably contributes to the different viral persistence in each of the anatomic regions of the head and neck. As in our study, Kreimer et al. [40] and Ndyae et al. [37] also found a low HPV18 prevalence in oropharynx tumors (1% and 0.7%, respectively), however, these studies reported a higher HPV18 prevalence in oral cancer (8% and 5.9%, respectively). These differences could be explained by the effect on HPV prevalence of different covariates such as geographical location, lifestyles (alcohol, tobacco or sexual activity), sample size, types of samples and methods used for HPV detection.

To the best of our knowledge, this is the first meta-analysis evaluating the association between salivary HPV and oral and/or oropharyngeal cancer. The pooled OR showed that oral and oropharyngeal cancer patients had an almost five-fold higher risk of HPV infection than controls. A previous meta-analysis evaluating the presence of HPV in oral and oropharyngeal cancer detected by different methods (histopathology, serum analysis, and cytopathology using OralCDx or oral swishes) reported a significant association with an OR of 2.82 [36]. Overall, our results indicate that salivary HPV causes a higher risk of oral and oropharyngeal carcinogenesis. In addition, we also conducted different subgroup analysis to evaluate the impact of HPV infection on cancer risk according to anatomic tumor location and HPV genotypes. We stratified the salivary HPV studies by anatomical location observing a stronger association between salivary HPV and oropharynx tumors compared to oral cavity tumors. Similarly, Shaik et al. performed a comprehensive metanalysis of HPV-associated head and neck cancers, reporting the highest association for oropharyngeal cancer, with an OR of 14.66, whereas oral cavity and laryngeal cancers had ORs of 4.06 and 3.23, respectively [46]. In addition, we evaluated type-specific salivary HPV risk associated with oral and oropharyngeal cancer. Compared to oncogenic potential, salivary HR-HPV types were associated with an increased risk of oral and oropharyngeal carcinomas. Thus, salivary HPV16 was significantly associated with oral cancer, confirming the findings reported in previous studies [43,47]. Like our study, Hobbs et al. reported a weak statistically significant association between HPV16 and oral cancer, with an OR of 2.0 [45]. On the contrary, a higher association (OR = 9) was reported by Zhu et al., suggesting the potential oncogenic role of HPV16 in oral carcinogenesis in Chinese population [43]. However, in our study, a stronger association was found between salivary HPV16 and oropharyngeal cancer, presenting an OR of 38.50, which suggests the role of HPV16 in the etiology of oropharyngeal cancer. Unlike other meta-analysis [47,48], our study did not analyze association based on specific subsites of the oropharynx. In this sense, a consistent association between HPV16 infection and tonsil cancer has previously been described [47], which seems to indicate a different oncogenic role for HPV infection in the different subsites of oropharynx.

All the studies included in the present meta-analysis addressed HPV status in oral exfoliated cells collected from saliva with or without oral rinses. In this sense, the first association between oral HPV and oral cancer was reported by Smith et al. [49]. These authors evaluated HPV status in oral exfoliated cells collected by oral rinses from 93 patients and 205 controls finding significantly increased risk (OR = 3.70) of cancer in positive oral HPV patients regardless of alcohol and tobacco use [49]. According to the evidence, salivary HPV DNA represents a promising approach for identifying oral HPV infection. Several authors have shown a significant correlation between HPV DNA detected in tissue and positivity for HPV DNA in saliva, suggesting the potential value of this biofluid for detecting HPV and thus predicting HPV-related head and neck carcinomas [1,50]. Furthermore, salivary HPV DNA has demonstrated to be a good marker for detecting HPV in oropharyngeal cancer, as a high agreement between salivary HPV16 DNA infection and tumor p16 expression has been observed [51–53]. However, a recent study revealed a lower sensitivity for identifying p16-positive oral cancer patients through salivary HPV, which may indicate a limited involvement of HPV16 in oral carcinogenesis [54]. Interestingly, our study reviewed the different salivary HPV genotypes identified in oral and oropharyngeal carcinomas, providing additional evidence on the co-existence of multiple HPV types during carcinogenesis. In this matter, saliva analysis represents a great opportunity for the identification and characterization of novel HPVs involved in head and neck cancer.

Our study has several strengths. It is the first meta-analysis highlighting the association between salivary HPV infection and oral and/or oropharyngeal cancer. Moreover, we examined both the overall and the specific prevalence of salivary HPV DNA in oral and/or oropharyngeal cancer. In addition, we performed a comprehensive literature review without language restrictions and the results of our study were in concordance with the scientific evidence. However, the present study is not exempt from limitations. Firstly, the studies included in our meta-analysis were heterogeneous, which could be explained by different factors such as ethnicity, sample size, geographic region, anatomic tumor location, method of HPV detection and different HPV genotypes. Although we performed a subgroup analysis by anatomic tumor location and HPV genotypes, we were unable to elucidate the potential sources contributing to this heterogeneity. Secondly, data such as age, smoking, drinking, sexual habits or diet were not provided by the studies in our sample, hampering the assessment of these confounding variables. Thirdly, some studies included in our analysis could be biased due to the fact that cases and controls were not matched for demographic variables such as age, sex and lifestyle habits. In addition, although almost all these studies analyzed HPV16 and HPV18, we observed high variability regarding HPV genotypes and HPV detection methods, which could substantially affect the results of our analysis.

5. Conclusions

To the best of our knowledge, this is the first meta-analysis addressing the association between salivary HPV infection and oral and oropharyngeal carcinoma. The findings of this meta-analysis provide additional evidence that salivary HPV is associated with oral and oropharyngeal cancer, suggesting that salivary HPV infection is a risk factor for oral and oropharyngeal cancer. However, to validate our findings, future research should focus on prospective cohort studies that explore the occurrence of salivary HPV infection in oral and oropharyngeal cancer. In addition, it is necessary to analyze confounding variables that might be associated with an increased risk of HPV infection in oral and oropharyngeal cancer.

Supplementary Materials:
Table S1: The Newcastle–Ottawa Scale (NOS) for assessing the quality of included studies, Figure S1: funnel plot for studies (of 12 studies) on the association between salivary HPV16 and oral and oropharyngeal cancer, Figure S2: funnel plot for studies (of 10 studies) on the association between salivary HPV18 and oral and oropharyngeal cancer, Figure S3: funnel plot for studies (of 12 studies) on the association between salivary HR-HPV and oral and oropharyngeal cancer, Figure S4: funnel plot for studies (of five studies) on the association between salivary LR-HPV and oral and oropharyngeal cancer, Figure S5: funnel plot for studies (of eight studies) on the association between salivary HPV and oropharyngeal cancer, Figure S6: funnel plot for studies (of seven studies) on the association between salivary HPV16 and oropharyngeal cancer, Figure S7: funnel plot for studies (of five studies) on the association between salivary HPV18 and oropharyngeal cancer, Figure S8: funnel plot for studies (of five studies) on the association between salivary HR-HPV and oropharyngeal cancer, Figure S9: funnel plot for studies (of three studies) on the association between salivary LR-HPV and oropharyngeal cancer, Figure S10: funnel plot for studies (of 12 studies) on the association between salivary HPV and oral cancer, Figure S11: funnel plot for studies (of eight studies) on the association between salivary HPV16 and oral cancer, Figure S12: funnel plot for studies (of seven studies) on the association between salivary HPV18 and oral cancer, Figure S13: funnel plot for studies (of nine studies) on the association between salivary HR-HPV and oral cancer, and Figure S14: funnel plot for studies (of two studies) on the association between salivary LR-HPV and oral cancer.

Author Contributions: Conceptualization, Ó.R.-G., R.L.-L. and M.M.S.-C.; methodology, Ó.R.-G., M.M.S.-C., Á.S.-B., and C.M.-R.; software, Á.S.-B. and C.M.-R.; validation, Ó.R.-G. and M.M.S.-C.; formal analysis, Á.S.-B. and C.M.-R.; investigation, Ó.R.-G. and M.M.S.-C.; resources, Ó.R.-G. and A.R.-F.; data curation, Á.S.-B. and C.M.-R.; writing—original draft preparation, Ó.R.-G. and M.M.S.-C.; writing—review and editing, Ó.R.-G., M.M.S.-C., L.M.-R., R.L.-L., S.A.-L. and L.L.-M.; visualization, Ó.R.-G. and M.M.S.-C.; supervision, M.M.S.-C. and R.L.-L.; project administration, M.M.S.-C. and R.L.-L.; funding acquisition, M.M.S.-C. All authors have read and agreed to the published version of the manuscript.

References

1. Smith, E.M.; Ritchie, J.M.; Summersgill, K.F.; Hoffman, H.T.; Wang, D.H.; Haugen, T.H.; Turek, L.P. Human papillomavirus in oral exfoliated cells and risk of head and neck cancer. *J. Natl. Cancer Inst.* **2004**, *96*, 449–455. [CrossRef] [PubMed]
2. D'Souza, G.; Kreimer, A.R.; Viscidi, R.; Pawlita, M.; Fakhry, C.; Koch, W.M.; Westra, W.H.; Gillison, M.L. Case-control study of human papillomavirus and oropharyngeal cancer. *N. Engl. J. Med.* **2007**, *356*, 1944–1956. [CrossRef] [PubMed]
3. Murtaza, M.; Dawson, S.J.; Tsui, D.W.Y.; Gale, D.; Forshew, T.; Piskorz, A.M.; Parkinson, C.; Chin, S.F.; Kingsbury, Z.; Wong, A.S.C.; et al. Non-invasive analysis of acquired resistance to cancer therapy by sequencing of plasma DNA. *Nature* **2013**, *497*, 108–112. [CrossRef] [PubMed]
4. Fakhry, C.; Westra, W.H.; Li, S.; Cmelak, A.; Ridge, J.A.; Pinto, H.; Forastiere, A.; Gillison, M.L. Improved survival of patients with human papillomavirus-positive head and neck squamous cell carcinoma in a prospective clinical trial. *J. Natl. Cancer Inst.* **2008**, *100*, 261–269. [CrossRef]
5. O'Rorke, M.A.; Ellison, M.V.; Murray, L.J.; Moran, M.; James, J.; Anderson, L.A. Human papillomavirus related head and neck cancer survival: A systematic review and meta-analysis. *Oral Oncol.* **2012**, *48*, 1191–1201. [CrossRef]
6. Tommasino, M. The human papillomavirus family and its role in carcinogenesis. *Semin. Cancer Biol.* **2014**, *26*, 13–21. [CrossRef]
7. Sabatini, M.E.; Chiocca, S. Human papillomavirus as a driver of head and neck cancers. *Br. J. Cancer* **2020**, *122*, 306–314. [CrossRef]
8. IARC Working Group on the Evaluation of Carcinogenic Risks to Humans. Human papillomaviruses. *IARC Monogr. Eval. Carcinog. Risks Hum.* **2007**, *90*, 1–636.
9. Schiffman, M.; Castle, P.E.; Jeronimo, J.; Rodriguez, A.C.; Wacholder, S. Human papillomavirus and cervical cancer. *Lancet (Lond. Engl.)* **2007**, *370*, 890–907. [CrossRef]
10. Faber, M.T.; Sand, F.L.; Albieri, V.; Norrild, B.; Kjaer, S.K.; Verdoodt, F. Prevalence and type distribution of human papillomavirus in squamous cell carcinoma and intraepithelial neoplasia of the vulva. *Int. J. Cancer* **2017**, *141*, 1161–1169. [CrossRef]
11. Schlenker, B.; Schneede, P. The role of human papilloma virus in penile cancer prevention and new therapeutic agents. *Eur. Urol. Focus* **2019**, *5*, 42–45. [CrossRef] [PubMed]
12. Lin, C.; Franceschi, S.; Clifford, G.M. Human papillomavirus types from infection to cancer in the anus, according to sex and HIV status: A systematic review and meta-analysis. *Lancet Infect. Dis.* **2018**, *18*, 198–206. [CrossRef]
13. Tumban, E. A current update on human papillomavirus-associated head and neck cancers. *Viruses* **2019**, *11*, 922. [CrossRef] [PubMed]
14. IARC Working Group on the Evaluation of Carcinogenic Risks to Humans. Biological agents. Volume 100 B. A review of human carcinogens. *IARC Monogr. Eval. Carcinog. Risks Hum.* **2012**, *100 (Pt B)*, 1–441.
15. Hübbers, C.U.; Akgül, B. HPV and cancer of the oral cavity. *Virulence* **2015**, *6*, 244–248. [CrossRef]
16. Kobayashi, K.; Hisamatsu, K.; Suzui, N.; Hara, A.; Tomita, H.; Miyazaki, T. A review of HPV-related head and neck cancer. *J. Clin. Med.* **2018**, *7*, 241. [CrossRef]
17. Tuna, M.; Amos, C.I. Next generation sequencing and its applications in HPV-associated cancers. *Oncotarget* **2017**, *8*, 8877–8889. [CrossRef]
18. Moher, D.; Liberati, A.; Tetzlaff, J.; Altman, D.G. Preferred reporting items for systematic reviews and meta-analyses: The PRISMA Statement. *PLoS Med.* **2009**, *6*, e1000097. [CrossRef]
19. Wells, G.A.; Shea, B.; O'Connell, D.; Peterson, J.; Welch, V.; Losos, M.; Tugwell, P. The Newcastle-Ottawa

Scale (NOS) for Assessing the Quality of Nonrandomized Studies in Meta-Analysis. Available online: http://www.ohri.ca/programs/clinical_epidemiology/oxford.asp (accessed on 18 February 2020).

20. Egger, M.; Davey Smith, G.; Schneider, M.; Minder, C. Bias in meta-analysis detected by a simple, graphical test. *BMJ* **1997**, *315*, 629–634. [CrossRef]
21. Begg, C.B.; Mazumdar, M. Operating characteristics of a rank correlation test for publication bias. *Biometrics* **1994**, *50*, 1088–1101. [CrossRef]
22. Kulkarni, S.S.; Kulkarni, S.S.; Vastrad, P.P.; Kulkarni, B.B.; Markande, A.R.; Kadakol, G.S.; Hiremath, S.V.; Kaliwal, S.; Patil, B.R.; Gai, P.B. Prevalence and distribution of high risk human papillomavirus (HPV) types 16 and 18 in carcinoma of cervix, saliva of patients with oral squamous cell carcinoma and in the general population in Karnataka, India. *Asian Pac. J. Cancer Prev.* **2011**, *12*, 645–648. [PubMed]
23. Goot-Heah, K.; Kwai-Lin, T.; Froemming, G.R.A.; Abraham, M.T.; Nik Mohd Rosdy, N.M.M.; Zain, R.B. Human papilloma virus 18 detection in oral squamous cell carcinoma and potentially malignant lesions using saliva samples. *Asian Pac. J. Cancer Prev.* **2012**, *13*, 6109–6113. [CrossRef]
24. Modak, H.; Sayad, T.; Fernandes, N. Molecular detection of HPV 16 in saliva of patients with oral squamous cell carcinoma and in the normal population of Southwesterly Indians. *Int. J. Adv. Biol. Res.* **2016**, *6*, 25–29.
25. Ramesh, P.S.; Devegowda, D.; Naik, P.R.; Doddamani, P.; Nataraj, S.M. Evaluating the feasibility of nested PCR as a screening tool to detect HPV infection in saliva of oral squamous cell carcinoma subjects. *J. Clin. Diagnostic Res.* **2018**, *12*, BC22–BC25. [CrossRef]
26. Rosenthal, M.; Huang, B.; Katabi, N.; Migliacci, J.; Bryant, R.; Kaplan, S.; Blackwell, T.; Patel, S.; Yang, L.; Pei, Z.; et al. Detection of HPV related oropharyngeal cancer in oral rinse specimens. *Oncotarget* **2017**, *8*, 109393–109401. [CrossRef]
27. Chen, K.M.; Stephen, J.K.; Ghanem, T.; Stachler, R.; Gardner, G.; Jones, L.; Schweitzer, V.P.; Hall, F.; Divine, G.; Worsham, M.J. Human papilloma virus prevalence in a multiethnic screening population. *Otolaryngol. Neck Surg.* **2013**, *148*, 436–442. [CrossRef]
28. Dang, J.; Bruce, G.A.; Zhang, Q.; Kiviat, N.B. Identification and characterization of novel human papillomaviruses in oral rinse samples from oral cavity and oropharyngeal cancer patients. *J. Oral Biosci.* **2019**, *61*, 190–194. [CrossRef]
29. Hansson, B.G.; Rosenquist, K.; Antonsson, A.; Wennerberg, J.; Schildt, E.-B.; Bladström, A.; Andersson, G. Strong association between infection with human papillomavirus and oral and oropharyngeal squamous cell carcinoma: A population-based case-control study in southern Sweden. *Acta Otolaryngol.* **2005**, *125*, 1337–1344. [CrossRef]
30. Nordfors, C.; Vlastos, A.; Du, J.; Ahrlund-Richter, A.; Tertipis, N.; Grün, N.; Romanitan, M.; Haeggblom, L.; Roosaar, A.; Dahllöf, G.; et al. Human papillomavirus prevalence is high in oral samples of patients with tonsillar and base of tongue cancer. *Oral Oncol.* **2014**, *50*, 491–497. [CrossRef]
31. Laprise, C.; Madathil, S.A.; Schlecht, N.F.; Castonguay, G.; Soulières, D.; Nguyen-Tan, P.F.; Allison, P.; Coutlée, F.; Hier, M.; Rousseau, M.C.; et al. Human papillomavirus genotypes and risk of head and neck cancers: Results from the HeNCe Life case-control study. *Oral Oncol.* **2017**, *69*, 56–61. [CrossRef]
32. Auguste, A.; Gaëte, S.; Herrmann-Storck, C.; Michineau, L.; Joachim, C.; Deloumeaux, J.; Duflo, S.; Luce, D. Prevalence of oral HPV infection among healthy individuals and head and neck cancer cases in the French West Indies. *Cancer Causes Control.* **2017**, *28*, 1333–1340. [CrossRef] [PubMed]
33. Hettmann, A.; Demcsák, A.; Bach, Á.; Decsi, G.; Dencs, Á.; Pálinkó, D.; Rovó, L.; Terhes, G.; Urbán, E.; Buzás, K.; et al. Prevalence and genotypes of human papillomavirus in saliva and tumor samples of head and neck cancer patients in Hungary. *Infect. Genet. Evol.* **2018**, *59*, 99–106. [CrossRef] [PubMed]
34. Khyani, I.A.M.; Qureshi, M.A.; Mirza, T.; Farooq, M.U. Salivary detection of human papilloma virus 16 & 18 in pre-malignant and malignant lesions of oral cavity: Is it feasible in Pakistani context of socio-cultural taboos? *Pak. J. Med. Sci.* **2015**, *31*, 1104–1109. [PubMed]
35. SahebJamee, M.; Boorghani, M.; Ghaffari, S.R.; AtarbashiMoghadam, F.; Keyhani, A. Human papillomavirus in saliva of patients with oral squamous cell carcinoma. *Med. Oral Patol. Oral Cir. Bucal* **2009**, *14*, e525–e528. [CrossRef]
36. Chaitanya, N.C.; Allam, N.S.; Gandhi Babu, D.B.; Waghray, S.; Badam, R.K.; Lavanya, R. Systematic meta-analysis on association of human papilloma virus and oral cancer. *J. Cancer Res. Ther.* **2016**, *12*, 969–974. [CrossRef]

37. Ndiaye, C.; Mena, M.; Alemany, L.; Arbyn, M.; Castellsagué, X.; Laporte, L.; Bosch, F.X.; de Sanjosé, S.; Trottier, H. HPV DNA, E6/E7 mRNA, and p16INK4a detection in head and neck cancers: A systematic review and meta-analysis. *Lancet Oncol.* **2014**, *15*, 1319–1331. [CrossRef]
38. Haeggblom, L.; Ramqvist, T.; Tommasino, M.; Dalianis, T.; Näsman, A. Time to change perspectives on HPV in oropharyngeal cancer. A systematic review of HPV prevalence per oropharyngeal sub-site the last 3 years. *Papillomavirus Res. (Amst. Neth.)* **2017**, *4*, 1–11. [CrossRef]
39. Guo, L.; Yang, F.; Yin, Y.; Liu, S.; Li, P.; Zhang, X.; Chen, D.; Liu, Y.; Wang, J.; Wang, K.; et al. Prevalence of human papillomavirus type-16 in head and neck cancer among the Chinese Population: A Meta-Analysis. *Front. Oncol.* **2018**, *8*, 619. [CrossRef]
40. Kreimer, A.R.; Clifford, G.M.; Boyle, P.; Franceschi, S. Human papillomavirus types in head and neck squamous cell carcinomas worldwide: A systematic review. *Cancer Epidemiol. Biomark. Prev.* **2005**, *14*, 467–475. [CrossRef]
41. Smitha, T.; Mohan, C.V.; Hemavathy, S. Prevalence of human papillomavirus16 DNA and p16INK4a protein in oral squamous cell carcinoma: A systematic review and meta-analysis. *J. Oral Maxillofac. Pathol.* **2017**, *21*, 76–81. [CrossRef]
42. Termine, N.; Panzarella, V.; Falaschini, S.; Russo, A.; Matranga, D.; Lo Muzio, L.; Campisi, G. HPV in oral squamous cell carcinoma vs head and neck squamous cell carcinoma biopsies: A meta-analysis (1988–2007). *Ann. Oncol.* **2008**, *19*, 1681–1690. [CrossRef] [PubMed]
43. Zhu, C.; Ling, Y.; Dong, C.; Zhou, X.; Wang, F. The relationship between oral squamous cell carcinoma and human papillomavirus: A meta-analysis of a Chinese population (1994–2011). *PLoS ONE* **2012**, *7*, e36294. [CrossRef]
44. Clifford, G.; Franceschi, S. Members of the human papillomavirus type 18 family (alpha-7 species) share a common association with adenocarcinoma of the cervix. *Int. J. Cancer* **2008**, *122*, 1684–1685. [CrossRef] [PubMed]
45. Grabowska, A.K.; Riemer, A.B. The invisible enemy—How human papillomaviruses avoid recognition and clearance by the host immune system. *Open Virol. J.* **2012**, *6*, 249–256. [CrossRef] [PubMed]
46. Shaikh, M.H.; McMillan, N.A.J.; Johnson, N.W. HPV-associated head and neck cancers in the Asia Pacific: A critical literature review & meta-analysis. *Cancer Epidemiol.* **2015**, *39*, 923–938. [PubMed]
47. Hobbs, C.G.L.; Sterne, J.A.C.; Bailey, M.; Heyderman, R.S.; Birchall, M.A.; Thomas, S.J. Human papillomavirus and head and neck cancer: A systematic review and meta-analysis. *Clin. Otolaryngol.* **2006**, *31*, 259–266. [CrossRef]
48. Saulle, R.; Semyonov, L.; Mannocci, A.; Careri, A.; Saburri, F.; Ottolenghi, L.; Guerra, F.; La Torre, G. Human papillomavirus and cancerous diseases of the head and neck: A systematic review and meta-analysis. *Oral Dis.* **2015**, *21*, 417–431. [CrossRef]
49. Smith, E.M.; Hoffman, H.T.; Summersgill, K.S.; Kirchner, H.L.; Turek, L.P.; Haugen, T.H. Human papillomavirus and risk of oral cancer. *Laryngoscope* **1998**, *108*, 1098–1103. [CrossRef]
50. Zhao, M.; Rosenbaum, E.; Carvalho, A.L.; Koch, W.; Jiang, W.; Sidransky, D.; Califano, J. Feasibility of quantitative PCR-based saliva rinse screening of HPV for head and neck cancer. *Int. J. Cancer* **2005**, *117*, 605–610. [CrossRef]
51. Chai, R.C.; Lim, Y.; Frazer, I.H.; Wan, Y.; Perry, C.; Jones, L.; Lambie, D.; Punyadeera, C. A pilot study to compare the detection of HPV-16 biomarkers in salivary oral rinses with tumour p16(INK4a) expression in head and neck squamous cell carcinoma patients. *BMC Cancer* **2016**, *16*, 178. [CrossRef]
52. Martin-Gomez, L.; Fulp, W.J.; Schell, M.J.; Sirak, B.; Abrahamsen, M.; Isaacs-Soriano, K.A.; Lorincz, A.; Wenig, B.; Chung, C.H.; Caudell, J.J.; et al. Oral gargle-tumor biopsy human papillomavirus (HPV) agreement and associated factors among oropharyngeal squamous cell carcinoma (OPSCC) cases. *Oral Oncol.* **2019**, *92*, 85–91. [CrossRef] [PubMed]
53. Tang, K.D.; Baeten, K.; Kenny, L.; Frazer, I.H.; Scheper, G.; Punyadeera, C. Unlocking the potential of saliva-based test to detect HPV-16-driven oropharyngeal cancer. *Cancers* **2019**, *11*, 473. [CrossRef] [PubMed]
54. Tang, K.D.; Menezes, L.; Baeten, K.; Walsh, L.J.; Whitfield, B.C.S.; Batstone, M.D.; Kenny, L.; Frazer, I.H.; Scheper, G.C.; Punyadeera, C. Oral HPV16 prevalence in oral potentially malignant disorders and oral cavity cancers. *Biomolecules* **2020**, *10*, 223. [CrossRef] [PubMed]

6

Surface Alterations Induced on Endodontic Instruments by Sterilization Processes, Analyzed with Atomic Force Microscopy

Mario Dioguardi [1,*], Vito Crincoli [2], Luigi Laino [3], Mario Alovisi [4], Enrica Laneve [1], Diego Sovereto [1], Bruna Raddato [1], Khrystyna Zhurakivska [1], Filiberto Mastrangelo [1], Domenico Ciavarella [1], Lucio Lo Russo [1] and Lorenzo Lo Muzio [1]

1 Department of Clinical and Experimental Medicine, University of Foggia, Via Rovelli 50, 71122 Foggia, Italy; enrica.laneve@unifg.it (E.L.); diego_sovereto.546709@unifg.it (D.S.); brunaraddato@gmail.com (B.R.); khrystyna.zhurakivska@unifg.it (K.Z.); filiberto.mastrangelo@unifg.it (F.M.); domenico.ciavarella@unifg.it (D.C.); lucio.lorusso@unifg.it (L.L.R.); lorenzo.lomuzio@unifg.it (L.L.M.)

2 Department of Basic Medical Sciences, Neurosciences and Sensory Organs, Division of Complex Operating Unit of Dentistry, "Aldo Moro" University of Bari, Piazza G. Cesare 11, 70124 Bari, Italy; vito.crincoli@uniba.it

3 Multidisciplinary Department of Medical-Surgical and Odontostomatological Specialties, University of Campania "Luigi Vanvitelli", 80121 Naples, Italy; luigi.laino@unicampania.it

4 Department of Surgical Sciences, Dental School, University of Turin, 10124 Turin, Italy; mario.alovisi@unito.it

* Correspondence: mario.dioguardi@unifg.it

Abstract: Endodontic canal disinfection procedures that use sodium hypochlorite, and subsequently, heat sterilization procedures can alter the surface of endodontic instruments, described as corrosion and micropitting. These phenomena can be visualized on the surface of the instruments by SEM and atomic force microscopy analyses. The endodontic instruments used in probing, pre-enlargement, and shaping phases are made of steel alloy or nickel-titanium alloy (NiTi) and are subject to torsional, flexor, and cyclic fatigue; indeed, reuse of these instruments must be done with the knowledge that these instruments are subject to fracture following stress caused during their use. Fracture of the instrument within the canal is an eventuality that can lead to failure of the treatment, and therefore it is important to try to reduce situations that can contribute to the fracture. This review was performed based on the PRISMA protocol. Studies were identified through bibliographic research using electronic databases. A total of 1036 records were identified on the PubMed and Scopus databases. After screening the articles, restricted by year of publication (1979 to 2019), there were 946 records. With the application of the eligibility criteria (all the articles pertaining to the issue of sterilization in endodontics), there were 228 articles. There were 104 articles after eliminating overlaps. There were 50 articles that discussed the influence of sterilization procedures on the surface characteristics of endodontic instruments, and 26 articles that measured parameters on surface alteration. Applying the inclusion and exclusion criteria resulted in a total of eleven articles for quantitative analysis. Four articles were in reference to the primary outcome, eight articles to secondary outcome, and five articles to tertiary outcome. The meta-analysis showed a statistically significant surface alteration effect after five autoclaves and after immersion in the canal irrigants after 10 min.

Keywords: autoclave; endodontic sterilization; atomic force microscopy; NiTi alloy; endodontics; corrosion

---

1. Introduction

Endodontic instruments are commonly used in dental practice to perform endodontic treatments of vital and necrotic teeth, endodontic retreatments, pulpotomies, pulpectomy and specification procedures. Depending on the phase of treatment, endodontic instruments are divided into instruments for probing the endodontic canal for the pre-enlargement, and glidepath for shaping the canal or instruments for the closure and three-dimensional sealing of endodontic canals [1,2]. Many of these tools are reusable after performing cleaning, disinfection, and sterilization procedures by autoclaving [3].

Endodontic canal disinfection procedures that use sodium hypochlorite [4], and subsequently, heat sterilization procedures, can alter the surface of endodontic instruments, described as corrosion and micropitting, phenomena [5] that can be visualized by SEM and atomic force microscopy analyses.

The endodontic instruments used in the probing, pre-enlargement, and shaping phases are made of steel alloy or nickel-titanium alloy (NiTi) and are subject to torsional, flexor, and cyclic fatigue, indeed the reuse of these instruments must be done with the knowledge that these tools are subject to fracture following stress caused during their use [6]. Fracture of the instrument within the canal is an eventuality that can lead to failure of the treatment, and therefore it is important to try to reduce situations that can contribute the fracture.

On the surface subject to fatigue, surface alterations can give rise to microcrack which can lead to fracture of the instrument, and also reduce the cutting capacity of the blades on the endodontic files [7]. Therefore, in order to maintain the same cutting efficiency, the endodontist has to exert greater pressure on the instrument with an increase in torsional fatigue stress [6].

An atomic force microscope is an instrument capable of analyzing the surface of instruments. It consists of a cantilever with a pointed tip (tip) mounted on the end, typically composed of silicon or silicon nitride and having a radius of curvature of the "order of nanometers". The sample to be scanned, through the Vand Der Waals forces, interacts with the tip of the detector by flexing it. There are several methods to detect any cantilever movement. The majority of atomic force microscopy (AFM) systems use laser beam detection, which is an optical system with position sensitive detectors called photodiodes. The laser light is reflected by the cantilever on the position-sensitive photodiode. Very small forces are produced between the probe and the surface to be scanned, and these are the forces that allow the AFM system to record the deflection of the cantilever. The cantilever deflection is called "cantilever rigidity". This rigidity can be measured by Hooke's law. Rigidity is recorded visually and can be viewed on the computer in real time. The surface scan of endodontic instruments is used both in non-contact mode and in contact mode and, in general, the scanned surfaces start at 3 mm from the tip of the instrument up to 6 mm. The parameters which are considered with AFM for the analysis of a surface are the arithmetic mean roughness(AMR) of the maximum height (MH) and root mean square (RMS). The atomic force microscopy, therefore, provides detailed information with measurable parameters of possible alterations and irregularities present on the surface of an instrument [8].

Surface alterations can represent a problem in the use of endodontic instruments. A study by Ylmaz, in 2018, identified surface alterations described as surface roughness with statistically significant results for instruments constructed with new M-wire and EDM alloys [9].

One problem of reusing endodontic instruments that are subject to fatigue is the deterioration they suffer that results from their use in the dental canal for the removal of dentin, as well as the corrosive action by the root canal irrigants such as sodium hypochlorite, and subsequently, the action of the temperature and steam induced by the autoclave sterilization process. The surface alterations are well described in a study by Inan, in 2007, on the universal ProTaper, after clinical use and sterilization [10].

Fayyad and Mahran, in a 2013 study, demonstrated by AFM analysis that the alterations on Twisted Files [11], Hero Shaper, RaCe, and GTX instruments were statistically significant after immersion in 5% sodium hypochlorite, however, the alterations were not statistically significant after EDTA immersion. In contrast, Ametrano et al., in 2010, reported significant results for instruments immersed in EDTA [12]. Other studies have report conflicting data, such as the study conducted by Casella, in 2011, in which there was no variation in corrosion resistance for some instruments (K FILE and GT-rotary) unlike the K3 knife immersed in 5% sodium hypochlorite [13]. In addition, studies conducted at the Sem da Razavianet, in 2015, reported an increase in roughness directly related to the number of sterilization cycles performed on endodontic instruments [14].

In contrast, there is debate within the scientific community regarding whether there are statistically significant surface alterations induced by the autoclave or the canal irrigants. This review aims to try to clarify this aspect by investigating the literature to extrapolate the data on surface alterations in endodontic instruments in order to statistically analyze them in a meta-analysis.

Previous systematic reviews on this topic have not included the effect of surface alterations of endodontic instruments subjected to heat sterilization. There is only one systematic review that analyzes the variations in torsional properties subjected to autoclave sterilization.

This review could help endodontists who perform endodontic therapy and reuse endodontic instruments daily. Awareness of the greater or lesser risk of potential fracture triggered by surface variations due to heat or use of canal irrigants on the instruments could be helpful.

2. Materials and Methods

This systematic review was conducted based on the Prisma protocol.

The study was constructed using the following PICO elements for questions: Population (endodontic instruments); intervention (surface alterations induced by sterilization processes and root canal irrigation); control (new endodontic instruments not subject to sterilization; and outcome (surface alterations induced by the sterilization process by autoclave, and by root canal irrigants such as sodium hypochlorite and EDTA).

The following PICO question was formulated: To what extent, statistically significant, the sterilization processes and the used canal irrigants alter the surface of the rotating endodontic instruments with respect to the control?

After an initial selection phase of article identification in the databases, the potentially eligible articles were qualitatively evaluated in order to investigate the surface alterations of endodontic instruments resulting from the sterilization of instruments and disinfection of endodontic canals.

2.1. Eligibility Criteria

This literature review took into consideration in vitro and clinical studies that concerned the subject of sterilization and the influence of the latter on the physical and chemical properties of endodontic instruments. In particular, articles that dealt with the corrosive phenomena and surface alterations considered by microscopy methods (atomic force microscopy), conducted in recent years, and published with abstracts in English, were considered potentially eligible.

Articles from the last 40 years were chosen, because disinfection and sterilization procedures have changed in light of new discovered infectious contaminants, such as HIV and HCV viruses and the prong of spongiform encephalopathy. Furthermore, the methods used to manufacture the instruments have changed with the introduction of new alloys and new instruments. Therefore, in summary, potentially eligible articles included studies that investigated the influence of sterilization and disinfection procedures on endodontic canals, as well as on the physical and chemical characteristics of endodontic instruments, however, articles published more than 40 years ago and those that did not present an abstract in English were excluded.

Finally, the articles that were potentially eligible were subjected to a full text analysis to verify their use for a qualitative and quantitative analysis.

The inclusion and exclusion criteria applied in the full text analysis are the following:

- Include all those studies that describe the alterations induced by the sterilization methods of the endodontic instruments, analyzed using atomic force microscopy;

- Include all the articles that describe the alterations induced by root canal irrigants (sodium hypochlorite and EDTA), analyzed using atomic force microscopy;
- The exclusion criteria are to exclude all those studies that do not report data (average and standard deviation) on surface irregularities (AMR, MH, and RMS).

2.2. *Research Methodology*

The studies were identified through a bibliographic research on electronic databases.

The literature search was conducted using the search engines "PubMed" and "Scopus". The search on the providers was conducted between 12 September 2019 and 18 September 2019 and the last search for a partial update of the literature was conducted on 1 October 2019.

The following search terms were used on PubMed and Scopus: "Endodontic sterilization" PubMed 333 and Scopus 269; "endodontic autoclave" PubMed 38 and Scopus 52; "atomic force microscopy" AND "endodontic" PubMed 21 and Scopus 33; "roughness" AND "endodontic" Pub Med 42 and Scopus 67; "roughness" AND "ethylenediaminetetraacetic acid" PubMed 15 and Scopus 40; "roughness" AND "sodium hypochlorite" PubMed 1 and Scopus 1; "sodium hypochlorite" AND "atomic force microscopy" PubMed 40 and Scopus 80; "atomic force microscopy" AND "NiTi rotary instruments" PubMed 1 and Scopus 2 (Table 1).

2.3. *Screening Methodology*

The records obtained were, subsequently, examined by two independent reviewers (M.D. and S.D), and a third reviewer (E.L.) acted as a decision maker in situations of doubt. The screening included the analysis of the title and the abstract to eliminate the recordings not related to the topics of the review. After the screening phase, the overlaps were removed and the complete texts of the articles were analyzed, from which the ones eligible for the qualitative analysis and the inclusion in the meta-analysis for the three results were identified. The results sought by the two reviewers were:

(1) Primary outcome, variations of the root mean square root (RMS) of endodontic instruments subjected to five autoclave cycles as compared with non-autoclaved control;

(2) Secondary outcome, variations of the root mean square (RMS) of endodontic instruments exposed to sodium hypochlorite 5% as compared with the control group;

(3) Tertiary outcome, variations of the root mean square (RMS) of the endodontic instruments described at EDTA 10% as compared with the control group.

The fourth reviewer, with supervisory duties, was L.Lo.M. The K agreement between the two screening reviewers was 0.8464 (Table 2). The K agreement was based on the formulas of the *Cochrane Handbook for Systematic Reviews* [15].

The Newcastle–Ottawa scale for case-control studies was used to assess the risk of bias in the included studies. The quantitative analysis was performed with the Rev Manager software 5.3 (Cochrane Collaboration, Copenhagen, Denmark [16].

Table 1. Complete overview of the search methodology.

Database-Provider	Key Words	Search Details	Number of Records	Number of Records after Restriction by Year of Publication (Last 40 Years)	Number of Articles Remaining after the Elimination of Records not Related to the Issue of Sterilization Influence on Endodontic Instruments	Articles After Remove Overlaps Articles	Number of Articles Dealing with the Problem of the Influence of Sterilization Procedures on the Surface Characteristics of Endodontic Instruments	Number of Articles that Have Analyzed the Surface Alterations with Methods Different from the Atomic Force Microscopy	Number of Articles that Analyzed Surface Alterations with Atomic Force Microscopy	Numbers of Articles Included in the Quantitative Analysis for the 3 Outcomes
PubMed	"endodontic sterilization"	"endodontic" [All Fields] AND ("sterilization"[All Fields] OR "sterilization", reproductive"[MeSH Terms] OR ("sterilization"[All Fields] AND "reproductive"[All Fields]) OR "reproductive sterilization"[All Fields] OR "sterilization"[All Fields] OR "sterilization"[MeSH Terms])	333	291	46					
PubMed	"endodontic autoclave"	"endodontic" [All Fields] AND "autoclave" [All Fields]	38	38	25					
PubMed	"atomic force microscopy" AND "endodontic"	"atomic force microscopy" [All Fields] AND "endodontic" [All Fields]	21	21	9					
PubMed	"roughness" AND "endodontic"	"roughness" [All Fields] AND "endodontic" [All Fields]	42	41	11					
PubMed	"roughness" AND "ethylenediaminetetraacetic acid"	"roughness" [All Fields] AND ("ethylenediaminetetraacetic" [All Fields] AND "acid" [All Fields])	15	15	2					
PubMed	"roughness" AND "sodium hypochlorite"	"roughness" [All Fields] AND ("sodium" [All Fields] AND "hypochlorite" [All Fields])	1	1	1					
PubMed	"sodium" "hypochlorite" AND "atomic force microscopy"	"sodium hypochlorite" [All Fields] AND "atomic force microscopy" [All Fields]	40	40	13					
PubMed	"atomic force microscopy" AND "NiTi rotary instruments"	"atomic force microscopy" [All Fields] AND "NiTi rotary instruments" [All Fields]	1	1	1					
Scopus	"endodontic sterilization"	TITLE-ABS-KEY (endodontic AND sterilization)	269	225	56					
Scopus	"endodontic autoclave"	TITLE-ABS-KEY (endodontic AND autoclave)	52	52	25					
Scopus	"atomic force microscopy" AND "endodontic"	TITLE-ABS-KEY ("atomic force microscopy" AND "endodontic")	33	33	13					
Scopus	"roughness" AND "endodontic"	TITLE-ABS-KEY ("roughness" AND "endodontic")	67	65	12					
Scopus	"roughness" AND sodium "hypochlorite"	TITLE-ABS-KEY ("roughness" AND "sodium" AND "hypochlorite")	1	1	1					
Scopus	"roughness" AND "ethylenediaminetetraacetic acid"	TITLE-ABS-KEY ("roughness" AND "ethylenediaminetetraacetic acid")	40	40	2					
Scopus	"sodium hypochlorite" AND "atomic force microscopy"	TITLE-ABS-KEY ("sodium hypochlorite" AND "atomic force microscopy")	80	80	9					
Scopus	"atomic force microscopy" AND "NiTi rotary instruments"	TITLE-ABS-KEY ("atomic force microscopy" AND "NiTi rotary instruments")	2	2	2					
Total records			1036	946	228	104	50	24	26	11

Table 2. K agreement calculation, Po = 0.94 (proportion of agreement), Pe = 0.6092 (agreement expected), K agreement = 0.8464 (<0 no agreement, 0.0 to 0.20 slight agreement, 0.21 to 0.40 fair agreement, 0.41 to 0.60 moderate agreement, 0.61 to 0.80 substantial agreement, and 0.81 to 1.00 almost perfect agreement). The K agreement was calculated from the 50 articles and included eleven articles with the application of the inclusion and exclusion criteria.

/	/	**Reviewer 2**	**Reviewer 2**	**Reviewer 2**	
		Include	Exclude	Unsure	Total
Reviewer 1	include	11	0	0	11
Reviewer 1	exclude	2	36	0	38
Reviewer 1	unsure	1	0	0	1
	total	14	36	0	50

3. Results

A total of 1036 records were identified on the PubMed and Scopus databases (Table 1). After screening the articles, with the restriction by year of publication (1979 to 2019), there were 946 records. With the application of the eligibility criteria (all the articles pertaining to the issue of sterilization in endodontics), there were 228 articles. There were 104 articles after eliminating overlaps. There were 50 articles that discussed the influence of sterilization procedures on the surface characteristics of endodontic instruments, and 26 that measured parameters on surface alteration.

Applying the inclusion and exclusion criteria resulted in a total of eleven articles for quantitative analysis.

Four articles were in reference to the primary outcome, eight to the secondary outcome, and five to the tertiary outcome. The entire selection and screening procedures are described in the flow chart (Figure 1).

3.1. *Study Characteristics and Data Extraction*

The studies included for quantitative analysis were:

- First outcome: Yılmaz et al., 2017 [9]; Spagnuolo et al., 2012 [17]; Inan et al., 2007 [10]; and Can Saglam et al., 2015 [18];
- Second outcome: Uslu et al., 2018 [19]; Can Saglam et al., 2015 [18]; Fayyad et al., 2013 [11]; Ametrano et al., 2010 [12]; Topuz et al., 2008 [20]; Cai et al., 2017 [21]; Saglam et al., 2012 [22]; and Prasad et al., 2014 [23];
- Third outcome: Uslu et al., 2018 [19]; Fayyad et al., 2013 [11]; Ametrano et al., 2010 [12]; Cai et al., 2017 [21]; and Prasad et al., 2014 [23].

The extracted data included the magazine (author, data, and journal); the endodontic instrumentation object of measurement (name, taper, and diameter at tip); the method of sterilization by heat (temperature, pressure, and time); the number autoclave cycles or irrigants; the number of instruments (control and experimental); the number of surfaces scanned by the instrument; the number of total scans; the size of the scanning surface; and the data concerning the root mean square (RMS) ± standard deviation.

The data extracted for the tree outcomes are shown in Tables 3 and 4.

3.2. *Risk of Bias*

The risk of bias was assessed through the Newcastle–Ottawa case-control scale. The results are reported in detail in Table 5. For each category, a value of one to three was assigned (one = low and three = high).

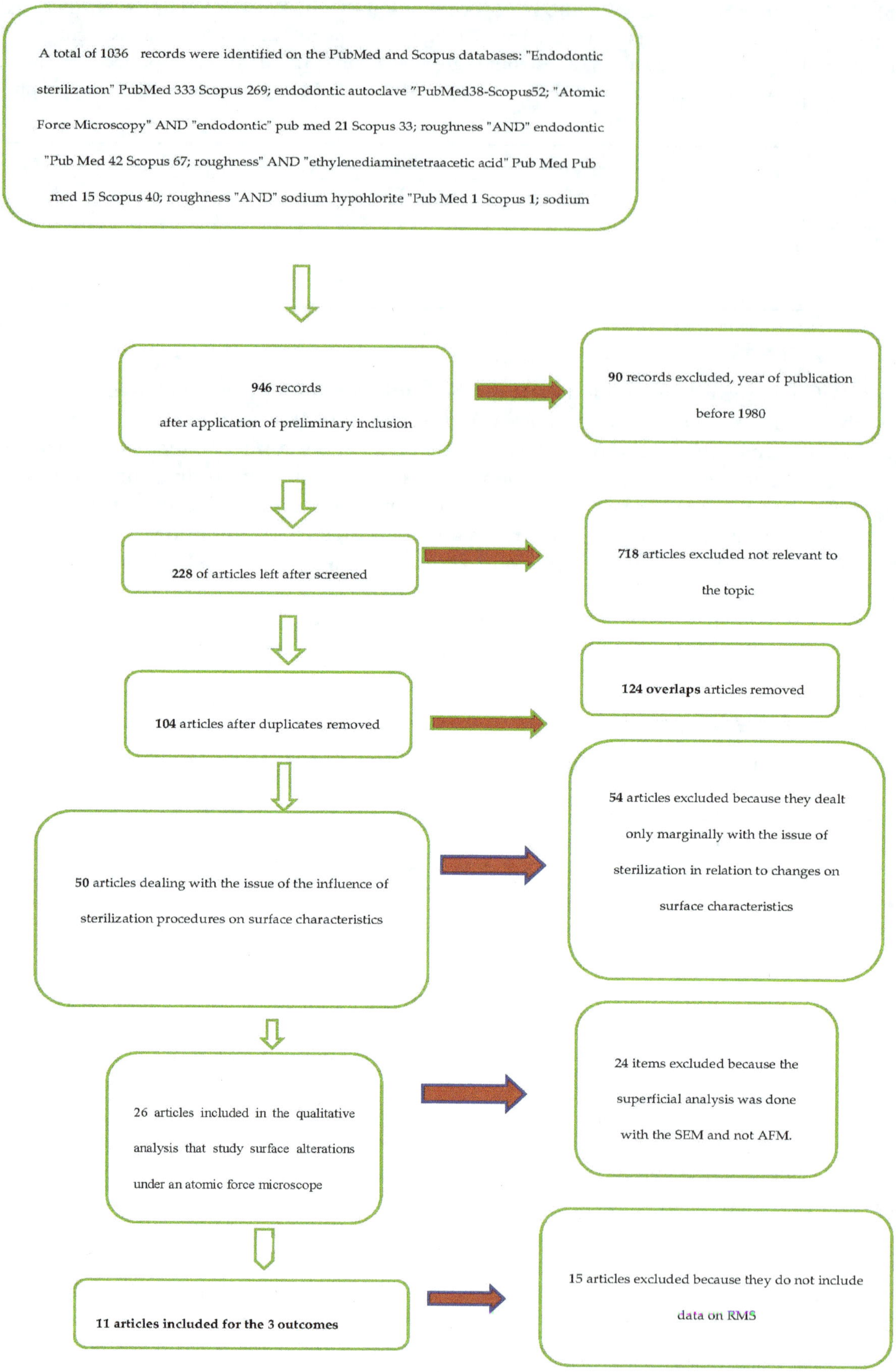

Figure 1. Flow chart of the different phases of the systematic review.

Table 3. Primary outcome (extraction of data relating to the root mean square detected on the surface of the endodontic instruments subjected to atomic force microscopy examination, with respect to control and after 5 cycles of autoclaving).

Autor, Data, Journal	Sterilization Method (Autoclave Temperature, Pressure Exposure Time)	Endodontic Instruments (Diameter and Taper at the Tip)	Autoclave Cycles	Number of Instruments	Surfaces Scanned by Instrument	Number of Total Scans	Scanning Surface	Root Mean Square (RMS) ± Standard Deviation
Yılmaz et al., 2017, Clin. Oral. Investig. [9]	Autoclave 134 °C, 30 psi for 20 min	HyFlex EDM (25/08)	0	2	15	30	5 × 5 µm	48.62 ± 7.76 nm
			5	2	15	30	5 × 5 µm	57.84 ± 6.94 nm
Spagnuolo et al., 2012, Int. Endod. J. [17]	Autoclave 121 °C, 15 psi, for 15 min	ProTaper F2 (25/08)	0	15	15	225	15 × 15 µm	203.75 ± 35.81 nm
			5	15	15	225	15 × 15 µm	715.22 nm ± 37.71
Can Saglam et al., 2015, Microsc. Res. Tech. [18]	Autoclave 121 °C for 20 min	ProTaper retreatment D1 (30/09)	0	1	11	11	2 × 2 µm	1.33 ± 0.558 nm
			5	1	11	11	2 × 2 µm	1.75 ± 0.940 nm
Inan et al., 2007, J. Endod. [10]	Autoclave 134 °C for 18 min	ProTaper F2 (25/08)	0	1	11	11	1 × 1 µm	1.46 ± 0.45 nm
			1	1	11	11	1 × 1 µm	7.29 ± 0.88 nm

Table 4. Extracted data relating to the secondary outcome and tertiary outcome, the data extracted are the root mean square (RMS), the total number of surfaces scanned, the endodontic instruments being scanned by the atomic force microscopy, and the irrigants used with the relative concentrations.

Autor, Data, Journal	Endodontic Instruments (Diameter and Taper at the Tip)	Irrigant Used (Concentration and Exposure Time)	Number of Instruments	Surfaces Scanned by Instrument	Number of Total Scans	Scanning Surface	Root Mean Square (RMS) ± Standard Deviation
Uslu et al. 2018, Microsc. Res. Tech. [19]	HyFlex EDM (25/.08)	control	4	20	80	5 × 5 µm	42.44 ± 4.51 nm
		NaOCl 5.25% for 5 min	4	20	80	5 × 5 µm	57.05 ± 8.55 nm
		EDTA 17% for 5 min	4	20	80	5 × 5 µm	60.65 ± 7.27 nm
Can Saglam et al., 2015, Microsc. Res. Tech. [18]	ProTaper retreatment D1 (30/09)	Control	1	11	11	2 × 2 µm	1.33 ± 0.558 nm
		NaOCl 2% for 5 min	1	11	11	2 × 2 µm	2.24 ± 0.555 nm
Fayyad et al , 2013, Int. Endod. J. [11]	RaCe	control	4	15	60	20 × 20 µm	83.3 ± 3.1 nm
		NaOCl 5.25% for 5 min	2	15	30	20 × 20 µm	92.3 ± 23.5 nm
		EDTA 17% for 5 min	2	15	30	20 × 20 µm	90 ± 7.5 nm
Ametrano et al., 2011, Int. Endod. J. [12]	ProTaper F2 (25/08)	control	1	20	20	1 × 1 µm	2.88 ± 0.72 nm
		NaOCl 5.25% for 5 min	1	20	20	1 × 1 µm	4.10 ± 1.13 nm
		EDTA 17% for 5 min	1	20	20	1 × 1 µm	4.79 ± 0.74 nm
Topuz et al., 2008, Oral. Surg. Oral. Med. Oral. Pathol. Oral. Radiol. Endod. [20]	RaCe rotary NiTi files (30.06)	control	1	11	11	1 × 1 µm	2.06 ± 0.49 nm
		NaOCl 5.25% for 5 min	1	11	11	1 × 1 µm	6.99 ± 2.18 nm
Saglam et al. Microsc. Res. Tech. 2012 [22]	ProTapar f3 (30.08)	control	1	12	12	5 × 5 µm	1.31 ± 0.558 nm
		NaOCl 5% for 10 min	1	12	12	5 × 5 µm	3.20 ± 1.280 nm
Prasad et al., 2014, J. Conserv. Dent. [23]	iRaCe-R3	control	1	9	9	1 × 1 µm	1.35 ± 0.29 nm
		NaOCL 5%	1	9	9	1 × 1 µm	4.74 ± 1.09 nm
		EDTA 17%	1	9	9	1 × 1 µm	3.90 ± 0.58 nm
Cai et al., 2017, Int. Endod. J. [21]	HyFlex (25.06)	control	1	15	15	1 × 1 µm	10.12 ± 1.88 nm
		NaOCl 5.25% for 10 min	1	15	15	1 × 1 µm	9.35 ± 2.05 nm
		control	1	15	15	1 × 1 µm	10.47 ± 2.34 nm
		EDTA 17% for 10 min	1	15	15	1 × 1 µm	13.88 ± 3.78 nm

Table 5. Assessment of risk of bias within the studies (Newcastle–Ottawa scale) with scores 7 to 12 = low quality, 13 to 20 = intermediate quality, and 21 to 24 = high quality.

	Selection				Comparability	Exposure			Score
Reference	**Definition of Cases**	**Representativeness of Cases**	**Selection of Controls**	**Definition of Controls**	**Comparability of Cases and Controls on the Basis of the Design or Analysis**	**Ascertainment of Exposure**	**Same Method of Ascertainment for Cases and Controls**	**Non-Response Rate**	
Cai et al., 2017 [21]	3	3	3	3	3	3	3	0	21
Prasad et al., 2014 [23]	2	2	2	2	2	2	3	0	15
Saglam et al., 2012 [22]	3	2	3	3	3	3	3	0	20
Topuz et al., 2008 [20]	3	2	3	3	3	3	3	0	20
Ametrano et al., 2011 [12]	2	2	2	2	3	3	3	0	17
Fayyad et al., 2013 [11]	2	2	2	2	2	3	3	0	16
Can Saglam et al., 2015 [18]	3	2	3	3	3	3	3	0	20
Uslu et al., 2018 [19]	3	3	3	3	3	3	3	0	21
Inan et al., 2007 [10]	3	2	3	3	3	3	3	0	20
Yılmaz et al., 2017 [9]	3	3	3	3	3	3	3	0	21
Spagnuolo et al., 2012 [17]	3	3	3	3	3	3	3	0	21

The risk of bias within the individual studies was low enough that the methods of investigation adopted for the controls were identical to the cases included in the meta-analysis. The Prasad study [23] was the only study of the exposure time of endodontic instruments to canal irrigants that was not well defined, exposing the study to a bias.

The risk of bias between the various studies was considered high, and therefore partly limited the importance of the results. The heterogeneity of the studies depended mainly on the diversity of the instruments, which were similar, in some cases, only in terms of tip diameter, taper, and type of metal alloy.

The heterogeneity of the studies was represented by funnel plots of the four outcomes, as shown in Figure 2.

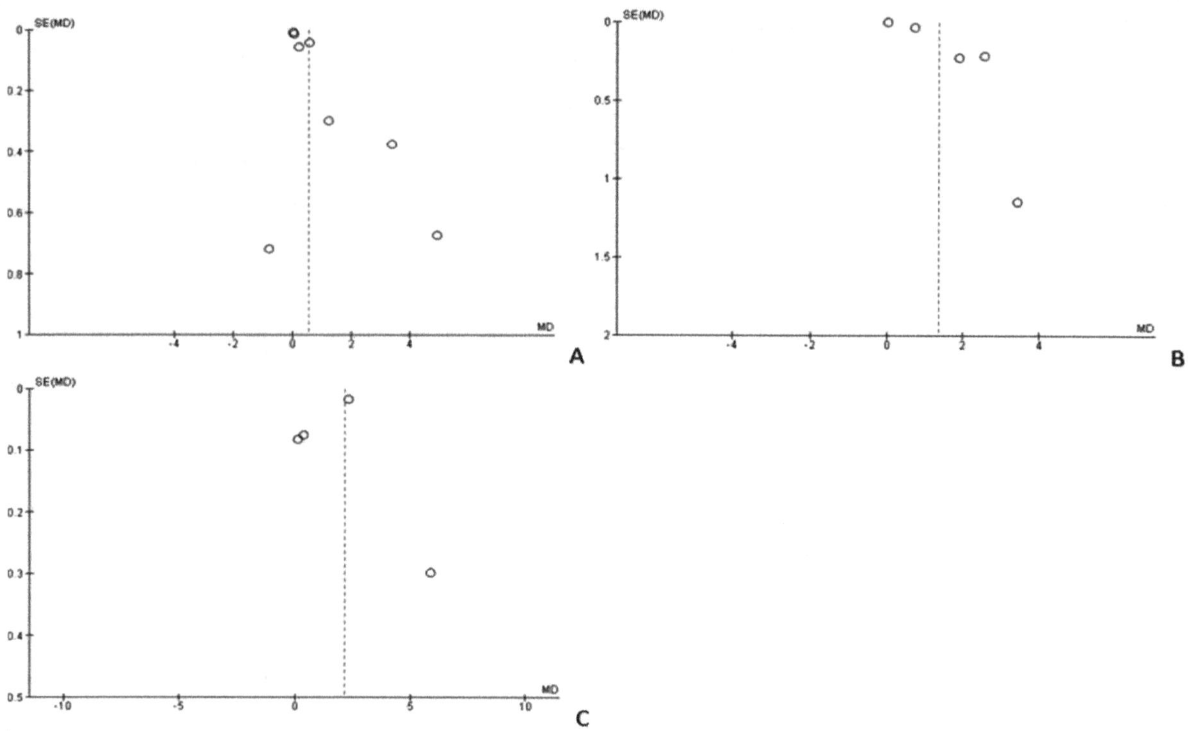

Figure 2. Funnel plots of the evaluation of heterogeneity for the (**A**) first, (**B**) second, (**C**) third outcomes.

3.3. Data Analysis

The statistical analysis of the data was performed using the Rev Manager 5.3 software (Copenhagen, 153 Denmark, The Nordic Cochrane Centre, The Nordic Cochrane Collaboration, 2014) and the results were represented by forest plots for each of the outcomes.

For the primary outcome, variations of the root mean square root (RMS) of endodontic instruments subjected to five autoclave cycles as compared with the non-autoclaved control, the comparison showed high heterogeneity of the studies, with an I2 equal to 100%. For this reason, a random effects model was used. Overall, for the primary outcome, meta-analysis was favorable for the control group. The studies that present data with a statistically significant difference are Inan et al., 2007 [10] and Spagnuolo et al., 20012 [17]. The studies by Ylmaz et al., 2018 [9] and Can Saglam et al., 2015 [22] are exactly at the center of the line of no effect. The studies by Ylzam and Can Saglam are exactly at the center of the line of no effect, however, the remaining two studies are favorable for the group subjected to control, their confidence intervals do not intercept the line of no effect (Figure 3).

Study or Subgroup	autoclave Mean	SD	Total	Control Mean	SD	Total	Weight	Mean Difference IV, Random, 95% CI
Can Saglam 2015	0.4375	0.235	11	0.3325	0.1395	11	25.2%	0.10 [-0.06, 0.27]
Inan I 2007	7.29	0.88	11	1.46	0.45	11	24.3%	5.83 [5.25, 6.41]
Spagnuolo 2012	3.17875	0.1676	225	0.9055	0.19515	225	25.3%	2.27 [2.24, 2.31]
Yilmaz 2018	2.3136	0.2776	30	1.9448	0.3104	30	25.2%	0.37 [0.22, 0.52]
Total (95% CI)			**277**			**277**	**100.0%**	**2.11 [0.65, 3.57]**

Heterogeneity: Tau² = 2.19; Chi² = 1363.03, df = 3 (P < 0.00001); I² = 100%
Test for overall effect: Z = 2.83 (P = 0.005)

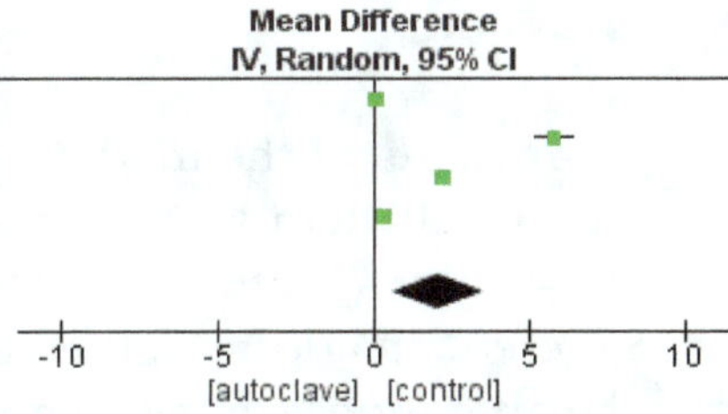

Figure 3. Forest plot of the random effects model of the meta-analysis of the primary outcome.

For the secondary outcome, variations of the root mean square (RMS) of endodontic instruments exposed to sodium hypochlorite 5% as compared with the control group, the comparison showed high heterogeneity among the studies, with an I2 equal to 98%. For this reason, for the second outcome, a random effects model was applied to avoid minimizing the roles of smaller-dimension studies. For the second outcome, the forest plot is in favor of the subject group control.

The studies that reported statistically significant data in favor of the control group are Ametrano, 2011; Prasad, 2014; Topuz, 2008; and Uslu, 2018. The Cai's study was the only study that was in favor of the group subjected to sodium hypochlorite, even though its confidence interval crosses the line of no effect. The other studies report statistically insignificant data (Figure 4).

Study or Subgroup	NaOCl Mean	SD	Total	Control Mean	SD	Total	Weight	Mean Difference IV, Random, 95% CI
Ametrano 2011	4.1	1.13	20	2.88	0.72	20	7.4%	1.22 [0.63, 1.81]
Cai 2017	9.35	2.05	15	10.12	1.88	15	1.8%	-0.77 [-2.18, 0.64]
Can Saglam 2015	0.56	0.13875	11	0.3325	0.1395	11	20.0%	0.23 [0.11, 0.34]
Fayyad 2013	0.23075	0.05875	30	0.20825	0.00775	60	21.5%	0.02 [0.00, 0.04]
Prasad 2014	4.74	1.09	9	1.35	0.29	9	5.3%	3.39 [2.65, 4.13]
Saglam 2012	0.128	0.0512	12	0.0524	0.02232	12	21.4%	0.08 [0.04, 0.11]
Topuz 2008	6.99	2.18	11	2.06	0.49	11	2.0%	4.93 [3.61, 6.25]
Uslu 2018	2.282	0.342	80	1.6976	0.1804	80	20.7%	0.60 [0.50, 0.67]
Total (95% CI)			**188**			**218**	**100.0%**	**0.54 [0.35, 0.74]**

Heterogeneity: Tau² = 0.05; Chi² = 314.28, df = 7 (P < 0.00001); I² = 98%
Test for overall effect: Z = 5.42 (P < 0.00001)

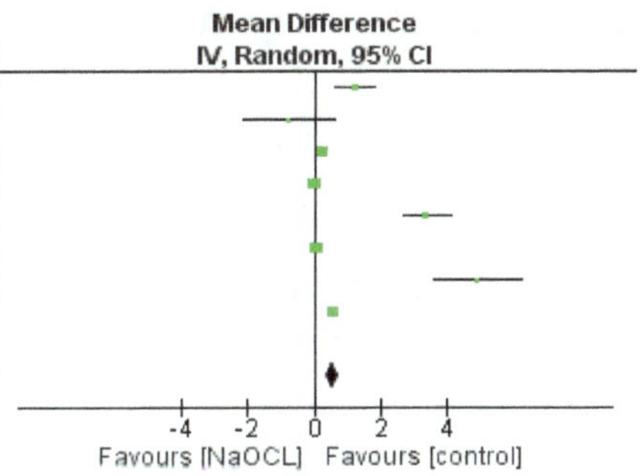

Figure 4. Forest plot of the random effects model of the meta-analysis of the secondary outcome.

For the tertiary outcome, variations of the root mean square (RMS) of the endodontic instruments exposed to EDTA 10% as compared with the control group, the comparison showed high heterogeneity between the studies, with an I2 of 99%, and therefore a random effects model was applied. For the tertiary outcome, the forest plot is in favor of the control group except for the study by Fayyad which is positioned in the line of no effect (Figure 5).

Study or Subgroup	EDTA Mean	SD	Total	Control Mean	SD	Total	Weight	Mean Difference IV, Random, 95% CI
Ametrano 2011	4.79	0.74	20	2.88	0.72	20	22.0%	1.91 [1.46, 2.36]
Cai 2017	13.88	3.78	15	10.47	2.34	15	5.7%	3.41 [1.16, 5.66]
Fayyad 2013	0.225	0.01875	30	0.20825	0.00775	60	25.1%	0.02 [0.01, 0.02]
Prasad 2014	3.9	0.58	9	1.35	0.29	9	22.3%	2.55 [2.13, 2.97]
Uslu 2018	2.426	0.2908	80	1.6976	0.1804	80	25.0%	0.73 [0.65, 0.80]
Total (95% CI)			**154**			**184**	**100.0%**	**1.37 [0.76, 1.98]**

Heterogeneity: Tau² = 0.30; Chi² = 666.09, df = 4 (P < 0.00001); I² = 99%
Test for overall effect: Z = 4.41 (P < 0.0001)

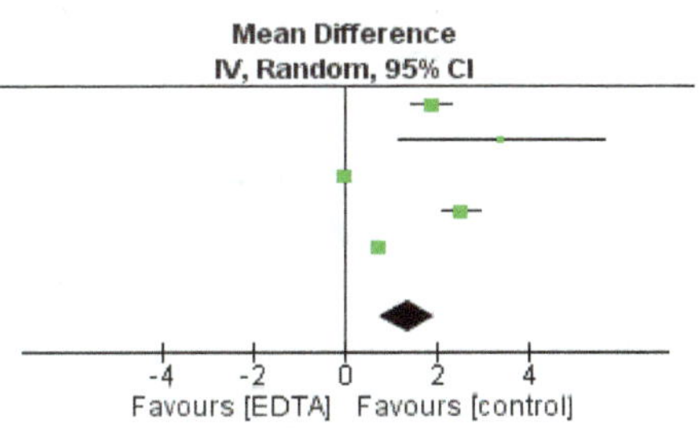

Figure 5. Forest plot of the random effects model of the meta-analysis of the tertiary outcome.

4. Discussion

The results of the meta-analysis for the three outcomes are in agreement in establishing that the superficial alterations induced by autoclave, from the sodium hypochlorite and from the EDTA, are statistically significant surface alterations that represent points where instrument fractures can be triggered. In addition, the alterations induced on the surface analyzed by SEM and AFM show that the alterations can also be expressed on the cutting surface, altering, in a pejorative sense, the cutting efficacy.

For the first outcome, the studies, in the literature, that supported a statistically significant alteration are:

1. In 2007, Inan reported statistically significant data for all the instruments of the ProTaper series (S1, S2, F1, F2), and reported that the superficial deterioration induced by the autoclave is greater for ProTaper finished than for ProTaper shaping;
2. In 2012, Spagnuolo confirmed, in agreement with Inan's data, that multiple cycles (autoclave sterilization) modified the surface topography and chemical composition of conventional NiTi (F2 ProTaper) and TiN-coated (alpha kit) instruments, in a statistically significant way (after five autoclave cycles).

Sodium hypochlorite certainly alters the surface of NiTi instruments and innumerable studies are in agreement such as Uslu et al., 2018 [19]; Ametrano et al., 2010 [12]; Topuz et al., 2008 [20]; and Prasad et al., 2014 [23]. Furthermore, a study conducted by Yokoyama et al., 2004 [24] stated that the action of sodium hypochlorite causes a worsening of the surface in endodontic instruments that facilitates their rupture following flexor and torsional stress.

The statistical analysis, in a similar way but with fewer studies, also confirms that the EDTA determines an increase in surface irregularities in a statistically significant way, and studies that confirm it after 10 min of exposure are well highlighted in the forest plot (Figure 5). Studies that are in contrast to the present meta-analysis report conflicting data regarding the action of EDTA on the surface. It seems that for exposures less than 5 min they do not alter the surface, however, according to Bonaccorsa et al. [25], a passivation phenomenon could lead to the creation of a complex between the metallic ions and the EDTA at a PH lower than four which renders the instrument resistant.

5. Conclusions

In conclusion, based on the present systematic analysis we affirm that autoclave induces a statistically significant corrosive phenomena, called micropitting, after five cycles of autoclave and determined by the heat, and comparatively, hypochlorite determines corrosion after only 5 min of exposure and EDTA after 10 min of exposure.

Superficial alterations, which are widely discussed in the literature, can determine the triggering of fractures in instruments subjected to cyclic fatigue and torsional fatigue. Therefore, it is important for endodontist to have knowledge of such corrosive phenomena, induced by irrigants such as sodium hypochlorite and EDTA, on instruments that can be reused and autoclaved.

Author Contributions: Conceptualization, M.D., D.S., and B.R.; methodology, K.Z. and M.D.; software, M.A. validation, M.D., and L.L.M.; formal analysis, D.S., M.D., and V.C.; investigation, L.L. and M.D.; resources, L.L.M.; data curation, E.L. and M.D.; writing—original draft preparation, M.D.; writing—review and editing, M.D., L.L.M., L.L.R., D.C., and F.M.

Acknowledgments: All the acknowledgements go to Lorenzo Lo Muzio, Director of the Dental Clinic and President of the Department of Clinical and Experimental Medicine of the University of Foggia, who gave fundamental technical support in the writing of this article.

References

1. Inan, U.; Keskin, C. Torsional Resistance of ProGlider, Hyflex EDM, and One G Glide Path Instruments. *J. Endod.* **2019**. [CrossRef]
2. Troiano, G.; Dioguardi, M.; Cocco, A.; Zhurakivska, K.; Ciavarella, D.; Muzio, L.L. Increase in [corrected] the glyde path diameter improves the centering ability of F6 Skytaper. *Eur. J. Dent.* **2018**, *12*, 89–93. [CrossRef] [PubMed]
3. Laneve, E.; Raddato, B.; Dioguardi, M.; Di Gioia, G.; Troiano, G.; Lo Muzio, L. Sterilisation in Dentistry: A Review of the Literature. *Int. J. Dent.* **2019**, *2019*, 6507286. [CrossRef] [PubMed]
4. Dioguardi, M.; Di Gioia, G.; Illuzzi, G.; Laneve, E.; Cocco, A.; Troiano, G. Endodontic irrigants: Different methods to improve efficacy and related problems. *Eur. J. Dent.* **2018**, *12*, 459–466. [CrossRef] [PubMed]
5. Berutti, E.; Angelini, E.; Rigolone, M.; Migliaretti, G.; Pasqualini, D. Influence of sodium hypochlorite on fracture properties and corrosion of ProTaper Rotary instruments. *Int. Endod. J.* **2006**, *39*, 693–699. [CrossRef] [PubMed]
6. Dioguardi, M.; Sovereto, D.; Aiuto, R.; Laino, L.; Illuzzi, G.; Laneve, E.; Raddato, B.; Caponio, V.C.A.; Dioguardi, A.; Zhurakivska, K.; et al. Effects of Hot Sterilization on Torsional Properties of Endodontic Instruments: Systematic Review with Meta-Analysis. *Materials* **2019**, *12*, 2190. [CrossRef] [PubMed]
7. Shen, Y.; Coil, J.M.; McLean, A.G.; Hemerling, D.L.; Haapasalo, M. Defects in nickel-titanium instruments after clinical use. Part 5: Single use from endodontic specialty practices. *J. Endod.* **2009**, *35*, 1363–1367. [CrossRef]
8. Ozyurek, T.; Yilmaz, K.; Uslu, G.; Plotino, G. The effect of root canal preparation on the surface roughness of WaveOne and WaveOne Gold files: Atomic force microscopy study. *Restor. Dent. Endod.* **2018**, *43*, e10. [CrossRef]
9. Yilmaz, K.; Uslu, G.; Ozyurek, T. Effect of multiple autoclave cycles on the surface roughness of HyFlex CM and HyFlex EDM files: An atomic force microscopy study. *Clin. Oral Investig.* **2018**, *22*, 2975–2980. [CrossRef]
10. Inan, U.; Aydin, C.; Uzun, O.; Topuz, O.; Alacam, T. Evaluation of the surface characteristics of used and new ProTaper Instruments: An atomic force microscopy study. *J. Endod.* **2007**, *33*, 1334–1337. [CrossRef]
11. Fayyad, D.M.; Mahran, A.H. Atomic force microscopic evaluation of nanostructure alterations of rotary NiTi instruments after immersion in irrigating solutions. *Int. Endod. J.* **2014**, *47*, 567–573. [CrossRef] [PubMed]
12. Ametrano, G.; D'Anto, V.; Di Caprio, M.P.; Simeone, M.; Rengo, S.; Spagnuolo, G. Effects of sodium hypochlorite and ethylenediaminetetraacetic acid on rotary nickel-titanium instruments evaluated using atomic force microscopy. *Int. Endod. J.* **2011**, *44*, 203–209. [CrossRef] [PubMed]
13. Casella, G.; Rosalbino, F. Corrosion behaviour of NiTi endodontic instrument. *Corros. Eng. Sci. Technol.* **2011**, *46*, 521–523. [CrossRef]
14. Razavian, H.; Iranmanesh, P.; Mojtahedi, H.; Nazeri, R. Effect of Autoclave Cycles on Surface Characteristics of S-File Evaluated by Scanning Electron Microscopy. *Iran. Endod. J.* **2016**, *11*, 29–32. [CrossRef]
15. Higgins, J.P.T.; Green, S. *Cochrane Collaboration. Cochrane Handbook for Systematic Reviews of Interventions*; Wiley-Blackwell: Chichester, UK; Hoboken, NJ, USA, 2008; 649p.
16. Lo, C.K.; Mertz, D.; Loeb, M. Newcastle-Ottawa Scale: Comparing reviewers' to authors' assessments. *BMC Med. Res. Methodol.* **2014**, *14*, 45. [CrossRef] [PubMed]
17. Spagnuolo, G.; Ametrano, G.; D'Anto, V.; Rengo, C.; Simeone, M.; Riccitiello, F.; Amato, M. Effect of autoclaving on the surfaces of TiN -coated and conventional nickel-titanium rotary instruments. *Int. Endod. J.* **2012**, *45*, 1148–1155. [CrossRef] [PubMed]
18. Can Saglam, B.; Gorgul, G. Evaluation of surface alterations in different retreatment nickel-titanium files: AFM and SEM study. *Microsc. Res. Tech.* **2015**, *78*, 356–362. [CrossRef]
19. Uslu, G.; Ozyurek, T.; Yilmaz, K. Effect of Sodium Hypochlorite and EDTA on Surface Roughness of HyFlex CM and HyFlex EDM Files. *Microsc. Res. Tech.* **2018**, *81*, 1406–1411. [CrossRef]
20. Topuz, O.; Aydin, C.; Uzun, O.; Inan, U.; Alacam, T.; Tunca, Y.M. Structural effects of sodium hypochlorite solution on RaCe rotary nickel-titanium instruments: An atomic force microscopy study. *Oral Surg. Oral Med. Oral Pathol. Oral Radiol. Endod.* **2008**, *105*, 661–665. [CrossRef]
21. Cai, J.J.; Tang, X.N.; Ge, J.Y. Effect of irrigation on surface roughness and fatigue resistance of controlled memory wire nickel-titanium instruments. *Int. Endod. J.* **2017**, *50*, 718–724. [CrossRef]

22. Saglam, B.C.; Kocak, S.; Kocak, M.M.; Topuz, O. Effects of irrigation solutions on the surface of ProTaper instruments: A microscopy study. *Microsc. Res. Tech.* **2012**, *75*, 1534–1538. [CrossRef] [PubMed]
23. Prasad, P.S.; Sam, J.E.; Arvind Kumar, K. The effect of 5% sodium hypochlorite, 17% EDTA and triphala on two different rotary Ni-Ti instruments: An AFM and EDS analysis. *J. Conserv. Dent.* **2014**, *17*, 462–466. [CrossRef] [PubMed]
24. Yokoyama, K.; Kancko, K.; Yabuta, E.; Asaoka, K.; Sakai, J. Fracture of nickel-titanium superelastic alloy in sodium hypochlorite solution. *Mater. Sci. Eng. A* **2004**, *369*, 43–48. [CrossRef]
25. Bonaccorso, A.; Tripi, T.R.; Rondelli, G.; Condorelli, G.G.; Cantatore, G.; Schafer, E. Pitting corrosion resistance of nickel-titanium rotary instruments with different surface treatments in seventeen percent ethylenediaminetetraacetic Acid and sodium chloride solutions. *J. Endod.* **2008**, *34*, 208–211. [CrossRef]

7

Salivary Biomarkers and their Correlation with Pain and Stress in Patients with Burning Mouth Syndrome

Pia Lopez-Jornet [1,*], Candela Castillo Felipe [2], Luis Pardo-Marin [3], Jose J. Ceron [3], Eduardo Pons-Fuster [4] and Asta Tvarijonaviciute [3]

1 Department Stomatology School of Medicine, Biomedical Research Institute (IMIB-Arrixaca), Faculty of Medicine and Odontology, University of Murcia, 30008 Adv Marques de los Velez s/n, Spain
2 Department Stomatology School of Medicine, Faculty of Medicine and Odontology, University of Murcia; 30008 Murcia, Span; candela.casti@gmail.com
3 Interdisciplinary Laboratory of Clinical Analysis, Interlab-UMU, Regional Campus of International Excellence 'Campus Mare Nostrum', University of Murcia, Espinardo, 30100 Murcia, Spain; lpm1@um.es (L.P.-M.); jjceron@um.es (J.J.C.); asta@um.es (A.T.)
4 Biomedical Research Institute (IMIB-Arrixaca), Faculty of Medicine and Odontology, University of Murcia, 30008 Murcia, Span; edupfl5@hotmail.com
* Correspondence: majornet@um.es

Abstract: Objective: To evaluate a panel of salivary analytes involving biomarkers of inflammation, stress, immune system and antioxidant status in patients with burning mouth syndrome (BMS) and to study their relationship with clinical variables. Materials and Methods: A total of 51 patients with BMS and 31 controls were consecutively enrolled in the study, with the recording of oral habits, the severity of pain using a visual analogue scale (VAS), the Hospital Anxiety and Depression (HAD) score and the Oral Health Impact Profile-14 (OHIP14) score. Resting whole saliva was collected with the drainage technique, followed by the measurement of 11 biomarkers. Results: The salivary flow was higher in patients with BMS. Among all the biomarkers studied, significantly higher levels of alpha-amylase, immunoglobulin A (IgA), and macrophage inflammatory protein-4 (MIP4) and lower levels of uric acid and ferric reducing activity of plasma (FRAP) were observed in the saliva of patients with BMS as compared to the controls ($p < 0.05$ in all cases). Positive correlations were found between pain, oral quality of life and anxiety scores and salivary biomarkers. Conclusions: BMS is associated with changes in salivary biomarkers of inflammation, oxidative stress and stress, being related to the degree of pain and anxiety.

Keywords: saliva; IgA; alpha-amylase; uric acid; stress; inflammation

1. Introduction

The International Association for the Study of Pain (IASP) defines burning mouth syndrome (BMS) as an intraoral burning or dysesthetic sensation that manifests daily for more than two hours over three months, with no evidence of clinical lesions [1]. The epidemiological data on BMS are largely contradictory, in part because of a lack of strict compliance with the diagnostic criteria of the disorder. Nevertheless, BMS is estimated to affect 4% of the general population and 18–33% of all postmenopausal women [2–6]. The symptoms are generally focused on the tongue and lips and are almost always bilateral. The palate and other locations within the oral cavity are less commonly affected. Although much has been published about BMS, its underlying etiopathogenesis is largely unknown, and complex interactions among local, systemic and psychogenic factors are believed to be involved [2,7,8]. For these reasons, BMS is poorly diagnosed, and in many cases management is deficient, a situation that causes frustration for both physicians and patients [3,5]. In the same way as with other chronic pain syndromes, BMS is characterized by associated psychological problems. Changes in personality and mood state, particularly anxiety and depression, are a typical finding in patients with BMS [2,9].

The use of saliva as a sample for clinical analysis has increased in recent decades. Saliva is a body fluid that reflects the physiological condition of the body. It can be easily collected using non-invasive and relatively inexpensive methods [4,5], and it is gaining attention as a source of biomarkers in different oral and systemic pathologies [10]. In BMS an increase in amylase (a marker of the adrenergic system) and immunoglobulin A (IgA) (a marker of the immune system) have been found [11–14]. However, to the authors' knowledge, there have been no studies in which a panel of analytes reflecting possible pathogenic and psychological factors were evaluated in this disease, and also compared with the degree of stress and pain.

The objective of this study was to evaluate how a panel of biomarkers of inflammation represented by complement C4 (CC4), α1-antitrypsin (a1AT), C-reactive protein (CRP), macrophage inflammatory protein-4 (MIP4), pigment epithelium-derived factor (PEDF), serum amyloid P (SAP), haptoglobin (Hp), a panel of biomarkers of oxidative stress integrated by uric acid and ferric reducing activity of plasma (FRAP), the salivary alpha-amylase (sAA) as a marker of the adrenergic system and total immunoglobulin A (IgA) as a marker of the innate immune system can be altered in patients with BMS, and study their possible relation with the degree of pain and stress of the patients was measured by visual analogue scale (VAS) and the Hospital Anxiety and Depression (HAD) score. Also, the possible influence of oral health was evaluated.

2. Material and Methods

2.1. Study Design and Subjects

A cross-sectional study was carried out with data compiled between January 2018 and September 2019 in the Dental Clinic of the University of Murcia (Murcia, Spain). All the patients were informed about the study and gave consent to participation in the trial, which was approved by the local Clinical Research Ethics Committee (Ref.: 2203/2018). The following inclusion criteria were established: patients over 18 years of age with a diagnosis of BMS based on exhaustive oral examination, laboratory findings and the patient profile and symptoms [15], presenting continuous symptoms of oral burning or pain persisting for at least two hours per day, lasting longer than three months, without paroxysms and not following any unilateral nerve trajectory, and with no clinical mucosal alterations. The patients underwent blood testing to confirm the absence of alterations (including blood count, glucose, serum iron, ferritin and transferrin, folic acid and vitamin B12 levels). Cancer patients and individuals with known liver or kidney disease were excluded, as were those with oral diseases other than BMS such as Sjögren's syndrome or ongoing infection, thyroid diseases, coagulation disorders, psychiatric disease, and pregnant or nursing women.

The healthy controls were recruited from the Dental School of the University of Murcia and consisted of patients with the same sociosanitary characteristics and matched for age and gender. Following the procurement of written informed consent, a structured questionnaire was administered to confirm the absence of significant medical conditions. The study was carried out following the STROBE (Strengthening the Reporting of Observational studies in Epidemiology) guidelines.

In all cases, patients were not included in the study if their samples showed hemolysis as determined by visual inspection [16,17].

2.2. Data Collection

A structured interview was used to collect sociodemographic and clinical information as well as data referring to smoking and alcohol consumption. The patients were evaluated by a trained professional (C.C.F.) who conducted the interviews and explorations, administered the questionnaires and collected the saliva samples.

An extraoral and intraoral exploration was carried out, documenting the presence of caries and missing teeth. Pain intensity was scored using a visual analogue scale (VAS) (0 = no pain and 10 = worst possible pain) [18].

The Hospital Anxiety and Depression (HAD) scale [19] was used to assess the emotional state of the participants. This instrument consists of two subscales relating to anxiety (HAD-A) and depression (HAD-D). Concerning the interpretation of the HAD scale, scores of > 10 indicate the probable presence of anxiety or depression, scores of ≤ 7 indicate no significant anxiety or depression, and scores of 8–10 are of borderline significance.

The evaluation of the oral quality of life, in turn, was based on the Oral Health Impact Profile-14 (OHIP14) score [20].

2.3. Saliva Collection

Resting whole saliva was collected using a standardized method [18]. To avoid possible contamination from other sources, the patients were instructed to rinse the mouth thoroughly before saliva sample collection. The subjects were required to avoid heavy physical exercise one hour before sampling. Unstimulated saliva was obtained using the draining method for 5 min. The samples were collected at about the same time in all subjects (8:00 to 11:00 a.m.). The saliva was vortexed and centrifuged (3000× *g* for 10 min at 4 °C) immediately after collection, and the supernatant was transferred into polypropylene tubes and stored at −80 °C until analysis.

2.4. Biochemical Analysis

Complement C4, a1AT, CRP, MIP4, PEDF and SAP in saliva were analyzed using a commercially available kit (Human Neurodegenerative Disease Magnetic Bead Panel 2, Neuroscience Multiplex Assay; Life Science, Darmstadt, Germany) according to the manufacturer's instructions. Values were calculated based on a standard curve constructed for the assay. Saliva total protein quantification was done using a commercially available colorimetric kit for measuring urine and low-complexity region (LCR) proteins (protein in urine and CSF, Spinreact, Barcelona, Spain) and validated for human saliva [21]. Uric acid was measured using a colorimetric commercial kit (Uric acid, Beckman Coulter Inc., Fullerton, CA, USA) following the International Federation of Clinical Chemistry and Laboratory Medicine (IFCC) method [21]. Total IgA was evaluated with a commercial ELISA kit (Bethyl, Montgomery, TX, USA) previously validated for use with human saliva samples [18]. FRAP (ferric reducing ability of plasma) measurement was based on the method described by Benzie and Strain [22] with some modifications [23]. Hp levels were measured in saliva using a homemade immunoassay as previously described [24]. Salivary alpha-amylase (sAA) activity was measured using a colorimetric commercial kit (Alpha-Amylase, Beckman Coulter Inc., Fullerton, CA, USA) following the IFCC method as previously reported and validated [25].

2.5. Statistical Analysis

For the descriptive statistical analysis of the sample, the basic descriptive methods were used, with calculation of the frequencies, mean, median, standard deviation (SD) and 25th and 75th percentile values. The comparison of means between groups was based on the Student's t-test or Mann–Whitney test, depending on the data distribution as verified with the Kolmogorov–Smirnov test, and the homogeneity of groups was confirmed. Clinical scores, smoking and alcohol consumption habits, as well as sex distribution among the two groups, were explored using the chi-square test. The correlations between variables were checked using the partial correlation corrected by age and sex. Previous studies that also analyzed biomarkers in saliva in patients with burning mouth syndrome, such as sAA and total IgA, have been able to detect differences with 30 or fewer individuals in each group considering $\alpha = 0.05$ and $\beta = 0.20$ [11]. Based on these data we assumed that the study was sufficiently powered ($n_{controls} = 31$; $n_{BMS} = 51$) to achieve our aims. Differences and associations among groups were considered statistically significant when $p < 0.05$.

3. Results

The study sample consisted of 82 consecutively enrolled individuals (71 females and 11 males), of which 51 were diagnosed with BMS while the remaining 31 constituted the control group. Table 1 describes the characteristics of each group. Statistically significant differences were not detected in sex, age or smoking and alcohol consumption habits between the two groups of patients ($p > 0.05$).

Table 1. General characteristics of participants.

Variable	Controls	SBA	*p*
Sex, *n* (%)			0.083 [c]
Women	26 (76.5)	45 (88.2)	
Men	5 (14.7)	6 (11.8)	
Age, mean (SD) years	58.3 (11.05)	59.12 (12.29)	0.765 [a]
Smoking, *n* (%)			0.292 [c]
Yes	10 (32.3)	11 (21.6)	
No	18 (58.1)	29 (56.9)	
Former smoker	3 (9.7)	11 (21.6)	
Alcohol consumption, *n* (%)			0.212 [c]
Less than once a week	21 (61.8)	31 (60.8)	
Daily	2 (5.9)	9 (17.6)	
Weekends only	11 (32.4)	11 (21.6)	
Tooth brushing, *n* (%)			0.236 [c]
No	0 (0)	1 (2)	
Less than once a day	1 (3.2)	1 (2)	
Once a day	7 (22.6)	5 (9.8)	
Twice a day	14 (45.2)	18 (35.3)	
≥3 times a day	9 (29)	26 (51)	
Dental floss, *n* (%)			**0.006** [c]
No	23 (74.2)	22 (43.1)	
Yes	8 (25.8)	29 (56.9)	
Mouthwashes, *n* (%)			0.080 [c]
No	28 (90.3)	38 (74.5)	
Yes	3 (9.7)	13 (25.5)	
Missing teeth, mean (SD)	2.1 (2.82)	5.8 (8.3)	**0.004** [b]
Missing teeth groups, *n* (%)			0.098 [c]
1–5	29 (93.5)	39 (76.5)	
6–9	0 (0)	5 (9.8)	
<10	2 (6.5)	7 (13.7)	

Table 1. *Cont.*

Variable	Controls	SBA	p
Caries, mean (SD)	0.42 (0.99)	0.2 (1.13)	0.121 [b]
OHIP14, mean (SD)	14.33 (1.37)	33.1 (9.02)	**<0.001** [b]
HAD-A, mean (SD)	3.77 (2.3)	8.71 (3.82)	**<0.001** [b]
HAD-D, mean (SD)	2.9 (2.4)	4.1 (3.6)	0.292 [b]
VAS, mean (SD)	0 (0)	8.12 (1.77)	**<0.001** [b]
VAS groups, n (%)			
Mild		1 (2.0)	
Moderate		16 (31.4)	
Severe		34 (66.7)	

a, Student's t-test; b, Mann–Whitney test; c, Pearson's chi-square. Bold type denotes statistical significance.

Concerning oral hygiene and health, the controls and patients with BMS did not present statistically significant differences in habits related to tooth brushing and use of mouthwashes, while patients with BMS used more dental floss than controls ($p < 0.01$). In turn, controls presented a comparatively greater number of caries, though the difference was not statistically significant ($p > 0.05$), and significantly fewer missing teeth compared with the BMS group ($p < 0.01$).

Of the clinical variables, the mean burning sensation score in patients with BMS was greater than 8, while it was equal to 0 in healthy controls. The OHIP14 score was 2.3-fold higher in the BMS group as compared with the control group ($p = 0.001$).

Concerning the psychological profile as evaluated by the HAD scale, the anxiety scores among the patients were 2.3-fold higher than in controls ($p < 0.001$). While HAD-D, although being 1.4-fold higher in patients, did not show statistically significant differences between the two groups ($p > 0.05$).

Resting whole saliva flow was 1.4-fold greater in the BMS group as compared to healthy controls ($p < 0.05$) (Figure 1a and Table S1). The study of biomarkers in resting whole saliva yielded significant differences between the cases (patients with BMS) and controls for sAA ($p < 0.01$) and IgA ($p < 0.05$) (Figure 1a,b and Table S1).

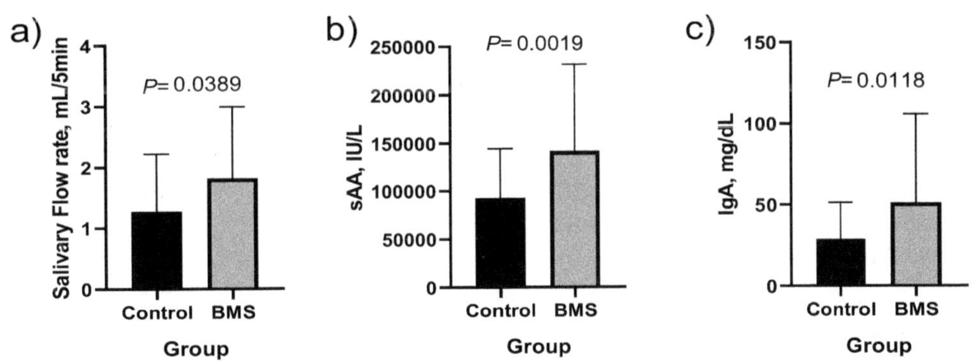

Figure 1. Salivary flow rate (**a**), salivary alpha-amylase (sAA; (**b**)) and immunoglobulin A (IgA; (**c**)) in healthy controls ($n = 31$) and patients with burning mouth syndrome (BMS; $n = 51$). Differences of medians and means±SD for salivary flow are 0.54 and 0.75 ± 0.41, for sAA they are 48,660 and 109,536 ± 41,492 and for IgA they are 22.47 and 34.01 ± 12.72.

When absolute values of salivary biomarkers were corrected by salivary flow, sAA, IgA and MIP4 showed statistically higher concentrations in patients with BMS as compared with healthy controls (Figure 2 and Table S1). When values were corrected by total protein content, statistically significantly higher levels in patients with BMS were observed for sAA and lower for uric acid and FRAP (Figure 3 and Table S1).

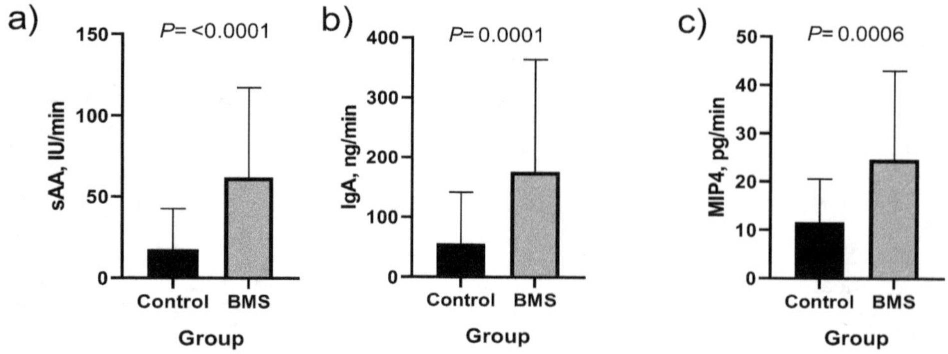

Figure 2. Salivary alpha-amylase (sAA; (**a**)), immunoglobulin A (IgA; (**b**)) and macrophage inflammatory protein-4 (MIP4; (**c**)) corrected by salivary flow in healthy controls ($n = 31$) and patients with burning mouth syndrome (BMS; $n = 51$). Difference of medians and means ± SD for sAA are 44.0 and 47.4 ± 15.91, for IgA are 119.9 and 147.6 ± 38.4 and for MIP4 are 13.0 and 33.6 ± 27.2.

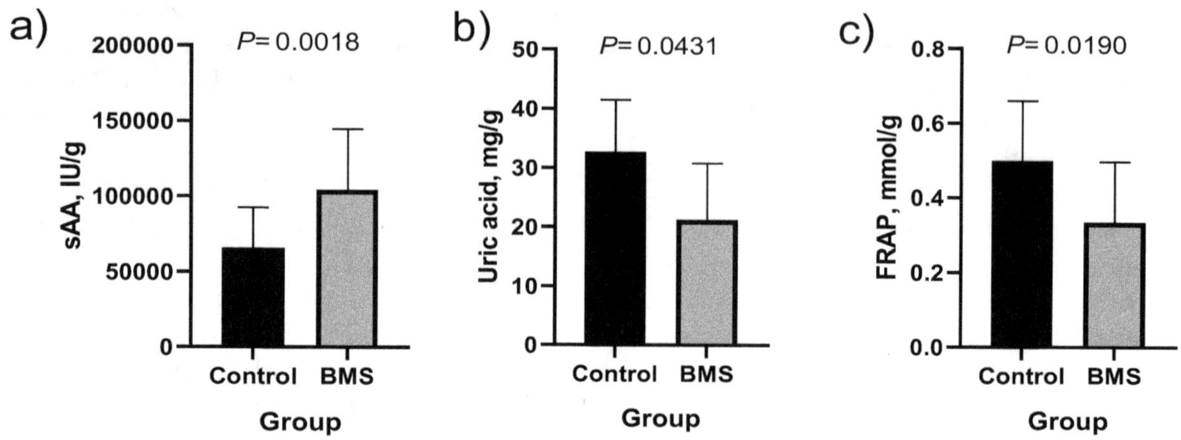

Figure 3. Salivary alpha amylase [sAA; (**a**)], uric acid (**b**) and ferric reducing activity [FRAP; (**c**)] corrected by salivary total protein content in healthy controls ($n = 31$) and patients with burning mouth syndrome (BMS; $n = 51$). Difference of medians and means ± SD for sAA are 38,525 and 33,653 ± 15,365, for uric acid are −11.5 and −7585 ± 4593 and for FRAP are −0.17 and −0.1413 ± 0.06614.

Partial correlation data are given in Table S2. When absolute values were evaluated, a positive correlation was detected between VAS and total proteins ($r = 0.241; p < 0.05$), sAA ($r = 0.260; p < 0.05$) and IgA ($r = 0.334; p < 0.01$); HAD-A was correlated with total proteins ($r = 0.251; p < 0.05$), IgA ($r = 0.302; p < 0.05$), PEDF ($r = 0.351; p < 0.01$) and MIP4 ($r = 0.267; p < 0.05$) and HAD-D with IgA ($r = 0.261; p < 0.05$), PEDF ($r = 0.363; p < 0.01$) and MIP4 ($r = 0.271; p < 0.05$); OHIP14 was correlated with IgA ($r = 0.273; p < 0.05$).

After data were corrected by salivary flow, statistically significant correlations remained between VAS and sAA ($r = 0.269; p < 0.05$) and IgA ($r = 0.367; p < 0.01$); between HAD-A and IgA ($r = 0.338; p < 0.01$), PEDF ($r = 0.297; p < 0.05$) and MIP4 ($r = 0.264; p < 0.05$); between HAD-D and PEDF ($r = 0.386; p = 0.01$) and MIP4 ($r = 0.269; p < 0.05$) and between OHIP14 and IgA ($r = 0.313; p < 0.01$).

After data were corrected by salivary flow, negative correlations appeared between sAA and OHIP14 ($r = -0.242; p < 0.05$) and between HAD-A and FRAP ($r = 0.250; p < 0.05$) and CRP ($r = -0.243; p < 0.05$).

4. Discussion

Burning mouth syndrome is a clinically relevant form of chronic orofacial pain [1–3]. The diagnosis of the syndrome remains a challenge for health professionals due to the discrepancy between the intensity of pain as reported by the patient and the absence of objective clinical lesions. In this study we therefore focused on the identification of potential biomarkers capable of reflecting the physiopathological changes involving pain, psychological stress and inflammation that occur in the context of the disease. Of 11 biomarkers evaluated in the present study, three—sAA, IgA and MIP4—were found to be increased, and two—uric acid and FRAP—were found to be decreased in the saliva of patients with BMS versus controls, suggesting that these patients can present with alterations in immune response, pro-inflammatory status and oxidative stress that are related to pain sensation and psychological stress.

In the present study, a higher salivary flow rate was detected in patients with BMS as compared with healthy controls. In the scientific literature, controversy exists regarding this topic since some authors did not detect changes in salivary flow between controls and patients with BMS [12–14], while others observed lower flow rates in patients with BMS [9,11,26]. Similarly, different authors reported divergent results related to total protein content in the saliva of patients with BMS, as some of them detected decreased [27], increased [12,14] or unchanged (present study) salivary total protein content in these patients when compared with controls. The characteristics of the method or device used to collect the samples and the analytical assays used may have influenced the results obtained and, therefore, the differences among the different studies. It is therefore important to follow the same guidelines for sample collection and processing to enable comparison of the results from different studies.

Since components present in saliva have different origins, i.e., are locally secreted by salivary glands or oral mucosa, or pass from blood among other, and can be affected by non-uniform salivary flow rate, the need to correct values of salivary biomarker by flow rate, total protein content or salivary osmolarity versus use of their absolute value is being increasingly acknowledged and studied by different authors [25,28]. In this study we aimed to evaluate the results without any adjustment, and we also corrected salivary flow or total protein content to gain knowledge about the possible effect that these corrections can have in this particular disease. When levels of biomarkers without any adjustment by saliva flow or protein content were compared between healthy and diseased patients, statistically significant changes were detected only in sAA and IgA. Correction by salivary flow rate allowed identification of the increased levels of MIP4 in the saliva of patients with BMS but also yielded higher differences between the studied groups for IgA in accordance with previously reported data [29]. When values were corrected by total protein content the presence of oxidative stress in patients with BMS was detected, as levels of uric acid and FRAP were lower compared to controls. Therefore, in BMS, correcting salivary values by flow rate and total protein content would be recommended in this disease since it can detect additional changes in salivary analytes that are correlated with the clinical condition of the patient.

sAA is considered to be a sensitive biomarker of stress-related changes that reflect the activity of the sympathetic nervous system (SNS) [30]. Most patients with BMS experience chronic pain and have a poorer quality of life than do healthy individuals [9]. Furthermore, chronic pain characterizing BMS was associated with psychological problems, specifically personality and mood changes, anxiety and depression. The results of this study agree with these findings and previous reports that detected higher sAA levels in the saliva of patients with BMS [12,14] since patients included in the present study showed both higher anxiety scores and sAA levels; however, another study did not detect changes in sAA between healthy controls and patients with BMS, and differences in the severity of the disease in the population evaluated or in the assay used could be the cause of these differences [9]. A weak positive correlation between sAA (expressed in absolute concentrations and when corrected by flow) and burning sensation was detected, which could indicate that increases in this enzyme could be influenced in part by pain.

Salivary IgA was another biomarker that showed statistically significant differences among controls and patients in the studied population, being higher in patients with BMS. These data are consistent with those reported by other authors [12–14]. Furthermore, a higher difference between the two groups was detected when IgA was corrected by salivary flow resulting in an increase of 1.8-fold to 2.9-fold change between the two groups. IgA is an immune glycoprotein that acts as a defense against pathogens [31]. Nevertheless, different studies have suggested that changes in salivary IgA can also be associated with stress [32]. This hypothesis would be supported by the observed positive correlations between IgA in saliva and oral quality of life, burning sensation and anxiety in the studied population. In addition, MIP, a biomarker of the innate immune system [33], was also increased in patients with BMS and weakly positively correlated with anxiety and depression scores, suggesting that the immune system is implicated in the pathogenesis of BMS.

In the present study, when the results were corrected by protein content, patients with BMS had lower salivary FRAP and uric acid, suggesting the presence of oxidative stress, and in the case of FRAP, it was weakly correlated with HAD-A, which would indicate that this increase could be influenced by stress. The two markers are closely related since uric acid was the main component (up to 60%) of the FRAP assay [22]. Uric acid is considered to be the most important antioxidant molecule in saliva since it is responsible for approximately 70% of the total antioxidant capacity of this body fluid. As a reactive oxygen species scavenger, it helps stabilize arterial pressure and oxidative stress [21,34–36]. In turn, alterations in its levels in saliva were associated with acute stress [34] and different local and systemic pathologies such as oral lichen planus [37] or nephropathies [38]. Previous studies that evaluated salivary uric acid in patients with BMS did not find statistically significant changes as compared with healthy controls [16,20], although these studies did not make corrections for total protein content.

A limitation of the study is the fact that the measurements were limited to a single time-point. Variations of these markers in the same individual should be investigated in the context of future studies with a larger sample size to increase the power, and by employing multiple samplings over time, resulting in more accurate estimations. Furthermore, it would be of interest to apply the biomarkers that showed significant changes in a larger population to corroborate the results of this study. Finally, the possible blood contamination in saliva samples should have been evaluated using more sensitive methods, such as determination of hemoglobin or transferrin, although these methods were shown to be affected by different factors such as age, hormones and salivary flow among others [16]. Conversely, visual inspection was shown to be sufficient in the case of determining some of the analytes including oxidative stress markers in saliva without interfering with the results [17].

5. Conclusions

In conclusion, patients with BMS showed changes in biomarkers associated with stress such as sAA and IgA, with the immune system such as MIP4 and oxidative stress such as uric acid and FRAP in saliva as compared with healthy controls, which are related to clinical variables including burning sensation and anxiety. Moreover, in this particular disease, the study of the absolute values but also the values corrected by flow and total protein would be recommended. Overall, biomarkers that were shown to change differently between groups could potentially help clinicians not only with diagnosis but also in objectively evaluating the severity of this disease, although further large-scale studies should first be performed to collaborate our findings.

Author Contributions: Conceptualization, P.L.-J., C.C.F. and A.T.; Methodology, P.L.-J., C.C.F. and A.T.; Software, L.P.-M., J.J.C. and A.T.; Validation, P.L.-J., C.C.F. and E.P.-F.; Formal Analysis, P.L.-J., A.T., L.P.-M. and J.J.C.; Investigation, P.L.-J., C.C.F., L.P.-M. and A.T.; Resources, P.L.-J., C.C.F., J.J.C. and A.T.; Data Curation, P.L.-J. and C.C.F.; Writing-Original, P.L.-J., J.J.C. and A.T.; Draft Preparation, E.P.-F.; Writing-Review & Editing, P.L.-J., A.T. and J.J.C.; Supervision, All authors; Project Administration, P.L.-J. and A.T. All authors have read and agreed to the published version of the manuscript.

References

1. Scala, A.; Checchi, L.; Montevecchi, M.; Marini, I.; Giamberardino, M.A. Update on burning mouth syndrome: Overview and patient management. *Crit. Rev. Oral Biol. Med.* **2003**, *14*, 275–291. [CrossRef]
2. Olesen, J. Headache classification committee of the International Headache Society (IHS) the international classification of headache disorders, 3rd edition. *Cephalalgia* **2018**, *38*, 1–211.

3. Kohorst, J.J.; Bruce, A.J.; Torgerson, R.R.; Schenck, L.A.; Davis, M.D.P. The prevalence of burning mouth syndrome: A population-based study. *Br. J. Dermatol.* **2015**, *172*, 1654–1656. [CrossRef] [PubMed]
4. Klasser, G.D.; Fischer, D.J.; Epstein, J.B. Burning mouth syndrome: Recognition, understanding, and management. *Oral Maxillofac. Surg. Clin. N. Am.* **2008**, *20*, 255–271. [CrossRef] [PubMed]
5. López-Jornet, P.; Camacho-Alonso, F.; Andujar-Mateos, P.; Sánchez-Siles, M.; Gómez-García, F. Burning mouth syndrome: Update. *Med. Oral Patol. Oral Cir. Bucal* **2010**, *15*, e562-8. [CrossRef] [PubMed]
6. Ariyawardana, A.; Chmieliauskaite, M.; Farag, A.M.; Albuquerque, R.; Forssell, H.; Nasri-Heir, C.; Klasser, G.D.; Sardella, A.; Mignogna, M.D.; Ingram, M.; et al. World Workshop on Oral Medicine VII: Burning mouth syndrome: A systematic review of disease definitions and diagnostic criteria utilized in randomized clinical trials. *Oral Dis.* **2019**, *25*, 141–156. [CrossRef] [PubMed]
7. Jääskeläinen, S.K. Is burning mouth syndrome a neuropathic pain condition? *Pain* **2018**, *159*, 610–613. [CrossRef]
8. Ritchie, A.; Kramer, J.M. Recent advances in the etiology and treatment of burning mouth syndrome. *J. Dent. Res.* **2018**, *97*, 1193–1199. [CrossRef]
9. Kim, H.-I.; Kim, Y.-Y.; Chang, J.-Y.; Ko, J.-Y.; Kho, H.-S. Salivary cortisol, 17β-estradiol, progesterone, dehydroepiandrosterone, and α-amylase in patients with burning mouth syndrome. *Oral Dis.* **2012**, *18*, 613–620. [CrossRef]
10. Tvarijonaviciute, A.; Martinez-Subiela, S.; Lopez-Jornet, P.; Lamy, E. *Saliva in Health and Disease: The Present and Future of a Unique*; Springer: Berlin/Heidelberg, Germany, 2020; ISBN 9783030376802.
11. Imura, H.; Shimada, M.; Yamazaki, Y.; Sugimoto, K. Characteristic changes of saliva and taste in burning mouth syndrome patients. *J. Oral Pathol. Med.* **2016**, *45*, 231–236. [CrossRef]
12. Nagler, R.M.; Hershkovich, O. Sialochemical and gustatory analysis in patients with oral sensory complaints. *J. Pain* **2004**, *5*, 56–63. [CrossRef] [PubMed]
13. Granot, M.; Nagler, R.M. Association between regional idiopathic neuropathy and salivary involvement as the possible mechanism for oral sensory complaints. *J. Pain* **2005**, *6*, 581–587. [CrossRef] [PubMed]
14. Hershkovich, O.; Nagler, R.M. Biochemical analysis of saliva and taste acuity evaluation in patients with burning mouth syndrome, xerostomia and/or gustatory disturbances. *Arch. Oral Biol.* **2004**, *49*, 515–522. [CrossRef] [PubMed]
15. Silvestre, F.J.; Silvestre Rangil, J.; López Jornet, P. Burning mouth syndrome: A review and update. *Rev. Neurol.* **2015**, *60*, 463.
16. Kang, J.H.; Kho, H.S. Blood contamination in salivary diagnostics: Current methods and their limitations. *Clin. Chem. Lab. Med.* **2018**, *57*, 1115–1124. [CrossRef]
17. Kamodyová, N.; Baňasová, L.; Janšáková, K.; Koborová, I.; Tóthová, Ľ.; Stanko, P.; Celec, P. Blood contamination in Saliva: Impact on the measurement of salivary oxidative stress markers. *Dis. Markers* **2015**, *2015*, 479251. [CrossRef]
18. Lopez-Jornet, P.; Cayuela, C.A.; Tvarijonaviciute, A.; Parra-Perez, F.; Escribano, D.; Ceron, J. Oral lichen planus: Salival biomarkers cortisol, immunoglobulin A, adiponectin. *J. Oral Pathol. Med.* **2016**, *45*, 211–217. [CrossRef]
19. Zigmond, A.S.; Snaith, R.P. The hospital anxiety and depression scale. *Acta Psychiatr. Scand.* **1983**, *67*, 361–370. [CrossRef]
20. Montero-Martin, J.; Bravo-Pérez, M.; Albaladejo-Martínez, A.; Hernández-Martin, L.A.; Rosel-Gallardo, E.M. Validation the Oral Health Impact Profile (OHIP-14sp) for adults in Spain. *Med. Oral Patol. Oral Cir. Bucal* **2009**, *14*, 14.
21. González-Hernández, J.M.; Franco, L.; Colomer-Poveda, D.; Martinez-Subiela, S.; Cugat, R.; Cerón, J.J.; Márquez, G.; Martínez-Aranda, L.M.; Jimenez-Reyes, P.; Tvarijonaviciute, A. Influence of sampling conditions, salivary flow, and total protein content in uric acid measurements in Saliva. *Antioxidants* **2019**, *8*, 389. [CrossRef]
22. Benzie, I.F.F.; Strain, J.J. The Ferric Reducing Ability of Plasma (FRAP) as a measure of "Antioxidant Power": The FRAP assay. *Anal. Biochem.* **1996**, *239*, 70–76. [CrossRef] [PubMed]
23. Tvarijonaviciute, A.; Aznar-Cayuela, C.; Rubio, C.P.; Ceron, J.J.; López-Jornet, P. Evaluation of salivary oxidate stress biomarkers, nitric oxide and C-reactive protein in patients with oral lichen planus and burning mouth syndrome. *J. Oral Pathol. Med.* **2017**, *46*, 387–392. [CrossRef] [PubMed]

24. Tvarijonaviciute, A.; Zamora, C.; Ceron, J.J.; Bravo-Cantero, A.F.; Pardo-Marin, L.; Valverde, S.; Lopez-Jornet, P. Salivary biomarkers in Alzheimer's disease. *Clin. Oral Investig.* **2020**. [CrossRef] [PubMed]
25. Contreras-Aguilar, M.D.; Escribano, D.; Martínez-Subiela, S.; Martínez-Miró, S.; Rubio, M.; Tvarijonaviciute, A.; Tecles, F.; Cerón, J.J. Influence of the way of reporting alpha-amylase values in saliva in different naturalistic situations: A pilot study. *PLoS ONE* **2017**, *12*, e0180100. [CrossRef]
26. Lee, Y.C.; Hong, I.K.; Na, S.Y.; Eun, Y.G. Evaluation of salivary function in patients with burning mouth syndrome. *Oral Dis.* **2015**, *21*, 308–313. [CrossRef]
27. Tammiala-Salonen, T.; Söderling, E. Protein composition, adhesion, and agglutination properties of saliva in burning mouth syndrome. *Eur. J. Oral Sci.* **1993**, *101*, 215–218. [CrossRef]
28. Lindsay, A.; Costello, J.T. Realising the potential of urine and saliva as diagnostic tools in sport and exercise medicine. *Sport. Med.* **2016**, *47*, 1–21. [CrossRef]
29. Marcotte, H.; Lavoie, M.C. Oral microbial ecology and the role of salivary Immunoglobulin A. *Microbiol. Mol. Biol. Rev.* **1998**, *62*, 71–109. [CrossRef]
30. Ngamchuea, K.; Chaisiwamongkhol, K.; Batchelor-Mcauley, C.; Compton, R.G. Chemical analysis in saliva and the search for salivary biomarkers-a tutorial review. *Analyst* **2018**, *143*, 81–99. [CrossRef]
31. Yoo, E.M.; Morrison, S.L. IgA: An immune glycoprotein. *Clin. Immunol.* **2005**, *116*, 3–10. [CrossRef]
32. Yang, Y.; Koh, D.; Ng, V.; Lee, C.Y.; Chan, G.; Dong, F.; Goh, S.H.; Anantharaman, V.; Chia, S.E. Self perceived work related stress and the relation with salivary IgA and lysozyme among emergency department nurses. *Occup. Environ. Med.* **2002**, *59*, 836–841. [CrossRef] [PubMed]
33. De Nadaï, P.; Chenivesse, C.; Gilet, J.; Porte, H.; Vorng, H.; Chang, Y.; Walls, A.F.; Wallaert, B.; Tonnel, A.B.; Tsicopoulos, A.; et al. CCR5 usage by CCL5 induces a selective leukocyte recruitment in human skin xenografts In vivo. *J. Investig. Dermatol.* **2006**, *126*, 2057–2064. [CrossRef] [PubMed]
34. Goodman, A.M.; Wheelock, M.D.; Harnett, N.G.; Mrug, S.; Granger, D.A.; Knight, D.C. The hippocampal response to psychosocial stress varies with salivary uric acid level. *Neuroscience* **2016**, *339*, 396–401. [CrossRef] [PubMed]
35. Albert, U.; De Cori, D.; Aguglia, A.; Barbaro, F.; Bogetto, F.; Maina, G. Increased uric acid levels in bipolar disorder subjects during different phases of illness. *J. Affect. Disord.* **2015**, *173*, 170–175. [CrossRef]
36. Wen, S.; Cheng, M.; Wang, H.; Yue, J.; Wang, H.; Li, G.; Zheng, L.; Zhong, Z.; Peng, F. Serum uric acid levels and the clinical characteristics of depression. *Clin. Biochem.* **2012**, *45*, 49–53. [CrossRef]
37. Bakhtiari, S.; Toosi, P.; Samadi, S.; Bakhshi, M. Assessment of uric acid level in the saliva of patients with oral lichen planus. *Med. Princ. Pract.* **2017**, *26*, 57–60. [CrossRef]
38. Bilancio, G.; Cavallo, P.; Lombardi, C.; Guarino, E.; Cozza, V.; Giordano, F.; Palladino, G.; Cirillo, M. Saliva for assessing creatinine, uric acid, and potassium in nephropathic patients. *BMC Nephrol.* **2019**, *20*, 242. [CrossRef]

8

Association between Gingival Biotype and Facial Typology through Cephalometric Evaluation and Three-Dimensional Facial Scanning

Rosa Valletta [1], Ada Pango [1], Gregorio Tortora [1], Roberto Rongo [1], Vittorio Simeon [2], Gianrico Spagnuolo [1,*] and Vincenzo D'Antò [1]

1 Department of Neurosciences, Reproductive Sciences and Oral Sciences, Section of Orthodontics, University of Naples "Federico II", 80131 Naples, Italy; valletta@unina.it (R.V.); apangom@gmail.com (A.P.); gregorio.tortora@gmail.com (G.T.); roberto.rongo@gmail.com (R.R.); vincenzodanto@gmail.com (V.D.)
2 Department of Mental Health and Preventive Medicine, Medical Statistics Unit, University of Campania "Luigi Vanvitelli", 80138 Napoli, Italy; vittoriosimeon@gmail.com
* Correspondence: gspagnuo@unina.it

Featured Application: Patients with a reduced inferior facial height present, with lower frequency, a thin gingival biotype, and might be less susceptible to periodontal damage due to orthodontic treatment.

Abstract: In dentistry, the assessment of periodontal biotype is considered one of the most important parameters with which to plan treatment, and craniofacial morphology might affect it. The aim of this study was to investigate the association between facial typology and gingival biotype in patients by means of two-dimensional and three-dimensional evaluations of facial typology. This study included 121 participants searching for orthodontic treatment (43 M, 78 F; 20.4 ± 10.4). Gingival biotype was evaluated based on the transparency of the periodontal probe through the gingival margin of the mid-buccal sulcus for both upper (UGB) and lower (LGB) anterior teeth. SellionNasion^GonionGnation (SN^GoGn) and CondylionGonionMenton (CoGoMe^) angles were measured on two-dimensional cephalograms. Three-dimensional face scans were acquired by means of a three-dimensional facial scanner (3dMD system) and successively analyzed to assess the facial typology using the ratio between lower facial height (SNMe) and total facial height (NMe). A chi-squared test and regression analysis were used to evaluate the associations between gingival biotype and facial morphology ($p < 0.05$). The chi-squared test showed that there was no statistically significant association between facial typology and gingival biotype (UGB $p = 0.83$; LGB $p = 0.75$). The logistic regression showed an association between SNMe/NMe and the UGB ($p = 0.036$), and SNMe/NMe and LGB ($p = 0.049$). The decreased ratio of SNMe/NMe might be a protective factor for a thin gingival biotype.

Keywords: facial typology; gingival biotype; orthodontic diagnosis; cephalometric analysis; three-dimensional facial scans

---

1. Introduction

Gingivitis develops more frequently in patients undergoing orthodontic treatment mainly due to an inflammatory reaction following the accumulation of bacterial plaque [1–3].

Many authors have shown that gingival recessions can develop during or after orthodontic treatment [4,5]. Indeed, at the end of orthodontic therapy, the reported prevalence of gingival recessions ranges from 5% to 12% and in long-term follow-up (5 years) has been observed an increase to 47% [4–6].

A recent systematic review has established that the direction of dental movements and the buccal-lingual thickness of the gingiva can play an important role in altering soft tissues during orthodontic treatment. There is a high probability of recession during tooth movement in areas with less than 2 mm of gingival thickness [7]. This could affect the integrity of periodontal tissues and represent a risk factor when orthodontic treatments [8], implants [9], and restorative treatments are performed [10]. Gingival biotype is defined as the thickness of the gingiva in the labiolingual direction [9]. Studies have reported that gingival biotype is an important parameter that must be evaluated to reduce the risk of gingival recession [11].

Hence, the assessment of periodontal biotype is considered one of the most important parameters for outcomes focused on dental planning according to the classification of periodontal and peri-implant diseases and conditions [12].

Many features of the gingival phenotype are genetically determined; others seem to be influenced by age, sex, growth, tooth shape, and tooth position [13]. Moreover, it has been shown that among individuals and intra-individual there is variation in the width [14] and thickness of the vestibular gingiva [15].

Facial typology is classified as dolichofacial, mesofacial, or brachyfacial. A dolichofacial typology has excessive vertical facial growth and is usually associated with an increased SellaNasion^GonionGnathion (SN^GoGN) angle and increased vertical jaw relation (AnsPns^GoGn) [16,17]. A brachyfacial typology has reduced vertical growth and is usually accompanied by reduced SN^GoGn, reduced AnsPns^GoGn, and a decreased lower facial height (SNMe) total facial height (NMe) ratio [18].

The cephalometric evaluation of facial type is essential for orthodontic diagnosis because the amount and direction of jaw growth will significantly alter the need for orthodontic biomechanics [19].

Craniofacial morphology may also affect the gingival phenotype [13,20]. Some studies have evaluated the relationship of bone morphology to facial typology [21–23] and a correlation between facial and alveolar bone has already been demonstrated [24]. Indeed, in dolichofacial patients, the mandibular symphysis is high and thin, while in brachyfacial patients, the symphysis is low and thick [25]. As a consequence, before starting orthodontic treatment, it is important to evaluate and to diagnose both the gingival biotype and facial typology with the objective of decreasing the risk of periodontal destruction [26]. Only a few studies have instead evaluated the association between gingival thickness and craniofacial morphology [26].

Facial soft tissue is evaluated using several methodologies; two of the most representative methods, used to obtain three-dimensional (3D) scans, are laser scanners and 3D stereophotogrammetry [27–30]. The analysis of the face using 3D stereophotogrammetry is consistent and valid [31–34]. Hence, this is a reliable method with which to analyze facial soft tissues and avoid any X-ray exposure to the patient [34,35].

Including only patients seeking orthodontic treatment, the aim of this study was to investigate the association between gingival biotype and facial typology evaluated by means of a cephalometric and 3D facial analysis.

The null hypothesis was that there is no association between gingival biotype and facial typology.

2. Materials and Methods

2.1. Subjects

The study sample comprised 121 patients (43 males, 78 females; from 10 to 56 years old, median age 17.04, and interquartile range (IQR) 13.7–22.1) recruited among patients who had to start orthodontic treatment at the Section of Orthodontics and Temporomandibular Disorders of the University of Naples "Federico II".

All patients were fully informed about the nature of the study and signed their informed consent. The research protocol was approved by the Ethics Committee of the University of Naples Federico II (58/19).

The following selection criteria were applied: (1) patients > 8 years, (2) patients had had pre-orthodontic treatment, (3) patients had upper and lower permanent anterior teeth, and (4) patients had good oral hygiene.

Exclusion criteria included diseases requiring premedication to perform periodontal probing, systemic diseases that can influence the activity of periodontal disease, individuals taking drugs that affect periodontal status, patients with removable prostheses, and pregnant or breastfeeding women.

2.2. *Periodontal Assessment and Clinical Procedure*

Gingival biotype was evaluated based on the transparency of the periodontal probe through the gingival margin of the mid-buccal sulcus of both central and lateral incisors and canines, both maxillary and mandibular. If the outline of the probe could be seen through the gingival margin, it was categorized as "thin" (Figure 1); if not, it was categorized as "thick" (Figure 2) [36].

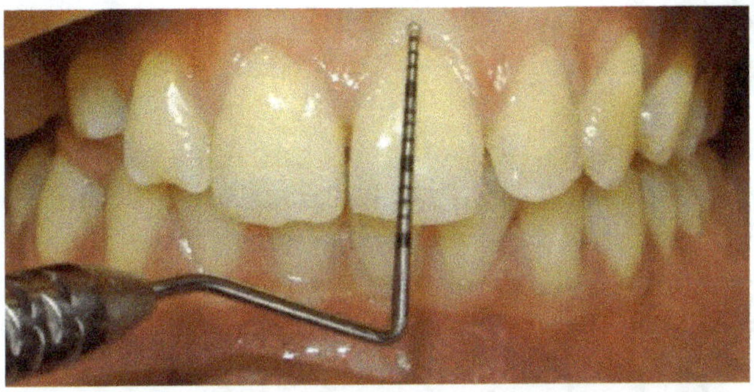

Figure 1. Thin biotype with North Carolina probe.

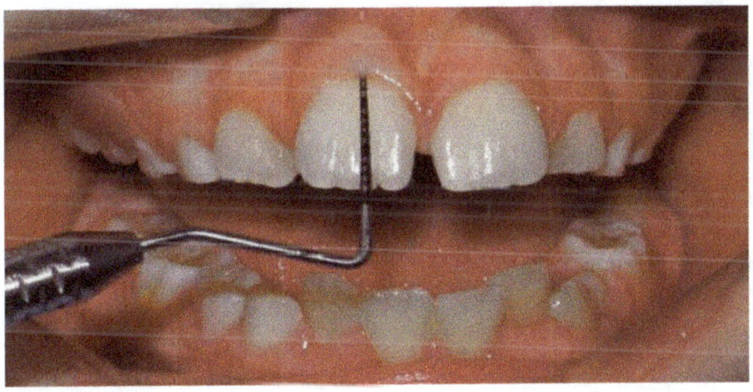

Figure 2. Thick biotype with North Carolina probe.

All the variables were recorded by one expert operator (periodontist) using a millimeter periodontal probe (15 mm North Carolina probe) inserted in the gingival sulcus with a force of about 0.25 Newton.

2.3. *D Facial Scans Acquisition Process*

The facial scanner 3dMD (3dMD LLC, Atlanta, GA, USA) was used in this study. The scanner was installed in a specific setting, with no lighting (neither natural nor artificial lighting) used during the acquisition.

The scanner configuration consisted of three pairs of stereo-cameras, two texture cameras, and four geometric cameras with lenses slightly convergent, as well as two projectors and three led panels positioned on the right and on the left.

The calibration of the system was the first step of the protocol acquisition. The operator invited the patient to look straight ahead with their head in a natural head position (NHP) for the total scanning time. The teeth were taken together with the eyes opened. After the participant had been properly positioned 90 cm away from the scanner, a video with the six cameras was recorded.

Successively, the scans were exported from the video as .obj images and analyzed using a 3dMDVultus (3dMD LLC, Atlanta, GA, USA). All images were stored on a secure computer in the School of Dentistry at the University of Naples.

2.4. Facial Typology Assessment with Two-Dimensional and Three-Dimensional Cephalometric Evaluation

Delta-Dent software (Outside Format, Spino D'Adda, Italy) was used to perform two-dimensional cephalometric tracings to evaluate facial typology.

For this study, cephalometric analysis was performed as shown in Figure 3a,b. Briefly, two cephalometric variables were assessed: the SN^GoGn (average value ± SD = 33° ± 2.5°) determined jaw divergence, which is the angle between the anterior cranial base (Sella-Nasion) and the mandibular plane (Gonion-Gnathion), and the CoGoMe^ angle (average value ± SD = 132° ± 6.0°) that measures the mandibular structure and is formed by the condylar axis (Condylion-Gonion) and the mandibular base (Gonion-Menton).

The sample was divided into three types of craniofacial morphology: brachyfacial, with a SN^GoGn equal to or lower than 27°, mesofacial, with a SN^GoGn between 27° and 37°, and dolichofacial, with a SN^GoGn equal to or greater than 37°.

In order to evaluate facial typology, six points (Figure 3a) were identified and traced on a lateral cephalogram: 'Sella' (S, the center of the sella turcica), 'Nasion' (N, the external point of the junction between the nasal and frontal bones), 'Gonion' (Go, the most inferior posterior point of the mandibular angle), 'Gnathion' (Gn, the point of the mandibular symphysis on the facial axis) 'Menton' (Me, the most inferior point of the mandibular symphysis), and 'Condylion' (Co, the highest and most posterior point on the contour of the mandibular condyle).

The facial scans were acquired and then analyzed using 3dMDVultus Software. On the facial scans, three landmarks were identified: N ('Soft Tissue Nasion', the midpoint on the soft tissue contour of the base of the nasal root at the level of the frontonasal suture), SN ('SubNasion', the midpoint on the nasolabial soft tissue contour between the columella crest and the upper lip), and Me ('Soft Tissue Menton', the most inferior midpoint on the soft tissue contour of the chin). Among these three points, two linear measurements were constructed for the analysis, namely, NMe (total facial height) and SNMe (inferior facial height), as shown in Figure 3c, and the ratio between them was calculated (SNMe/NMe).

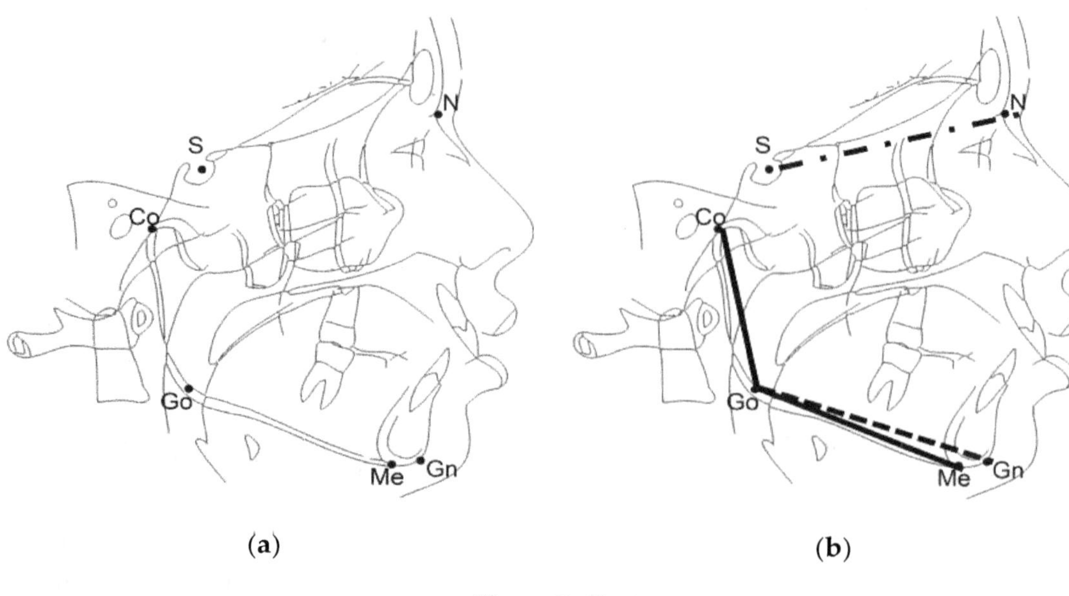

(a) (b)

Figure 3. *Cont.*

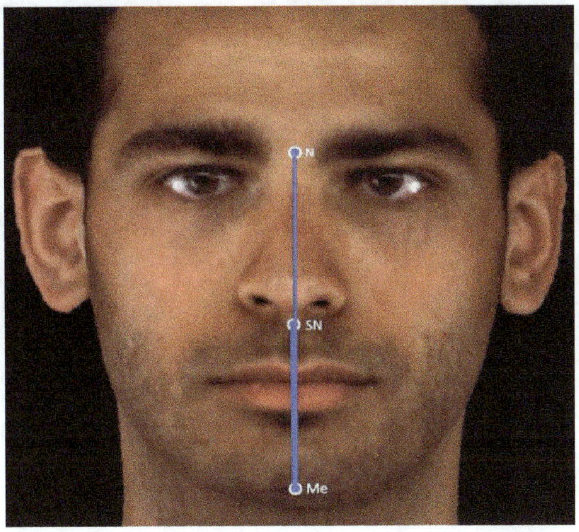

(c)

Figure 3. (**a–c**) Points, planes, and angles for the assessment of facial typology with cephalometry and facial scanner. (**a**) 'Sellion' (S, the center of the sella turcica), 'Nasion' (N, the external point of the junction between the nasal and frontal bones), 'Gonion' (Go, the most inferior posterior point of the mandibular angle), 'Gnathion' (Gn, the point of the mandibular symphysis on the facial axis) 'Menton' (Me, the most inferior point of the mandibular symphysis), 'Condylion' (Co, the highest and most posterior point on the contour of the mandibular condyle); (**b**) SN plane, GoGn plane, and CoGoMe angle; (**c**) N ('Soft Tissue Nasion', the midpoint on the soft tissue contour of the base of the nasal root at the level of the frontonasal suture), SN ('SubNasion', the midpoint on the nasolabial soft tissue contour between the columella crest and the upper lip), and Me ('Soft Tissue Menton', the most inferior midpoint on the soft tissue contour of the chin). NMe indicates total facial height and SNMe indicates inferior facial height.

2.5. *Sample Size*

The sample size was established based on the fact that a sample size of 100 patients reaches 80% of power (1-beta) to detect an effect size (W) of 0.31 (medium-large effect size) using a Chi-squared test with two degrees of freedom and a significance level (alpha) of 0.05.

2.6. *Statistical Analysis*

Descriptive statistics on age, gender, gingival biotype, and baseline characteristics were performed (Table 1). Continuous variables were reported as mean and SD or median and IQR, according to Shapiro-Wilk test, which was performed to evaluate variable distribution. Categorical variables were reported as count and percentage and were compared using the Chi-squared test (gingival biotype versus facial typology). Logistic regression analysis was used to assess the association between continuous variables (CoGoMeˆ and SNMe/NMe) and dichotomous variables (thin or thick biotype) used as dependent variables, including age as a covariate. The level of statistical significance was set at $p < 0.05$. Statistical analysis was performed using STATA version 14.0 (StataCorp. 2015. Stata Statistical Software: Release 14. StataCorp LP: College Station, TX, USA).

3. Results

The total sample consisted of 121 pre-orthodontic patients, comprising 43 males and 78 females which a median age of 17.04 (IQR = 13.7–22.1). Table 1 shows a description of the sample regarding age, sex, gingival biotype, and facial typology. Two-dimensional and 3D cephalometric data are reported in Table 2, and all were normally distributed.

Table 1. Characteristics of study subjects according to age, gender, gingival biotype, and facial typology.

Variables	N	Median (IQR)
Age	121	17.04 (13.7–22.1)
	Frequency	Percentage (%)
Gender		
Male	43	35.54
Female	78	63.64
Upper Gingival Biotype		
Thick	105	86.78
Thin	16	13.22
Lower Gingival Biotype		
Thick	63	52.07
Thin	58	47.93
Facial Typology SN^GoGn		
Brachyfacial	33	27.27
Mesofacial	59	48.76
Dolichofacial	29	23.97

Data are presented as median and interquartile range (IQR) or frequencies and percentages.

Table 2. Descriptive variables of the sample size.

Variables	Mean ± SD	P50	P25	P75
SN^Go-Gn	32.7° ± 8°	32.7°	28.1°	36.3°
CoGoMe^	123.2° ± 6.6°	122.8°	118.7°	127.4°
SNMe/SMe	0.514 ± 0.042	0.51	0.497	0.530

Data are presented as mean ± SD and IQR. SN^GoGn (mean ± SD = 33° ± 2.5°) is the angle between the anterior cranial base (Sella-Nasion) and the mandibular plane (Gonion-Gnathion). CoGoMe^ (average value ± SD = 132° ± 6.0°) is the angle between the condylar axis (Condylion-Gonion) and the mandibular base (Gonion-Menton). SNMe/NMe is the ratio between SNMe (inferior facial height) and NMe (total facial height).

The sample was divided into three groups according to SN^GoGn, and there were 33 (27.27%) brachyfacial patients, 59 (48.76%) mesofacial patients, and 29 (23.97%) dolichofacial patients, as shown in Table 1.

Regarding gingival biotype, most patients presented a thick gingival biotype (upper anterior teeth (UGB) 86.78%; lower anterior teeth (LGB) 52.07%), as seen in Table 1.

The Chi-squared test showed that there was no statistically significant association between SN^GoGn and gingival biotype (UGB $p = 0.83$; LGB $p = 0.75$; and gingival biotype $p = 0.77$, Table 3).

Similarly, the logistic regression analysis showed that CoGoMe^ was not associated with any variables of gingival biotype (UGB, $p = 0.340$; LGB, $p = 0.065$).

Finally, logistic regression analysis showed a statistically significant association of SNMe/NMe with the UGB (odds ratio = 0.843; 95% CI 0.719–0.989; $p = 0.036$) and of SNMe/NMe with LGB (odds ratio = 0.904; 95% CI 0.818–1.000; $p = 0.049$), showing that when the ratio of SNMe/NMe decreases, there is a minor risk of finding a thin biotype (Table 4).

Table 3. Classification of gingival biotype in patients with different facial typologies (classified according to SN^GoGn) using a 15 mm North Carolina probe.

Facial Typology (N)	Upper Gingival Biotype			
	Thick	Thin		*p* value
Brachyfacial (33)	29 (27.62%)	4 (25.00%)		0.83
Mesofacial (59)	50 (47.62%)	9 (56.25%)		
Dolichofacial (29)	26 (24.76%)	3 (18.75%)		
Total (121)	105 (100%)	16 (100%)		
	Lower Gingival Biotype			
	Thick	Thin		*p* value
Brachyfacial (33)	16 (25.40%)	17 (29.31%)		0.75
Mesofacial (59)	33 (52.38%)	26 (44.83%)		
Dolichofacial (29)	14 (22.22%)	15 (25.86%)		
Total (121)	63 (100%)	58 (100%)		
	Gingival Biotype			
	Thick/Thick	Thick/Thin	Thin/Thin	*p* value
Brachyfacial (33)	16 (25.40%)	13 (30.95%)	4 (25%)	0.77
Mesofacial (59)	33 (52.38%)	17 (40.48%)	9 (56.25%)	
Dolichofacial (29)	14 (22.22%)	12 (28.57%)	3 (18.75%)	
Total (121)	63 (100%)	42 (100%)	16 (100%)	

Data are presented as numbers, percentages, and *p* values.

Table 4. Logistic regression model for SNMe/NMe ratio × 100 with and without including age as a coviariate.

Model	Variable	*p* Value	Odds Ratio (OR)	95% IC
Upper biotype (SNMe/NMe)	SNMe/NMe	**0.036** *	0.843	0.719–0.989
Lower biotype (SNMe/NMe)	SNMe/NMe	**0.049** *	0.904	0.818–0.999
Upper biotype (SNMe/NMe × Age)	SNMe/NMe	**0.034** *	0.839	0.714–0.987
	Age	**0.620**	0.985	0.927–1.046
Lower biotype (SNMe/NMe × Age)	SNMe/NMe	**0.048** *	0.903	0.815–0.999
	Age	**0.207**	0.976	0.939–1.014

Data are presented as OR and IQR. * and bold text indicate statistically significant values ($p < 0.05$).

4. Discussion

The aim of this study was to investigate the association between facial typology and gingival biotype in pre-orthodontic patients in order to guarantee a better diagnosis and planning of orthodontic treatment.

We tested whether the facial typology measured on two-dimensional cephalograms (SN^GoGn and CoGoMe^) or on three-dimensional facial scans (SNMe/NMe) could affect gingival biotype. No association was found between facial typology assessed using the two-dimensional angles SN^GoGn or CoGoMe^ and maxillary and mandibular gingival biotype of the anterior regions. There is one study that correlates craniofacial morphology using magnetic resonance imaging (MRI) with tooth root exposure and periodontal attachment loss. The study used the ratio of facial width and length (facial index) to describe craniofacial morphology and showed that patients with long narrow faces were associated with higher loss of attachment [37].

A recent study performed by Kaya et al. has investigated the relationship between gingival phenotype and craniofacial morphology in the sagittal and vertical directions. In contrast to this research, an endodontic file, namely, transgingival probing, was used to assess gingival phenotype (<1 mm and >1 mm, thin and thick phenotype, respectively). These results demonstrated that there is no association between gingival thickness and craniofacial typology [26].

In this study, facial typology was also evaluated with three-dimensional facial scans to assess the association between SNMe/NMe and gingival thickness. Our analysis showed that facial proportions have a statistically significant association with gingival biotype. In particular, when the ratio of SNMe/NMe is decreased, there is a minor risk of finding a thin gingival biotype either in the upper or lower anterior regions.

This is the first study that has evaluated gingival thickness through the periodontal probe's translucency (thin and adequate biotype) with different vertical facial heights, and these findings support the hypothesis that there is no correlation between facial morphology and gingival thickness on lateral cephalograms [24]. Gingival thickness can be assessed by transgingival probing [38], ultrasonic measurement [39], or through the visibility of the probe [40,41]. Transgingival probing was not used because of the need for local anesthesia, which could induce a local volume increase and discomfort for patients [38]. Additionally, ultrasonic measurement was not preferred because of its repeatability with a coefficient of 1.20 mm [42]. Instead, the transparency of the probe through the gingival margin has been found to have a high reproducibility by De Rouck et al., showing 85% inter-examiner repeatability (k value = 0.7, p value = 0.002) [40]. Thus, this study used the periodontal probe visible through the gingiva after its placement in the facial sulcus of the anterior teeth [40].

The prevalence of malocclusion can vary between children and adolescents. However, the demand for orthodontic treatment is increasing [43–45], and greater attention has to be paid to periodontal aspects; indeed, orthodontic treatment can play an important role in periodontal changes [46]. The thickness of the gingiva is supposed to represent an indicator for reducing the risk of bone loss and gingival recession [47]. In fact, there are two studies which have indicated a statistically significant relationship between facial biotype and alveolar height and thickness with a greater risk of moving incisors beyond the anatomic limits of the alveolar bone by application of uncontrolled forces [6,48]. This uncontrolled movement can bring to: alveolar bone fenestrations, increasing susceptibility to gingival recession [49,50] and recession in the case of less than 2 mm of gingival thickness [7].

The current study presents several strengths. First, the periodontal assessments were performed in all of patients at the beginning of orthodontic treatment. This allows for an accurate diagnosis and treatment planning. In order to avoid bias due to differences in operator performance, only two trained clinicians performed the periodontal evaluations. Moreover, a new method to evaluate craniofacial morphology was introduced without exposure to the patients of further radiation. The study also has some limitations. Firstly, the sample size was relatively small to achieve a more reliable result. Secondly, only a few patients presented a thin UGB; however, this was in accordance with the normal prevalence of this biotype [26]. Further longitudinal studies are necessary to monitor the long-term effects of orthodontic treatment on gingival biotype in different facial typologies.

5. Conclusions

1. There is no association between facial typology (evaluated with SN^GoGn and CoGoMe) and gingival biotype.
2. When the ratio of SNMe/NMe is decreased, it represents a protective factor and a minor risk of finding a thin gingival biotype.

Author Contributions: Conceptualization, V.D., R.R. and R.V.; Methodology, A.P., R.R., V.S. and V.D.; Validation, A.P., G.S., G.T., and R.V.; Formal Analysis, A.P., G.T., R.R., and V.S.; Investigation, A.P., G.T. and R.R.; Resources, V.D. and R.V.; Data Curation, A.P., G.T., R.R. and V.S.; Writing–Original Draft Preparation, A.P., R.R. and V.D.; Writing–Review & Editing, G.T., V.S., G.S. and R.V.; Visualization, A.P., G.T., and R.R.; Supervision, G.S., V.D. and R.V.; Project Administration, A.P., V.D. and R.R.

References

1. Liu, P.; Liu, Y.; Wang, J.; Guo, Y.; Zhang, Y.; Xiao, S. Detection of fusobacterium nucleatum and fada adhesin gene in patients with orthodontic gingivitis and non-orthodontic periodontal inflammation. *PLoS ONE* **2014**, *9*, e85280. [CrossRef] [PubMed]
2. Bollen, A.; Cunha-cruz, J.; Bakko, W.; Huang, G.J.; Hujoel, P.P. The Effects of Orthodontic Therapy on Periodontal Health: A Systematic Review of Controlled Evidence. *J. Am. Dent. Assoc.* **2008**, *139*, 413–422. [CrossRef] [PubMed]
3. Tanner, A.C.R.; Sonis, A.L.; Lif Holgerson, P.; Starr, J.R.; Nunez, Y.; Kressirer, C.A.; Paster, B.J.; Johansson, I. White-spot lesions and gingivitis microbiotas in orthodontic patients. *J. Dent. Res.* **2012**, *91*, 853–858. [CrossRef] [PubMed]
4. Renkema, A.M.; Navratilova, Z.; Mazurova, K.; Katsaros, C.; Fudalej, P.S. Gingival labial recessions and the post-treatment proclination of mandibular incisors. *Eur. J. Orthod.* **2015**, *37*, 508–513. [CrossRef]
5. Renkema, A.M.; Fudalej, P.S.; Renkema, A.A.P.; Abbas, F.; Bronkhorst, E.; Katsaros, C. Gingival labial recessions in orthodontically treated and untreated individuals: A case-Control study. *J. Clin. Periodontol.* **2013**, *40*, 631–637. [CrossRef]
6. Morris, J.W.; Campbell, P.M.; Tadlock, L.P.; Boley, J.; Buschang, P.H. Prevalence of gingival recession after orthodontic tooth movements. *Am. J. Orthod. Dentofac. Orthop.* **2017**, *151*, 851–859. [CrossRef]
7. Kim, D.M.; Neiva, R. Periodontal Soft Tissue Non–Root Coverage Procedures: A Systematic Review From the AAP Regeneration Workshop. *J. Periodontol.* **2015**, *86*, S56–S72. [CrossRef]
8. Joss-Vassalli, I.; Grebenstein, C.; Topouzelis, N.; Sculean, A.; Katsaros, C. Orthodontic therapy and gingival recession: A systematic review. *Orthod. C. Res.* **2010**, *13*, 127–141. [CrossRef]
9. Kois, J.C. Predictable single-tooth peri-implant esthetics: Five diagnostic keys. *Compend. Contin. Educ. Dent.* **2004**, *25*, 895–896.
10. Ahmad, I. Anterior dental aesthetics: Gingival perspective. *Br. Dent. J.* **2005**, *199*, 195–202. [CrossRef]
11. Grover, V.; Bhardwaj, A.; Mohindra, K.; Malhotra, R. Analysis of the gingival biotype based on the measurement of the dentopapillary complex. *J. Indian Soc. Periodontol.* **2014**, *18*, 43. [CrossRef] [PubMed]
12. Papapanou, P.N.; Sanz, M.; Buduneli, N.; Dietrich, T.; Feres, M.; Fine, D.H.; Flemmig, T.F.; Garcia, R.; Giannobile, W.V.; Graziani, F.; et al. Periodontitis: Consensus report of workgroup 2 of the 2017 World Workshop on the Classification of Periodontal and Peri-Implant Diseases and Conditions. *J. Clin. Periodontol.* **2018**, *89*, S173–S182. [CrossRef] [PubMed]
13. Vandana, K.L.; Savitha, B. Thickness of gingiva in association with age, gender and dental arch location. *J. Clin. Periodontol.* **2005**, *32*, 828–830. [CrossRef] [PubMed]
14. Seibert, J.; Lindhe, J. Aestetics and periodontal therapy. In *Textbook of Clinical Periodontology*, 2nd ed.; Munksgaard: Copenhagen, Denmark, 1989; pp. 477–514.
15. Olsson, M.; Lindhe, J. Periodontal characteristics in individuals with varying form of the upper central incisors. *J. Clin. Periodontol.* **1991**, *18*, 78–82. [CrossRef]
16. Fields, H.; Proffit, W.; Nixon, W.; Phillips, C.; Stanek, E. Facial pattern differences in long-faced children and adults. *Am. J. Orthod.* **1984**, *85*, 217–223. [CrossRef]
17. Cangialosi, T.J. Additional criteria for sample division suggested. *Am. J. Orthod. Dentofac. Orthop.* **1989**, *96*, A24. [CrossRef]
18. Opdebeeck, H.; Bell, W. The short face syndrome. *Am. J. Orthod.* **1978**, *73*, 499–511. [CrossRef]
19. Schudy, F.F. The Rotation of The Mandible Resulting From Growth: Its Implications In Orthodontic Treatment. *Angle Orthod.* **1964**, *34*, 75–93.
20. Matarese, G.; Isola, G.; Ramaglia, L.; Dalessandri, D.; Lucchese, A.; Alibrandi, A.; Fabiano, F.; Cordasco, G. Periodontal biotype: Characteristc, prevalence and dimension related to dental malocclusion. *Minerva Stomatol.* **2016**, *65*, 231–238.
21. Al-Zo'ubia, I.A.; Hammadb, M.M.; Abu Alhaijac, E.S.J. Periodontal parameters in different dentofacial vertical patterns. *Angle Orthod.* **2008**, *78*, 1006–1014. [CrossRef]
22. Hornera, K.A.; Behrents, R.G.; Beom Kim, K.; Buschangd, P.H. Cortical bone and ridge thickness of hyperdivergent and hypodivergent adults. *Am. J. Orthod. Dentofac. Orthop.* **2012**, *142*, 170–178. [CrossRef] [PubMed]

23. Esfahanizadeh, N.; Daneshparvar, N.; Askarpour, F.; Akhoundi, N.; Panjnoush, M. Correlation Between Bone and Soft Tissue Thickness in Maxillary Anterior Teeth. *J. Dent. (Tehran)* **2016**, *13*, 302–308.
24. Sadek, M.M.; Sabet, N.E.; Hassan, I.T. Alveolar bone mapping in subjects with different vertical facial dimensions. *Eur. J. Orthod.* **2014**, *37*, 194–201. [CrossRef] [PubMed]
25. Björk, A. Prediction of mandibular growth rotation. *Am. J. Orthod.* **1969**, *55*, 585–599. [CrossRef]
26. Kaya, Y.; Alkan, Ö.; Alkan, E.A.; Keskin, S. Gingival thicknesses of maxillary and mandibular anterior regions in subjects with different craniofacial morphologies. *Am. J. Orthod. Dentofac. Orthop.* **2018**, *154*, 356–364. [CrossRef] [PubMed]
27. Baik, H.S.; Kim, S.Y. Facial soft-tissue changes in skeletal Class III orthognathic surgery patients analyzed with 3-dimensional laser scanning. *Am. J. Orthod. Dentofac. Orthop.* **2010**, *138*, 167–178. [CrossRef] [PubMed]
28. Kau, C.H.; Richmond, S.; Incrapera, A.; English, J.; Xia, J.J. Three-dimensional surface acquisition systems for the study of facial morphology and their application to maxillofacial surgery. *Int. J. Med. Robot. Comput. Assist. Surg.* **2007**, *3*, 97–110. [CrossRef]
29. Staderini, E.; Patini, R.; De Luca, M.; Gallenzi, P. Three-dimensional stereophotogrammetric analysis of nasolabial soft tissue effects of rapid maxillary expansion: A systematic review of clinical trials. *Acta Otorhinolaryngol. Ital.* **2018**, *38*, 399–408.
30. Antoun, J.S.; Lawrence, C.; Leow, A.; Rongo, R.; Dias, G.; Farella, M. A three-dimensional evaluation of Māori and New Zealand European faces. *Aust. Orthod. J.* **2014**, *30*, 169.
31. Aynechi, N.; Larson, B.E.; Leon-Salazar, V.; Beiraghi, S. Accuracy and precision of a 3D anthropometric facial analysis with and without landmark labeling before image acquisition. *Angle Orthod.* **2011**, *81*, 245–252. [CrossRef]
32. Plooij, J.M.; Swennen, G.R.J.; Rangel, F.A.; Maal, T.J.J.; Schutyser, F.A.C.; Bronkhorst, E.M.; Kuijpers-Jagtman, A.M.; Bergé, S.J. Evaluation of reproducibility and reliability of 3D soft tissue analysis using 3D stereophotogrammetry. *Int. J. Oral Maxillofac. Surg.* **2009**, *38*, 267–273. [CrossRef] [PubMed]
33. Toma, A.M.; Zhurov, A.; Playle, R.; Ong, E.; Richmond, S. Reproducibility of facial soft tissue landmarks on 3D laser-scanned facial images. *Orthod. Craniofac. Res.* **2009**, *12*, 33–42. [CrossRef] [PubMed]
34. Rongo, R.; Antoun, J.S.; Lim, Y.X.; Dias, G.; Valletta, R.; Farella, M. Three-dimensional evaluation of the relationship between jaw divergence and facial soft tissue dimensions. *Angle Orthod.* **2014**, *84*, 788–794. [CrossRef] [PubMed]
35. Young, N.M.; Sherathiya, K.; Gutierrez, L.; Nguyen, E.; Bekmezian, S.; Huang, J.C.; Hallgrimsson, B.; Lee, J.S.; Marcucio, R.S. Facial surface morphology predicts variation in internal skeletal shape. *Am. J. Orthod. Dentofac. Orthop.* **2016**, *149*, 501–508. [CrossRef]
36. Kan, J.Y.K.; Rungcharassaeng, K.; Umezu, K.; Kois, J.C. Dimensions of Peri-Implant Mucosa: An Evaluation of Maxillary Anterior Single Implants in Humans. *J. Periodontol.* **2003**, *74*, 557–562. [CrossRef]
37. Salti, L.; Holtfreter, B.; Pink, C.; Habes, M.; Biffar, R.; Kiliaridis, S.; Krey, K.F.; Bülow, R.; Völzke, H.; Kocher, T.; et al. Estimating effects of craniofacial morphology on gingival recession and clinical attachment loss. *J. Clin. Periodontol.* **2017**, *44*, 363–371. [CrossRef]
38. Ronay, V.; Sahrmann, P.; Bindl, A.; Attin, T.; Schmidlin, P.R. Current status and perspectives of mucogingival soft tissue measurement methods. *J. Esthet. Restor. Dent.* **2011**, *23*, 146–156. [CrossRef]
39. Eger, T.; Muller, H.-P.; Heinecke, A. Ultrasonic determination of gingival thickness subject variation and influence of tooth type and clinical features. *J. Clin. Periodontol.* **1996**, *23*, 839–845. [CrossRef]
40. De Rouck, T.; Eghbali, R.; Collys, K.; De Bruyn, H.; Cosyn, J. The gingival biotype revisited: Transparency of the periodontal probe through the gingival margin as a method to discriminate thin from thick gingiva. *J. Clin. Periodontol.* **2009**, *36*, 428–433. [CrossRef]
41. Cortellini, P.; Bissada, N.F. Mucogingival conditions in the natural dentition: Narrative review, case definitions, and diagnostic considerations. *J. Clin. Periodontol.* **2018**, *45*, S190–S198. [CrossRef]
42. Müller, H.P.; Könönen, E. Variance components of gingival thickness. *J. Periodontal Res.* **2005**, *40*, 239–244. [CrossRef] [PubMed]
43. Paduano, S.; Rongo, R.; Bucci, R.; Aiello, D.; Carvelli, G.; Ingenito, A.; Cantile, T.; Ferrazzano, G.F. Is there an association between various aspects of oral health in Southern Italy children? An epidemiological study assessing dental decays, periodontal status, malocclusions and temporomandibular joint function. *Eur. J. Paediatr. Dent.* **2018**, *19*, 176–180. [PubMed]

44. Asiri, S.N.; Tadlock, L.P.; Buschang, P.H. The prevalence of clinically meaningful malocclusion among US adults. *Orthod. Craniofac. Res.* **2019**, *22*, 321–328. [CrossRef]
45. Jawad, Z.; Bates, C.; Hodge, T. Who needs orthodontic treatment? Who gets it? And who wants it? *Br. Dent. J.* **2015**, *218*, 99–103. [CrossRef]
46. Alfuriji, S.; Alhazmi, N.; Alhamlan, N.; Al-Ehaideb, A.; Alruwaithi, M.; Alkatheeri, N.; Geevarghese, A. The effect of orthodontic therapy on periodontal health: A review of the literature. *Int. J. Dent.* **2014**, *2014*, 585048. [CrossRef]
47. Maynard, J.G. The rationale for mucogingival therapy in the child and adolescent. *Int. J. Periodontics Restor. Dent.* **1987**, *7*, 36–51.
48. Renkema, A.M.; Fudalej, P.S.; Renkema, A.; Kiekens, R.; Katsaros, C. Development of labial gingival recessions in orthodontically treated patients. *Am. J. Orthod. Dentofac. Orthop.* **2013**, *143*, 206–212. [CrossRef]
49. Holmesa, H.D.; Tennantb, M.; Goonewardenec, M.S. Augmentation of faciolingual gingival dimensions with free connective tissue grafts before labial orthodontic tooth movement: An experimental study with a canine model. *Am. J. Orthod. Dentofac. Orthop.* **2005**, *127*, 562–572. [CrossRef]
50. Wennström, J.L.; Lindhe, J.; Sinclair, F.; Thilander, B. Some periodontal tissue reactions to orthodontic tooth movement in monkeys. *J. Clin. Periodontol.* **1987**, *14*, 121–129. [CrossRef]

9

Sex Prediction Based on Mesiodistal Width Data in the Portuguese Population

João Albernaz Neves [1], Nathalie Antunes-Ferreira [2,3], Vanessa Machado [1,4], João Botelho [1,4,*], Luís Proença [5], Alexandre Quintas [2,3], José João Mendes [1,4] and Ana Sintra Delgado [1,4]

1 Clinical Research Unit (CRU), Centro de Investigação Interdisciplinar Egas Moniz (CiiEM), Egas Moniz, CRL, 2829-511 Caparica, Almada, Portugal; jalbernazneves@gmail.com (J.A.N.); vanessamachado558@gmail.com (V.M.); jmendes@egasmoniz.edu.pt (J.J.M.); anasintradelgado@gmail.com (A.S.D.)

2 Laboratório de Ciências Forenses e Psicológicas Egas Moniz (LCFPEM), Centro de Investigação Interdisciplinar Egas Moniz (CiiEM), Egas Moniz CRL, 2829-511 Caparica, Almada, Portugal; natantfer@gmail.com (N.A.-F.); alexandre.quintas@gmail.com (A.Q.)

3 Laboratory of Biological Anthropology and Human Osteology (LABOH), CRIA/FCSH, Universidade NOVA de Lisboa, 1069-061 Lisboa, Portugal

4 Orthodontics Department, Egas Moniz Dental Clinic (EMDC), Egas Moniz, CRL, 2829-511 Caparica, Almada, Portugal

5 Quantitative Methods for Health Research (MQIS), CiiEM, Egas Moniz, CRL, 2829-511 Caparica, Almada, Portugal; lproenca@egasmoniz.edu.pt

* Correspondence: jbotelho@egasmoniz.edu.pt

Abstract: Accurate sex prediction is a key step in creating a postmortem forensic profile as it excludes approximately half the population. It is our goal to develop a predictive model to establish sex through teeth mesiodistal widths in a Portuguese population. The pretreatment dental casts of 168 of Portuguese orthodontics subjects (59 males and 109 females) were included. Mesiodistal widths from right first molar to left first molar were measured on each pretreatment cast to the nearest 0.01 mm using a digital caliper. Overall, the mesiodistal widths of the upper and lower canines, premolars, and molars were found to be significantly different between females and males. Conversely, no significant differences between sexes were identified for incisors. A multivariate logistic regression model for sex prediction was developed and the teeth included in the final reduced model being the upper left canine (2.3), the lower right lateral incisor (4.2) and the lower right canine (4.3). There is a prevalence of sexual dimorphism in all teeth except the incisors. The canines present the most noticeable difference between sexes. The presented sex determination predictive model exhibits an overall correct classification of 75%, outperforming all available models for this purpose and therefore is a potential tool for forensic analysis in this population.

Keywords: forensic dentistry; sex determination; sexual dimorphism; dental measurements; predictive model; Portuguese population

---

1. Introduction

Forensic dentistry emerges as a part of forensic medicine and dental anthropology. This is the branch of dentistry that focuses on the issues of identifying human remains by direct comparison, bite mark identification, clinical malpractice, and forensic dental profiling, such as sex and age estimation, in cases of unknown human remains, in order to facilitate their subsequent identification [1,2].

Teeth are the hardest organ in the human body and very important in postmortem identification procedures. Although pelvic and cranial bones can be more accurate in identifying sex, they are rarely in optimal condition in extreme cases, such as natural disasters or mass graves, which may prevent accurate estimation through them. Teeth are considered quite useful in these scenarios as they are often recovered intact [3–6]. However, there may be some setbacks that prevent dental eruption of teeth useful for forensic identification [7–10].

Accurate sex prediction is a key step in creating a postmortem forensic profile as it excludes approximately half the population [11]. Several studies state that teeth have a high degree of sexual dimorphism [2,4,5,12,13]. Generally, male teeth are larger than female teeth, however data are not consensual and reverse dimorphism also occurs [4,12]. Sexual dimorphism may vary between different populations, possibly due to variations in the environment, available food resources, or genetic pool [3,14].

The most usual way to obtain data is from dental casts using a digital caliper. There are several measures to take into account and their analysis may be performed through direct comparison of measures, statistical analyses, or indexes.

Only two previous studies presented potential predictive sex models for Portuguese populations using dental measurements. Pereira et al. (2010) [1], using upper canine-to-canine teeth, rendered a combination of incisors mesiodistal and canine diagonal distances. As the proposed model was confined to only six teeth, it lacks a complete teeth analysis. On the other hand, Silva et al. (2015) [12] employed the mandibular canine index [15] with a modest success rate of 64.2%, concluding that this index should be restrictively applied to the Portuguese scenario in sex identification.

Given the lack of robust sex identification models for the Portuguese population, we aimed to use cast models of a previously studied sample (Machado et al., 2018) [16] to develop a new sex prediction model based on mesiodistal width measures. We hypothesize that there is a sex-based teeth dimorphism in this population and it is distinguishable through a predictive model; therefore our null hypothesis is that such dimorphism may not exist.

2. Materials and Methods

2.1. Study Design

This study used a previously reported sample [16] that has received approval by the Egas Moniz Ethics Committee (Number 600). Written informed consents were obtained from all participants during their first appointment at the Orthodontic Department of the Egas Moniz Dental Clinic.

This investigation follows the transparent reporting of a multivariable prediction model for individual prognosis or diagnosis (TRIPOD) reporting guidelines [17] for validation of prediction models (see supplementary material). This study was conducted on a triple-blind basis with respect to diagnosis and clinical outcome, data collection, and analysis.

2.2. Participants

The assessment tool consisted of pre-treatment dental casts, a part of standard orthodontic treatment planning, in dental stone selected from the archives of the Egas Moniz Dental Clinic Orthodontic Department (Almada, Portugal). From a total of 541 casts gathered from November 2010 to December 2017, 168 (59 males and 109 females) were selected according to the inclusion and exclusion criteria.

The inclusion criteria were: all teeth, from first molar in the right side to first molar in the left side in both upper and lower jaws, were fully erupted and present; no history of interproximal stripping; no proximal caries that might interfere with precise tooth measurement; no restorations, abrasions or attrition; no previous or ongoing orthodontic treatment; no abnormal tooth morphology or congenitally missing or impacted [16]. All patients failing to fulfil these criteria were excluded.

2.3. Dental Casts Analysis and Measurement Reproducibility

Dental cast measurements were performed by one researcher (VM) using a digital caliper to measure the mesiodistal tooth widths from the right first molar to the left first molar to the nearest 0.01 mm. The mesiodistal width of each tooth was measured at the widest distance between the mesial and distal contact points. The position of the caliper had to be perpendicular to the occlusal surface of the measured tooth [1,11,14,16,18–21].

Ten study casts were randomly chosen from the total of 168 and remeasured one week later by the same investigator (V.M.). Intraclass correlation coefficient (ICC) was calculated with an absolute agreement of ICC = 0.98.

2.4. *Statistical Analysis*

Data analysis was performed using IBM SPSS Statistics version 25.0 for Windows (Armonk, NY: IBM Corp.). Descriptive statistics as mean and standard deviation (SD) were determined for the mesiodistal width per tooth. Mean mesiodistal width for each tooth was compared according to sex and by Student's *t*-test. A multivariate stepwise adjusted logistic regression procedure was applied to derive a reduced predictive model for sex determination based on the mesiodistal widths for each tooth. To test the performance of the obtained model and compare it to previous ones, the sensitivity, specificity, accuracy, and precision were determined for all models when applied to the studied sample [22]. Performance measurement was assessed by binary area under the curve (AUC) and through receiver operating characteristics (ROC) analysis. The level of significance was set at 5%, in all statistical inference analyses.

3. Results

3.1. *Mesiodistal Width Per Tooth*

In the studied sample the mean age was 20.1 (±7.3) (see Machado et al., 2018 [16] for a detailed description). The mean mesiodistal width for each tooth, according to sex, is presented in Table 1. Overall, the mean mesiodistal widths of upper and lower canines, premolars, and molars were found to be significantly different between females and males. Regarding the incisors, no significant differences were found as a function of sex.

Table 1. Descriptive values of mesiodistal width (mm), presented as mean and standard deviation (SD) for each tooth, as a function of sex (n = 168).

Semi-Arch	Tooth Type	Tooth Code	Female (n = 109)		Male (n = 59)		*p*-Value *
			Mean (±SD)	Range (Min–Max)	Mean (±SD)	Range (Min–Max)	
Upper right	Molar	1.6	10.13 (±0.56)	8.50–12.52	10.40 (±0.60)	9.26–12.37	**0.004**
	Premolars	1.5	6.62 (±0.47)	5.51–8.04	6.40 (±0.52)	5.71–8.30	**0.008**
		1.4	6.93 (±0.47)	5.70–8.17	7.18 (±0.48)	6.35–8.50	**0.001**
	Canine	1.3	7.67 (±0.46)	6.40–8.90	7.97 (±0.57)	6.10–9.22	**<0.001**
	Incisors	1.2	6.64 (±0.61)	5.20–7.89	6.70 (±0.63)	5.25–8.55	0.565
		1.1	8.60 (±0.58)	7.00–10.05	8.68 (±0.66)	6.47–10.78	0.414
Upper left		2.1	8.62 (±0.54)	7.39–9.88	8.69 (±0.67)	6.47–10.66	0.437
		2.2	6.54 (±0.60)	4.73–7.89	6.71 (±0.65)	5.25–8.30	0.091
	Canine	2.3	7.65 (±0.46)	6.40–8.70	8.04 (±0.52)	6.83–9.22	**<0.001**
	Premolars	2.4	6.92 (±0.48)	5.70–8.17	7.17 (±0.50)	5.96–8.28	**0.002**
		2.5	6.62 (±0.47)	5.51–8.04	6.84 (±0.52)	5.70–8.30	**0.005**
	Molar	2.6	10.12 (±0.56)	8.50–12.52	10.33 (±0.59)	9.4–12.44	**0.018**
Lower right	Molar	4.6	10.63 (±0.61)	9.10–12.32	11.03 (±0.57)	9.82–12.17	**<0.001**
	Premolars	4.5	7.19 (±0.52)	6.04–8.93	7.36 (±0.54)	6.17–8.98	**0.050**
		4.4	7.08 (±0.43)	6.11–8.30	7.36 (±0.51)	6.22–8.50	**0.001**
	Canine	4.3	6.63 (±0.42)	5.84–8.15	7.01 (±0.48)	6.03–8.91	**<0.001**
	Incisors	4.2	5.89 (±0.43)	4.50–6.94	5.97 (±0.44)	4.98–6.95	0.253
		4.1	5.38 (±0.43)	4.50–7.60	5.46 (±0.43)	4.68–6.51	0.280
Lower left		3.1	5.38 (±0.44)	4.50–7.60	5.41 (±0.47)	3.73–6.37	0.708
		3.2	5.86 (±0.44)	4.50–6.78	5.99 (±0.42)	4.92–6.99	0.052
	Canine	3.3	6.63 (±0.41)	5.84–8.16	7.00 (±0.50)	6.14–8.95	**<0.001**
	Premolars	3.4	7.03 (±0.50)	5.65–8.30	7.35 (±0.52)	6.22–8.50	**<0.001**
		3.5	7.14 (±0.50)	6.04–8.70	7.37 (±0.58)	6.00–8.98	**0.008**
	Molar	3.6	10.62 (±0.57)	9.10–12.32	11.00 (±0.61)	9.76–12.17	**<0.001**

Note: * Student's *t*-test. Significant *p*-values ($p < 0.05$) denoted in bold.

3.2. *Sex Prediction Model Development*

In order to develop a model for sex prediction based on the teeth mesiodistal width, a multivariate logistic regression procedure was implemented considering a first stage that included all teeth that exhibited significant differences in the sex-based comparison: canines, premolars and molars. Then, a stepwise adjusted logistic regression procedure derived a reduced best fitting model that is depicted in Table 2. In this final optimized model, the upper left canine (2.3), the lower right lateral incisor (4.2) and the lower right canine (4.3) were the only teeth included.

Table 2. Final reduced logistic regression model (n = 168).

Variables	*B*	*p*-Value	EXP (B)	EXP (B) 95% CI	
				Lower	Upper
Tooth 2.3	1.208	0.019	3.35	1.22	9.22
Tooth 4.3	1.800	0.003	6.05	1.84	19.91
Tooth 4.2	−1.317	0.018	0.27	0.09	0.80
Constant	−14.546	<0.001	-	-	-

$R^2(N) = 0.268$, % correct classification = 75%; H&L: $X^2 = 6.767$ ($p = 0.562$); Note: outcome variable (sex) coded as male: 1, female: 0.

From the fitted model data, the following formula can be derived:

$$\ln(p/(1-p)) = -14.546 + 1.208x + 1.800y - 1.317z$$

where p is the probability of an individual being classified as male, with a lower cutoff value of 0.5, and with x, y, and z representing the mesiodistal width of the upper left canine (2.3), lower right canine (4.3) and lower right lateral incisor (4.2), respectively.

3.3. Comparison with Previous Models

The achieved model was then compared to the previous sex prediction tools by means of performance when applied to this sample (Table 3).

Table 3. Performance assessment of the different models when applied to the studied sample. Measures are presented as percentage. For AUC, estimation by a 95% confidence interval (95% CI) is also shown.

Model		Sensitivity (%)	Specificity (%)	Accuracy (%)	Precision (%)	AUC within ROC Analysis (95% CI)
Acharya et al., 2007 [23]	Model 1	85.3	50.8	73.2	76.2	0.642 (0.551–0.733)
	Model 2	13.8	93.2	41.7	78.9	0.637 (0.546–0.728)
Mitsea et al., 2014 [4]		65.1	45.8	58.3	68.9	0.681 (0.592–0.770)
Peckmann et al., 2016 [5]	Model 1	89.9	39.0	72.0	73.1	0.535 (0.445–0.625)
	Model 2	59.6	49.2	56.0	68.4	0.555 (0.463–0.646)
	Model 3	65.1	45.8	58.3	68.9	0.644 (0.553–0.736)
	Model 4	88.1	37.3	70.2	72.2	0.544 (0.452–0.636)
	Model 5	86.2	37.3	69.0	71.8	0.555 (0.463–0.646)
	Model 6	82.6	45.8	69.6	73.8	0.627 (0.535–0.719)
	Model 7	81.7	45.8	69.0	73.6	0.618 (0.525–0.710)
Neves et al., 2020		87.2	52.5	75.0	77.2	0.768 (0.693–0.843)

AUC—Area under the curve; ROC—Receiver operating characteristic.

4. Discussion

Sex estimation is a vital step in forensic medicine for body identification both in single and mass disaster events. In the Portuguese scenario, sex estimation models through dental hard tissues are scarce and previous proposed models lacked consistency and only accounted for a small subset of teeth. Therefore, we aimed to develop a potential model using mesiodistal widths of models cast previously for studies of orthodontic indexes. Then, we compared the performance of this model with other full-mouth mesiodistal models published elsewhere. Overall, our model outperformed all available strategies and might be used as a forensic tool for sex estimation in Portuguese samples.

As previously stated, sexual dimorphism may vary between populations, possibly due to a variety of reasons [3,14]. Therefore, this new model arises as a valuable tool to forensic dentistry.

Our results have prospective importance. (1) Until now, there were no models developed for the Portuguese population from complete models. (2) Dental hard tissues are of utmost interest because they are the most lasting tissue of human body, even in post-mortem difficult conditions. (3) This tool may be very useful in single or mass disasters or body identification cases in Portugal, especially due to the unpredictability of these situations. (4) These results confirm sexual dimorphism on teeth mesiodistal width in canines, premolars, and molars of the upper and lower arches.

Dental crown dimensions can be obtained through intraoral measurements [18], dental forms [4,11,13,14,16,19,24], or human remains [20,21]. The mesiodistal and buccolingual measurements of the crown were the two most commonly used and studied dimensions [1,11,14,18–21], followed by diagonal measurements (mesiobuccal-distolingual and distobuccal-mesiolingual) [1,21,25] and the canine mandibular index (expressed as the ratio between the mesiodistal dimension of the canines and the width of the intercanine arch [12,15,19,26]). These studies have shown that canine dimensions provide the highest sexual dimorphism [16,18,21,24,25], followed by premolars [21,25], first and second molars [20,21,25,27].

In this study, we analyzed the degree of sexual dimorphism in different teeth by measuring the maximum mesiodistal diameters of fully erupted permanent teeth from study casts. Overall, several teeth are sexually dimorphic and the crown mesiodistal dimensions were larger on average in males than in females. The results of this study confirm what was previously demonstrated, canine teeth are the most dimorphic teeth [1–5,7,19,21,24–26] but also molars present significant differences between sexes [11,13,23,25,28–30]. Within the elements that fit into our sex prediction model, the upper left canine, the lower right lateral incisor, and the lower right canine were the most appropriate and with better replicability.

Regarding the performance, our developed model outperformed previous published indexes in terms of AUC. In terms of accuracy and precision values, our model also outperformed the remaining models (75.0% and 77.2% for accuracy and precision, respectively). Furthermore, for sensitivity and specificity, this newly developed model presented the best combination of results, only being outperformed in sensitivity by Peckmann et al., 2016 [5] (model 4) and in specificity by Acharya et al., 2007 [23] (model 2).

Like other methodologies used in sex prediction, the amount and quality of evidence available for analysis are critical in forensic investigation. Some limitations of the applied methodology include any post-eruptive changes such as caries, interproximal wear, and interproximal restorations, which compromises the correct measurement of the teeth.

5. Strengths and Limitations

A possible limitation of this study is the fact that we have not accounted for second molars, mainly because the data that this analysis is derived from is an orthodontic population whose main purpose was to study a mesiodistal proportion measure. This measure, Bolton's analysis [31], only accounts for the mesiodistal width from the first molar to the first molar. Nevertheless, two previous large-base studies from this population revealed that second molars are one of the most commonly missing teeth, aside from first molars and premolars [32,33]. Interestingly, none of them accounted for the final model. Another possible limitation is the fact that the new model emerged from the same sample being studied, which may influence the results. The new model should be further investigated with a new sample in a future study.

6. Conclusions

Considering the limitations of this study, the present study found that there is a prevalence of sexual dimorphism in all teeth except the incisors and that the canines exhibit the most noticeable difference between sexes, followed by the first mandibular molars and premolars.

Through a stepwise adjusted logistic regression procedure, a suitable model for sex determination was developed. The reduced model was based on the upper left canine (2.3), the lower right lateral incisor (4.2), and the lower right canine (4.3) and achieved an accuracy of 75%.

Author Contributions: Conceptualization, V.M. and J.B.; methodology, J.A.N.; validation, J.B., V.M. and L.P.; formal analysis, L.P.; investigation, J.A.N.; resources, A.S.D.; writing—original draft preparation, J.A.N.; writing—review and editing, J.J.M., N.A.-F. and A.Q.; supervision, J.J.M., A.S.D., N.A.-F. and A.Q.; project administration, J.J.M. and A.S.D. All authors have read and agreed to the published version of the manuscript.

References

1. Pereira, C.; Bernardo, M.; Pestana, D.; Santos, J.C.; de Mendonça, M.C. Contribution of teeth in human forensic identification—Discriminant function sexing odontometrical techniques in Portuguese population. *J. Forensic Leg. Med.* **2010**, *17*, 105–110. [CrossRef]
2. Khamis, M.F.; Taylor, J.A.; Malik, S.N.; Townsend, G.C. Odontometric sex variation in Malaysians with application to sex prediction. *Forensic Sci. Int.* **2014**, *234*, 183.e1–183.e7. [CrossRef]
3. Işcan, M.Y.; Kedici, P.S. Sexual variation in bucco-lingual dimensions in Turkish dentition. *Forensic Sci. Int.* **2003**, *137*, 160–164. [CrossRef]
4. Mitsea, A.G.; Moraitis, K.; Leon, G.; Nicopoulou-Karayianni, K.; Spiliopoulou, C. Sex determination by tooth size in a sample of Greek population. *HOMO-J. Comp. Hum. Biol.* **2014**, *65*, 322–329. [CrossRef] [PubMed]
5. Peckmann, T.R.; Logar, C.; Garrido-Varas, C.E.; Meek, S.; Pinto, X.T. Sex determination using the mesio-distal dimension of permanent maxillary incisors and canines in a modern Chilean population. *Sci. Justice* **2016**, *56*, 84–89. [CrossRef] [PubMed]
6. Capitaneanu, C.; Willems, G.; Thevissen, P. A systematic review of odontological sex estimation methods. *J. Forensic Odontostomatol.* **2017**, *35*, 1–19. [PubMed]
7. Isola, G.; Anastasi, G.; Matarese, G.; Williams, R.; Cutroneo, G.; Bracco, P.; Piancino, M. Functional and molecular outcomes of the human masticatory muscles. *Oral Dis.* **2018**, *24*, 1428–1441. [CrossRef]
8. Isola, G.; Alibrandi, A.; Rapisarda, E.; Matarese, G.; Williams, R.C.; Leonardi, R. Association of vitamin D in patients with periodontitis: A cross-sectional study. *J. Periodontal Res.* **2020**, 1–11. [CrossRef]
9. Staderini, E.; Patini, R.; Guglielmi, F.; Camodeca, A.; Gallenzi, P. How to manage impacted third molars: Germectomy or delayed removal? A systematic literature review. *Medicina* **2019**, *55*, 79. [CrossRef]
10. Botelho, J.; Machado, V.; Proença, L.; Delgado, A.S.; Mendes, J.J. Vitamin D deficiency and oral health: A comprehensive review. *Nutrients* **2020**, *12*, 1471. [CrossRef]
11. Angadi, P.V.; Hemani, S.; Prabhu, S.; Acharya, A.B. Analyses of odontometric sexual dimorphism and sex assessment accuracy on a large sample. *J. Forensic Leg. Med.* **2013**, *20*, 673–677. [CrossRef] [PubMed]
12. Silva, A.M.; Pereira, M.L.; Gouveia, S.; Tavares, J.N.; Azevedo, Á.; Caldas, I.M. A new approach to sex estimation using the mandibular canine index. *Med. Sci. Law.* **2016**, *56*, 7–12. [CrossRef] [PubMed]
13. Prabhu, S.; Acharya, A.B. Odontometric sex assessment in Indians. *Forensic Sci. Int.* **2009**, *192*, 129.e1–129.e5. [CrossRef] [PubMed]
14. Brook, A.H.; Griffin, R.C.; Townsend, G.; Levisianos, Y.; Russell, J.; Smith, R.N. Variability and patterning in permanent tooth size of four human ethnic groups. *Arch. Oral Biol.* **2009**, *54*, 79–85. [CrossRef] [PubMed]
15. Rao, N.G.; Rao, N.N.; Pai, M.L.; Kotian, M.S. Mandibular canine index—A clue for establishing sex identity. *Forensic Sci. Int.* **1989**, *42*, 249–254. [CrossRef]
16. Machado, V.; Botelho, J.; Pereira, D.; Vasques, M.; Fernandes-Retto, P.; Proença, L.; Mendes, J.J.; Delgado, A. Bolton ratios in Portuguese subjects among different malocclusion groups. *J. Clin. Exp. Dent.* **2018**, *10*, e864–e868. [CrossRef]
17. Moons, K.G.M.; Altman, D.G.; Reitsma, J.B.; Ioannidis, J.P.A.; Macaskill, P.; Steyerberg, E.W.; Vickers, A.J.; Ransohoff, D.F.; Collins, G.S. Transparent reporting of a multivariable prediction model for individual prognosis or diagnosis (TRIPOD): Explanation and elaboration. *Ann. Intern. Med.* **2015**, *162*, W1–W73. [CrossRef] [PubMed]
18. Khangura, R.; Sircar, K.; Singh, S.; Rastogi, V. Sex determination using mesiodistal dimension of permanent maxillary incisors and canines. *J. Forensic Dent. Sci.* **2012**, *3*, 81. [CrossRef]
19. Phulari, R.S.; Rathore, R.; Talegaon, T.; Jariwala, P. Comparative assessment of maxillary canine index and

maxillary first molar dimensions for sex determination in forensic odontology. *J. Forensic Dent. Sci.* **2017**, *9*, 110. [CrossRef]

20. Zorba, E.; Moraitis, K.; Manolis, S.K. Sexual dimorphism in permanent teeth of modern Greeks. *Forensic Sci. Int.* **2011**, *210*, 74–81. [CrossRef]
21. Zorba, E.; Moraitis, K.; Eliopoulos, C.; Spiliopoulou, C. Sex determination in modern Greeks using diagonal measurements of molar teeth. *Forensic Sci. Int.* **2012**, *217*, 19–26. [CrossRef] [PubMed]
22. Glas, A.S.; Lijmer, J.G.; Prins, M.H.; Bonsel, G.J.; Bossuyt, P.M.M. The diagnostic odds ratio: A single indicator of test performance. *J. Clin. Epidemiol.* **2003**, *56*, 1129–1135. [CrossRef]
23. Acharya, A.B.; Mainali, S. Univariate sex dimorphism in the Nepalese dentition and the use of discriminant functions in gender assessment. *Forensic Sci. Int.* **2007**, *173*, 47–56. [CrossRef] [PubMed]
24. Mujib, A.B.R.; Tarigoppula, R.K.V.N.; Kulkarni, P.G. Gender determination using diagonal measurements of maxillary molar and canine teeth in davangere population. *J. Clin. Diagn. Res.* **2014**, *8*, 141–144. [CrossRef]
25. Viciano, J.; Lõpez-Lázaro, S.; Alemán, I. Sex estimation based on deciduous and permanent dentition in a contemporary spanish population. *Am. J. Phys. Anthropol.* **2013**, *152*, 31–43. [CrossRef]
26. Acharya, A.B.; Angadi, P.V.; Prabhu, S.; Nagnur, S. Validity of the mandibular canine index (MCI) in sex prediction: Reassessment in an Indian sample. *Forensic Sci. Int.* **2011**, *204*, 207.e1–207.e4. [CrossRef]
27. Acharya, A.B.; Prabhu, S.; Muddapur, M.V. Odontometric sex assessment from logistic regression analysis. *Int. J. Leg. Med.* **2011**, *125*, 199–204. [CrossRef]
28. Thapar, R.; Angadi, P.V.; Hallikerimath, S.; Kale, A.D. Sex assessment using odontometry and cranial anthropometry: Evaluation in an Indian sample. *Forensic Sci. Med. Pathol.* **2012**, *8*, 94–100. [CrossRef]
29. Filho, I.E.M.; Lopez-Capp, T.T.; Biazevic, M.G.H.; Michel-Crosato, E. Sexual dimorphism using odontometric indexes: Analysis of three statistical techniques. *J. Forensic Leg. Med.* **2016**, *44*, 37–42. [CrossRef]
30. Filipovic, G.; Kanjevac, T.; Cetenovic, B.; Ajdukovic, Z.; Petrovic, N. Sexual dimorphism in the dimensions of teeth in serbian population. *Coll. Antropol.* **2016**, *40*, 23–28. Available online: http://www.ncbi.nlm.nih.gov/pubmed/27301233 (accessed on 7 May 2020).
31. Bolton, W.A. Disharmony in tooth size and its relation to the analysis and treatment of malocclusion. *Angle Orthod.* **1985**, *28*, 113–130.
32. Machado, V.; Botelho, J.; Amaral, A.; Proença, L.; Alves, R.; Rua, J.; Cavacas, M.A.; Delgado, A.S.; Mendes, J.J. Prevalence and extent of chronic periodontitis and its risk factors in a Portuguese subpopulation: A retrospective cross-sectional study and analysis of Clinical Attachment Loss. *PeerJ* **2018**, *6*, e5258. [CrossRef] [PubMed]
33. Botelho, J.; Machado, V.; Proença, L.; Alves, R.; Cavacas, M.A.; Amaro, L.; Mendes, J.J. Study of Periodontal Health in Almada-Seixal (SoPHiAS): A cross-sectional study in the Lisbon Metropolitan Area. *Sci. Rep.* **2019**, *9*, 1–10. [CrossRef] [PubMed]

10

Salivary Levels of Titanium, Nickel, Vanadium and Arsenic in Patients Treated with Dental Implants

Piero Papi [1], Andrea Raco [1], Nicola Pranno [1,*], Bianca Di Murro [1], Pier Carmine Passarelli [2], Antonio D'Addona [2], Giorgio Pompa [1,†] and Maurizio Barbieri [3,†]

1 Department of Oral and Maxillo-Facial Sciences, "Sapienza" University of Rome, 00161 Rome, Italy; piero.papi@uniroma1.it (P.P.); a.raco@hotmail.it (A.R.); bianca.dimurro@uniroma1.it (B.D.M.); giorgio.pompa@uniroma1.it (G.P.)
2 Division of Oral Surgery and Implantology, Department of Head and Neck, Oral Surgery, and Implantology Unit, Institute of Clinical Dentistry, Fondazione Policlinico Universitario A. Gemelli IRCCS-Università Cattolica del Sacro Cuore, 00168 Rome, Italy; piercarminepassarelli@hotmail.it (P.C.P.); antonio.daddona@policlinicogemelli.it (A.D.)
3 Department of Earth Sciences, "Sapienza" University of Rome, 00161 Rome, Italy; maurizio.barbieri@uniroma1.it
* Correspondence: nicola.pranno@uniroma1.it
† These two authors contributed equally.

Abstract: Background: Recent articles have hypothesized a possible correlation between dental implants dissolution products and peri-implantitis. The null hypothesis tested in this case-control study was that there would be no differences in salivary concentrations of titanium (Ti), vanadium (V), nickel (Ni) and arsenic (As) ions among patients with dental implants, healthy (Group A) or affected by peri-implantitis (Group B), compared to subjects without implants and/or metallic prosthetic restorations (Group C). Methods: Inductively coupled plasma mass spectrometry was used to analyze saliva samples. One-way repeated-measure analysis of variance (ANOVA) was used to identify statistically significant differences in the salivary level of Ti, V, Ni and As between the three groups. Results: A total of 100 patients were enrolled in the study (42 males and 58 females), distributed in three groups: 50 patients in Group C, 26 patients in Group B and 24 patients Group B. In our study, concentrations of metallic ions were higher in Group A and B, compared to the control group, with the exception of vanadium. However, there were no statistically significant differences ($p > 0.05$) for metallic ions concentrations between Group A and Group B. Conclusions: Based on our results, there are no differences in titanium or other metals concentrations in saliva of patients with healthy or diseased implants.

Keywords: dental implants; saliva; corrosion; titanium; metallic ions

---

1. Introduction

Dental implants are usually made of commercially pure titanium or titanium-based alloys (Ti-6Al-4V), these metals, as well as showing great long-term success and survival rates [1,2], are known to be bio compatibles and chemically inert in the oral cavity and consequently considered corrosion-resistant. Corrosion is a state of metal's deterioration caused by oxidation or chemical action, thwarted by a titanium dioxide layer (TiO_2), spontaneously covering the implant surface in presence of oxygen and providing great resistance and stability to the implant [3,4]. Nevertheless, titanium alloys can be affected by this gradual degradation and the structural and mechanical integrity of the implant may be jeopardized and at risk of failure. Corrosion leads to titanium dissolution, release and dispersion of metal ions and particles into soft and hard tissues either, which may be a possible factor in peri-implant inflammatory processes [5,6].

The factors that trigger corrosion are acidification of the oral environment or the release of lactic acid by bacteria, such as *Streptococcus mutans*, and also chemical stimuli by fluorides (with a concentration range greater than 100 ppm) normally present in home and professional oral care products [7–9].

Titanium and other metals particles released by dental implants are not totally bioinert: they induce the release of mediating inflammation cytokines, such as tumor necrosis factor-alpha (TNF-α), interleukin 1 beta (IL-1β) and the secretion of RANKL. These present an immunogenic potential which—by acting as a secondary inflammatory stimulus in peri-implantitis—amplifies bone resorption [10]

Under physiological conditions, osteoprotegerin (OPG) secreted by the fibroblasts of the periodontal ligament and osteoblasts, subtracts the receptor activator of nuclear factor kappa-B ligand (RANKL) from the link with its true receptor activator of nuclear factor kappa-B (RANK), creating a real competitive inhibition, preventing differentiation from the pre-osteoclast into osteoclasts and subsequent bone resorption [11,12]. In the presence of inflammation, an up-regulation of RANKL is associated with a down-regulation of OPG, which is produced in minimal quantities. The RANKL produced will, therefore, bind the RANK present on the osteoclastic precursors, with consequent massive bone resorption [13,14]

Furthermore, other kinds of corrosion can occur, such as mechanical corrosion due to functional stresses of implants or the cracking or weakening of its prosthetic components [7,8].

Once ultimately dispersed in the peri-implant environment, metal ions and particles are no longer biocompatible and inert, and are, therefore considered a potential incentive to the inflammatory process in peri-implantitis [5]. A study in mice immune cells has demonstrated that Titanium ions release pro-inflammatory cytokines involved in bone resorption, demonstrating that peri-implantitis may be directly related to corrosion and, therefore, with metal ions dispersion [15].

Peri-implantitis treatment and risk factors are still controversial [16,17], with incontrovertible evidence just for periodontitis, inadequate plaque control and lack of supportive periodontal therapy [18–20].

Furthermore, smoking, excess cement and other systemic conditions have all been described as potential risk indicators, however there is inconclusive evidence to draft clear conclusions [18,21–26].

Recent articles have hypothesized a possible correlation between titanium dissolution products and peri-implantitis [27–29] therefore, the aims of this case-control study were to evaluate salivary metallic ions dissolution in patients with dental implants, healthy or affected by peri-implantitis.

The null hypothesis tested was that there would be no differences in the salivary concentrations of titanium (Ti), vanadium (V), nickel (Ni) and arsenic (As) ions among patients with dental implants, healthy or affected by peri-implantitis, compared to subjects without implants and/or metallic prosthetic restorations.

2. Material and Methods

2.1. Study Design

To address the research purpose, the authors designed a case-control study, conducted at the Departments of Oral and Maxillo-Facial Sciences, at "Sapienza" University of Rome.

2.2. Study Population

From May 2018 to May 2019, all subjects who underwent previous implant surgery since January 2008 at the Oral Surgery Unit, Policlinico Umberto I, "Sapienza" University of Rome were identified and consecutively evaluated.

Each patient received detailed descriptions of the study protocol and all subjects signed an informed consent form to be included in the study population, according to the World Medical Declaration of Helsinki. The Institution Review Board of "Sapienza" approved the study (Ref. 4939/2018).

Eligible patients were divided into two groups: subjects with clinically healthy implants (Group A) and patients with peri-implantitis (Group B).

Patients in group A were enrolled in the study based on the following inclusion and exclusion criteria:

- Single crown implants functioning for >1 year
- No clinical signs of pathologies of the oral mucosa
- Age ≥ 18 years
- Implants classified as clinically healthy
- No antibiotic treatment in the previous three months
- Non-smoker
- No uncontrolled systemic diseases
- Not pregnant or breastfeeding
- No metal reconstruction, crowns or other prosthetic restorations present in the oral cavity

Patients in Group B had to meet the following inclusion and exclusion criteria:

- Single crown implants functioning for >1 year
- No clinical signs of pathologies of the oral mucosa
- Age ≥ 18 years
- Implants with a diagnosis of peri-implantitis
- No antibiotic treatment in the previous three months
- Non-smoker
- No uncontrolled systemic diseases
- Not pregnant or breastfeeding
- No metal reconstruction, crowns or other prosthetic restorations present in the oral cavity

Furthermore, a third group of patients (Group C) without dental implants, derived from a population of subjects attending the Oral Surgery Unit from May 2018 to May 2019 for wisdom tooth removal, was enrolled in accordance with the following inclusion and exclusion criteria:

- Absence of dental implants
- No metal reconstruction, crowns or other prosthetic restorations present in the oral cavity
- Age ≥ 18 years
- No clinical signs of pathologies of the oral mucosa
- No antibiotic treatment in the previous three months
- Non-smoker
- No uncontrolled systemic diseases
- Not pregnant or breastfeeding

2.3. Clinical Examination

Patients' data collected included sex and age.

For each implant, the following clinical measurements were recorded at six sites per implant by using a periodontal probe (PCP-Unc 15, Hu-Friedy®, Chicago, IL, USA):

- Probing pocket depth (PPD) measured in millimeters
- Plaque index (PI) recorded with dichotomic values (present/absent)
- Mucosal redness recorded with dichotomic values (present/absent)

- Suppuration recorded with dichotomic values (present/absent)
- Bleeding on probing recorded with dichotomic values (present/absent)

2.4. Radiographic Assessment

Mesial and distal implant crestal bone levels were measured on standardized (Rinn Centratore XCP Evolution 2003, Dentsply, Rome, Italy) digital periapical X-rays for each implant using a calibrated software (SOPRO Imaging, Acteon Group, Norwich, UK). The implant length and width were used as references for calibration of measurements, with the bone level digitally evaluated by measuring the distance between the implant shoulder and the first visible bone contact on the implant.

Case definitions for epidemiological or disease surveillance studies of the 2017 World Workshop on the Classification of Periodontal and Peri-Implant Diseases and Conditions were adopted to establish the diagnosis of peri-implant diseases [30].

2.5. Saliva Collection

Five milliliters of saliva were collected from each patient using the unstimulated drainage method, or alternatively by leaving the saliva flow passively from the lower lip directly into designated sterile tubes.

Patients were advised not to take food or drink and to avoid oral hygiene procedures before saliva collection.

All samples were stored at a temperature of 1 °C, in order to block any biologic process still in place.

2.6. ICP-MS Analysis

Samples were analyzed using a Thermo Scientific XSERIES2 ICP-MS instrument (Thermo-Fisher Scientific, Waltham, MA, USA) at the Department of Earth Sciences at "Sapienza" University of Rome. Samples were processed as previously described [29]. The concentrations of Ti, V, Ni and As were quantified in μg/L.

2.7. Statistical Analysis

The required sample size was calculated using statistics software (GPower 3.1.9.2, Heinrich-Heine-Universität, Düsseldorf, Germany). A power analysis using the repeated measures ANOVA with three measurements, an alpha level of 0.05 and a medium effect size ($f = 0.56$) showed that 100 subjects would be adequate to obtain 95% power in detecting a statistical difference in the salivary level of Ti, assuming a loss to follow-up of 20% [31].

A database was created using Excel (Microsoft, Redmond, WA, USA). Descriptive statistics were calculated for each variable. The Shapiro–Wilk test was used to determine whether or not the data conformed to a normal distribution.

One-way repeated-measures ANOVA was used to identify statistically significant differences in the salivary level of Ti, V, Ni and As between three different groups: Control group, patients with healthy implant and patients with implant affected by peri-implantitis. Pairwise Tukey honestly significant difference (HSD) test for multiple comparisons.

The chi-squared test of homogeneity was used to evaluate the presence of differences in the proportion of males and females among the three groups.

Data were evaluated using standard statistical analysis software (version 20.0, Statistical Package for the Social Sciences, IBM Corporation, Armonk, NY, USA). A p value <0.05 was considered as statistically significant.

3. Results

A total of 100 patients were enrolled in the study (42 males and 58 females; age 49.02 ± 11.37 years). The patients were thus distributed in the three groups: 50 patients in Group C, 26 patients in Group B and 24 patients Group B. There were no significant differences in the proportions of males and females in the three groups ($p = 0.620$). Patients' demographics are reported in Table 1.

Table 1. Sample demographic.

Study Variable	Group A	Group B	Group C
Sample size	26	24	50
Male	11	11	20
Female	15	13	30
Age (y) ± SD (range)	63.13 ± 17.72	70.52 ± 8.24	46.57 ± 9.23
Dental implants (n)	26	24	NA
Functional loading (y) ± SD (range)	7.8 ± 2.62	9.88 ± 3.52	NA
Mean PPD (mm)	3.2 ± 0.44	4.66 ± 1.32	NA
Mean MBL (mm)	0.89 ± 0.32	1.95 ± 1.43	NA

SD, standard deviation; PPD, probing pocket depth; MBL, marginal bone loss; NA, not applicable.

3.1. *Titanium*

The mean concentration of Ti was 136.65 ± 263.28 µg/L in the Group C, 489.60 ± 227.86 µg/L in the Group A and 492.83 ± 313.90 in the Group B. Statistical significant differences in mean concentration were found between the Group C and the Group A ($p < 0.001$) and between the Group C and the Group B ($p < 0.001$) (Table 2).

3.2. *Nickel*

The mean concentration of Ni was 4.77 ± 8.33 µg/L in the Group C, 24.99 ± 12.47 µg/L in the Group A and 23.50 ± 10.12 in the Group B. Statistical significant differences in mean concentration were found between the Group C and the Group A ($p < 0.001$) and between the Group C and Group B ($p < 0.001$) (Table 2).

3.3. *Vanadium*

The mean concentration of V was 1.30 ± 4.28 µg/L in the Group C, 2.27 ± 2.43 µg/L in the Group A and 2.01 ± 1.35 in the Group B. The group means of V concentration were not statistically significant different ($p = 0.440$) (Table 2).

3.4. *Arsenic*

The mean concentration of As was 0.01 ± 0.01 µg/L in the Group C, 2.20 ± 1.88 µg/L in the Group A and 1.54 ± 2.07 in the Group B. Statistical significant differences in mean concentration were found between the Group C and the Group A ($p < 0.001$) and between the Group C and the Group B ($p < 0.001$) (Table 2).

Table 2. Difference in the mean concentration of titanium, nickel vanadium and arsenic in the three groups.

Multiple Comparisons							
Tukey's HSD							
Dependent Variable	(I) Groups	(J) Groups	Mean Difference (I-J)	Std. Error	Sig.	95% Confidence Interval	
						Lower Bound	Upper Bound
Titanium	Group C	Group A	−352.951280 *	59.517272	0.000	−494.61555	−211.28701
		Group B	−356.184613 *	61.127007	0.000	−501.68041	−210.68882
	Group A	Group C	352.951280 *	59.517272	0.000	211.28701	494.61555
		Group B	−3.233333	69.678791	0.999	−169.08426	162.61760
	Group B	Group C	356.184613 *	61.127007	0.000	210.68882	501.68041
		Group A	3.233333	69.678791	0.999	−162.61760	169.08426
Nickel	Group C	Group A	−20.215246 *	2.410887	0.000	−25.95369	−14.47680
		Group B	−18.728483 *	2.476093	0.000	−24.62213	−12.83483
	Group A	Group C	20.215246 *	2.410887	0.000	14.47680	25.95369
		Group B	1.486763	2.822503	0.858	−5.23142	8.20494
	Group B	Group C	18.728483 *	2.476093	0.000	12.83483	24.62213
		Group A	−1.486763	2.822503	0.858	−8.20494	5.23142
Vanadium	Group C	Group A	−0.965529	0.809320	0.460	−2.89189	0.96083
		Group B	−0.707260	0.831209	0.672	−2.68572	1.27120
	Group A	Group C	0.965529	0.809320	0.460	−0.96083	2.89189
		Group B	0.258269	0.947497	0.960	−1.99698	2.51352
	Group B	Group C	0.707260	0.831209	0.672	−1.27120	2.68572
		Group A	−0.258269	0.947497	0.960	−2.51352	1.99698
Arsenic	Group C	Group A	−2.193412 *	0.336286	0.000	−2.99385	−1.39298
		Group B	−1.525553 *	0.345382	0.000	−2.34764	−0.70347
	Group A	Group C	2.193412 *	0.336286	0.000	1.39298	2.99385
		Group B	0.667859	0.393701	0.212	−0.26924	1.60496
	Group B	Group C	1.525553 *	0.345382	0.000	0.70347	2.34764
		Group A	−0.667859	0.393701	0.212	−1.60496	0.26924

* The mean difference is significant at the 0.05 level. HSD, honestly significant difference.

4. Discussion

The aims of this study were to detect salivary metallic ions levels of Ti, V, Ni and As in patients with and without dental implants.

The metal concentration was measured by the use of ICP-MS, a versatile, rapid and extremely sensitive analytical technique used to determine different metallic and non-metallic inorganic substances present in concentrations lower than one part per billion.

Just a few studies have investigated the possible relationship of metallic ions dissolution and peri-implantitis, mainly focusing on titanium levels [27–29]

Safioti et al. first hypothesized a possible association between high titanium levels and implants affected by peri-implantitis, studying the metal concentration in submucosa plaque. The plaque samples were taken from the deepest points of the pockets of each implant through dental scalers (mini-five 1–2 Gracey) and then analyzed by ICP-MS. Results showed that implants with peri-implantitis had significantly ($p < 0.05$) higher titanium levels than healthy implants [27].

Olmedo et al. using the exfoliative cytology technique, measured the concentration of titanium particles in the peri-implant mucosa cells and found higher values in the group of patients affected by peri-implantitis compared to the group of patients with healthy implants [28,32].

In our study setting, attention was focused not only on titanium but also on other metals such as V, Ni and As.

Vanadium is ubiquitous: it is present in water and soil and its effects at systemic level are still debated: several authors have reported the use of vanadium in the treatment of diabetes mellitus, while others have correlated the long-term exposure with risk of cancer [33–36].

Nickel is known to be the cause of contact dermatitis and in general of allergic episodes, which can develop with serious consequences in the most sensitive subjects. Adverse reactions were documented in relation to orthodontic devices (brackets, arches) containing nickel. This element has a carcinogenic and mutagenic effects; therefore, exposure must be minimized [37–39].

Arsenic is one of the most widespread elements in nature: it can be found in soil, water, air and almost in all animal and plant tissues.

Arsenic poisoning can be acute (lethal) or chronic, caused by prolonged exposure even at low concentrations.

Martin-Camean et al. in 2014, in an in vivo study, evaluated the dissolution of different metal ions in the oral mucosa of subjects with orthodontic mini-implants. The epithelial cells of the oral mucosa were taken from each patient using a rubber brush. The samples were then analyzed through ICP-MS. The results reported only traces of vanadium, while the release of other elements occurred in the following growing order Cr < Ni < Ti < Cu < Al [40–42].

In our study, concentrations of metallic ions were higher in subjects with dental implants, either healthy or affected by peri-implantitis, compared to the control group, with the exception of vanadium.

Based on our results, metallic ions are detectable in the saliva of patients with dental implants; according to a recent systematic review conducted by Noronha Oliveira et al., degradation products—in the form of micro and nanoscale particles—can be found for different reasons, such as detachment from implant surface during surgical insertion, wear caused by micro-movements between contacting surfaces at implant connections, corrosive effects of therapeutic substances, like bleaching agents and fluorides or peri-implantitis treatment (mainly implantoplasty) [43].

In the present study, there were no statistically significant differences ($p > 0.05$) for metallic ions concentrations between patients with healthy dental implants and peri-implantitis subjects.

Our results are in contrast with the findings of Safioti et al. and Olmedo et al. [27,28]. However, in the above-mentioned articles, exclusion criteria did not limit enrollment to patients without other metallic prosthetic reconstructions and a control group without implants was not provided.

A recent systematic review by Gomes et al. [44] evaluated the diagnostic accuracy of biomarker levels in saliva to distinguish between healthy implants and implants affected by peri-implantitis. Based on their results, there was no clear evidence to support the use of salivary biomarkers (IL-6, IL-1β) in peri-implantitis detection. Pettersson et al. [45] performed gingival biopsies during surgical treatment of patients with severe periodontitis or peri-implantitis in order to evaluate titanium levels via ICP-MS. They found higher titanium values in peri-implantitis patients ($p < 0.001$) compared to periodontitis subjects, however samples were obtained after surgical treatment of dental implants and titanium release may be, therefore, exacerbated by ultrasonic scaling, as previously demonstrated by Eger et al. [46].

Furthermore, human samples from appropriate control groups (healthy implants and patients without metallic reconstructions) could not be obtained for ethical reasons.

Therefore, saliva collection and analysis through ICP-MS, as performed in the present study, seem a viable alternative to investigate data obtained by different populations.

5. Conclusions

Current evidence on the possible role of titanium or other metal particles in peri-implantitis pathogenesis is still controversial: in a recent critical review, Mombelli et al. concluded that there is poor specificity for the association of titanium particles and peri-implantitis, since metallic ions can be commonly detected in healthy and diseased peri-implant mucosa, as well as in gingiva of subjects without dental implants, being Tio2 used in multiple kinds of foods, toothpastes, cosmetics or medical pills [10].

Schwarz et al. in the latest World Workshop on the Classification of Periodontal and Peri-Implant Diseases and Conditions [18] stated that there was insufficient available evidence to consider titanium particles as a risk indicator for peri-implantitis.

Based on our results, concentrations of metallic ions were higher in subjects with dental implants, either healthy or affected by peri-implantitis, compared to the control group, with the exception of vanadium. No statistically significant differences were found in the metallic concentrations of healthy implants or peri-implantitis.

Future research should be orientated in conducting further studies, with a larger sample and a longitudinal design, to determine the role of titanium or other metals in peri-implantitis pathogenesis.

Author Contributions: P.P. and A.R. drafted the article, revised the paper and gave substantial contributions to the conception of the work; G.P. and A.D. gave substantial contributions to the conception of the work and revised the manuscript critically for important intellectual content. N.P. revised the paper, gave substantial contributions to the conception of the work and performed the statistical analysis. B.D.M. and P.C.P. revised the paper, gave substantial contributions to the conception of the work and recruited patients. M.B. gave substantial contributions to the conception of the work, revised the manuscript critically for important intellectual content and performed the ICP-MS analysis. All authors have read and agreed to the published version of the manuscript.

References

1. De Angelis, F.; Papi, P.; Mencio, F.; Rosella, D.; Di Carlo, S.; Pompa, G. Implant survival and success rates in patients with risk factors: Results from a long-term retrospective study with a 10 to 18 years follow-up. *Eur. Rev. Med. Pharmacol. Sci.* **2017**, *21*, 433–437. [PubMed]
2. Rossi, F.; Lang, N.P.; Ricci, E.; Ferraioli, L.; Baldi, N.; Botticelli, D. Long-term follow-up of single crowns supported by short, moderately rough implants—A prospective 10-year cohort study. *Clin. Oral Implant. Res.* **2018**, *29*, 1212–1219. [CrossRef] [PubMed]
3. Li, J.; He, X.; Zhang, G.; Hang, R.; Huang, X.; Tang, B.; Zhang, X. Electrochemical corrosion, wear and cell behavior of ZrO(2)/TiO(2) alloyed layer on Ti-6Al-4V. *Bioelectrochemistry* **2018**, *121*, 105–114. [CrossRef]
4. Zhang, R.; Wan, Y.; Ai, X.; Liu, Z.; Zhang, D. Corrosion resistance and biological activity of TiO(2) implant coatings produced in oxygen-rich environments. *Proc. Inst. Mech. Eng. Part H* **2017**, *231*, 20–27. [CrossRef]
5. Delgado-Ruiz, R.; Romanos, G. Potential Causes of Titanium Particle and Ion Release in Implant Dentistry: A Systematic Review. *Int. J. Mol. Sci.* **2018**, *19*, 3585. [CrossRef] [PubMed]
6. Apaza-Bedoya, K.; Tarce, M.; Benfatti, C.A.M.; Henriques, B.; Mathew, M.T.; Teughels, W.; Souza, J.C.M. Synergistic interactions between corrosion and wear at titanium-based dentalimplant connections: A scoping review. *J. Periodontal Res.* **2017**, *52*, 946–954. [CrossRef] [PubMed]
7. Maruthamuthu, S.; Rajasekar, A.; Sathiyanarayanan, S.; Muthukumar, N.; Palaniswamy, N. Electrochemical behaviour of microbes on orthodontic wires. *Curr. Sci.* **2005**, *89*, 988–996.
8. Chang, J.C.; Oshida, Y.; Gregory, R.L.; Andres, C.J.; Barco, T.M.; Brown, D.T. Electrochemical study on microbiology-related corrosion of metallic dental materials. *Bio-Med. Mater. Eng.* **2003**, *13*, 281–295.
9. Souza, J.C.M.; Henriques, M.; Oliveira, R.; Teughels, W.; Celis, J.P.; Rocha, L.A. Do oral biofilms influence the wear and corrosion behavior of titanium titanium? *Biofouling* **2010**, *26*, 471–478. [CrossRef] [PubMed]
10. Mombelli, A.; Hashim, D.; Cionca, N. What is the impact of titanium particles and biocorrosion on implant survival and complications? A critical review. *Clin. Oral. Implant. Res.* **2018**, *29*, 37–53. [CrossRef]
11. Boyce, B.F.; Xing, L. Functions of RANKL/RANK/OPG in bone modeling and remodeling. *Arch. Biochem. Biophys.* **2008**, *473*, 139–146. [CrossRef] [PubMed]
12. Walsh, M.C.; Choi, Y. Biology of the RANKL-RANK-OPG System in Immunity, Bone, and Beyond. *Front. Immunol.* **2014**, *5*, 511.
13. Wachi, T.; Shuto, T.; Shinohara, Y.; Matono, Y.; Makihira, S. Release of titanium ions from an implant surface and their effect on cytokine production related to alveolar bone resorption. *Toxicology* **2015**, *327*, 1–9. [CrossRef] [PubMed]
14. Cadosch, D.; Al-Mushaiqri, M.S.; Gautschi, O.P.; Meagher, J.; Simmen, H.P.; Filgueira, L. Biocorrosion and uptake of titanium by human osteoclasts. *J. Biomed. Mater. Res.* **2010**, *95*, 1004–1010. [CrossRef] [PubMed]

15. Nishimura, K.; Kato, T.; Ito, T. Influence of titanium ions on cytokine levels of murine splenocytes stimulated with periodontopathic bacterial lipopolysaccharide. *Int. J. Oral. Maxillofac. Implant.* **2014**, *29*, 472–477.
16. La Monaca, G.; Pranno, N.; Annibali, S.; Cristalli, M.P.; Polimeni, A. Clinical and radiographic outcomes of a surgical reconstructive approach in the treatment of peri-implantitis lesions: A 5-year prospective case series. *Clin. Oral Implant. Res.* **2018**, *29*, 1025–1037. [CrossRef]
17. Mencio, F.; De Angelis, F.; Papi, P.; Rosella, D.; Pompa, G.; Di Carlo, S. A randomized clinical trial about presence of pathogenic microflora and risk of peri-implantitis: Comparison of two different types of implant-abutment connections. *Eur. Rev. Med. Pharmacol. Sci.* **2017**, *21*, 1443–1451.
18. Schwarz, F.; Derks, J.; Monje, A.; Wang, H.L. Peri-implantitis. *J. Periodontol.* **2018**, *89*, 267–290. [CrossRef]
19. Pimentel, S.P.; Shiota, R.; Cirano, F.R.; Casarin, R.C.V.; Pecorari, V.G.A.; Casati, M.Z.; Haas, A.N.; Ribeiro, F.V. Occurrence of peri-implant diseases and risk indicators at the patient and implant levels: A multilevel cross-sectional study. *J. Periodontol.* **2018**, *89*, 1091–1100. [CrossRef]
20. Dreyer, H.; Grischke, J.; Tiede, C.; Eberhard, J.; Schweitzer, A.; Toikkanen, S.E.; Glöckner, S.; Krause, G.; Stiesch, M. Epidemiology and risk factors of peri-implantitis: A systematic review. *J. Periodontal Res.* **2018**, *53*, 657–681. [CrossRef]
21. Papi, P.; Di Murro, B.; Pranno, N.; Bisogni, V.; Saracino, V.; Letizia, C.; Polimeni, A.; Pompa, G. Prevalence of peri-implant diseases among an Italian population of patients with metabolic syndrome: A cross-sectional study. *J. Periodontol.* **2019**, *90*, 1374–1382. [CrossRef]
22. Papi, P.; Letizia, C.; Pilloni, A.; Petramala, L.; Saracino, V.; Rosella, D.; Pompa, G. Peri-implant diseases and metabolic syndrome components: A systematic review. *Eur. Rev. Med. Pharmacol. Sci.* **2018**, *22*, 866–875. [PubMed]
23. Kotsakis, G.A.; Lan, C.X.; Barbosa, J.; Lill, K.; Chen, R.Q.; Rudney, J.; Aparicio, C. Antimicrobial agents used in the treatment of peri-implantitis alter the physicochemistry and cytocompatibility of titanium surfaces. *J. Periodontol.* **2016**, *87*, 809–819. [CrossRef] [PubMed]
24. Gurgel, B.C.V.; Montenegro, S.C.L.; Dantas, P.M.C.; Pascoal, A.L.B.; Lima, K.C.; Calderon, P.D.S. Frequency of peri-implant diseases and associated factors. *Clin. Oral Implant. Res.* **2017**, *28*, 1211–1217. [CrossRef] [PubMed]
25. Dalago, H.; Schuldt Filho, G.; Rodrigues, M.; Renvert, S.; Bianchini, M. Risk indicators for peri-implantitis: A cross-sectional study with 916 implants. *Clin. Oral Implant. Res.* **2017**, *28*, 144–150. [CrossRef] [PubMed]
26. Renvert, S.; Aghazadeh, A.; Hallström, H.; Persson, G.R. Factors related to peri-implantitis—A retrospective study. *Clin. Oral Implant. Res.* **2014**, *25*, 522–529. [CrossRef] [PubMed]
27. Safioti, L.M.; Kotsakis, G.A.; Pozhitkov, A.E.; Chung, W.O.; Daubert, D.M. Increased levels of dissolved titanium are associated with peri-implantitis—A cross-sectional study. *J. Periodontol.* **2017**, *88*, 436–442. [CrossRef]
28. Olmedo, D.G.; Nalli, G.; Verdú, S.; Paparella, M.L.; Cabrini, R.L. Exfoliative cytology and titanium dental implants: A pilot study. *J. Periodontol.* **2013**, *84*, 78–83. [CrossRef]
29. Barbieri, M.; Mencio, F.; Papi, P.; Rosella, D.; Di Carlo, S.; Valente, T.; Pompa, G. Corrosion behavior of dental implants immersed into human saliva: Preliminary results of an in vitro study. *Eur. Rev. Med. Pharmacol. Sci.* **2017**, *21*, 3543–3548.
30. Berglundh, T.; Armitage, G.; Araujo, M.G. Peri-implant diseases and conditions: Consensus report of workgroup 4 of the 2017 World Workshop on the Classification of Periodontal and Peri-Implant Diseases and Conditions. *J. Clin. Periodontol.* **2018**, *45*, 286–291. [CrossRef]
31. Faul, F.; Erdfelder, E.; Lang, A.G.; Buchner, A. G*Power 3: A flexible statistical power analysis program for the social, behavioral, and biomedical sciences. *Behav. Res. Methods* **2007**, *39*, 175–191. [CrossRef]
32. Olmedo, D.; Fernandez, M.M.; Guglielmotti, M.B.; Cabrini, R.L. Macrophages related to dental implant failure. *Implant Dent.* **2003**, *12*, 75–80. [CrossRef] [PubMed]
33. Zwolak, I. Vanadium carcinogenic, immunotoxic and neurotoxic effects: A review of in vitro studies. *Toxicol. Mech. Methods* **2014**, *24*, 1–12. [CrossRef] [PubMed]
34. Domingo, J.L.; Gómez, M. Vanadium compounds for the treatment of human diabetes mellitus: A scientific curiosity? A review of thirty years of research. *Food Chem. Toxicol.* **2016**, *95*, 137–141. [CrossRef] [PubMed]
35. Imtiaz, M.; Rizwan, M.S.; Xiong, S.; Li, H.; Ashraf, M.; Shahzad, S.M.; Shahzad, M.; Rizwan, M.; Tu, S. Vanadium, recent advancements and research prospects: A review. *Environ. Int.* **2015**, *80*, 79–88. [CrossRef] [PubMed]

36. Gruzewska, K.; Michno, A.; Pawelczyk, T.; Belarczyk, H. Essentiality and toxicity of vanadium supplements in health and pathology. *J. Physiol. Pharmacol.* **2014**, *65*, 603–611.
37. Lu, L.; Vollmer, J.; Moulon, C.; Weltzien, H.U.; Marrack, P.; Kappler, J. Components of the ligand for a Ni++ reactive human T cell clone. *J. Exp. Med.* **2003**, *197*, 567–574. [CrossRef]
38. Saito, M.; Arakaki, R.; Yamada, A.; Tsunematsu, T.; Kudo, Y.; Ishimaru, N. Molecular mechanisms of nickel allergy. *Int. J. Mol. Sci.* **2016**, *17*, 202. [CrossRef]
39. Girolomoni, G.; Gisondi, P.; Ottaviani, C.; Cavani, A. Immunoregulation of allergic contact dermtitis. *J. Dermatol.* **2004**, *31*, 264–270. [CrossRef]
40. Martín-Cameán, A.; Jos, A.; Calleja, A.; Gil, F.; Iglesias, A.; Solano, E.; Cameán, A.M. Validation of a method to quantify titanium, vanadium and zirconium in oral mucosa cells by inductively coupled plasma-mass spectrometry (ICP-MS). *Talanta* **2014**, *118*, 238–244. [CrossRef]
41. Martín-Cameán, A.; Jos, A.; Puerto, M.; Calleja, A.; Iglesias-Linares, A.; Solano, E.; Cameán, A.M. In vivo determination of aluminum, cobalt, chromium, copper, nickel, titanium and vanadium in oral mucosa cells from orthodontic patients with mini-implants by inductively coupled plasma-mass spectrometry (ICP-MS). *J. Trace Elem. Med. Biol.* **2015**, *32*, 13–20. [CrossRef] [PubMed]
42. Martín-Cameán, A.; Molina-Villalba, I.; Jos, A.; Iglesias-Linares, A.; Solano, E.; Cameán, A.M.; Gil, F. Biomonitorization of chromium, copper, iron, manganese and nickel in scalp hair from orthodontic patients by atomic absorption spectrometry. *Environ. Toxicol. Pharmacol.* **2014**, *37*, 759–771. [CrossRef] [PubMed]
43. Noronha Oliveira, M.; Schunemann, W.V.H.; Mathew, M.T.; Henriques, B.; Magini, R.S.; Teughels, W.; Souza, J.C.M. Can degradation products released from dental implants affect peri-implant tissues? *J. Periodontal Res.* **2018**, *53*, 1–11. [CrossRef] [PubMed]
44. Gomes, A.M.; Douglas-de-Oliveira, D.W.; Oliveira Costa, F. Could the biomarker levels in saliva help distinguish between healthy implants and implants with peri-implant disease? A systematic review. *Arch. Oral Biol.* **2018**, *96*, 216–222. [CrossRef]
45. Pettersson, M.; Pettersson, J.; Johansson, A.; Molin Thorén, M. Titanium release in peri-implantitis. *J. Oral Rehabil.* **2019**, *46*, 179–188. [CrossRef] [PubMed]
46. Eger, M.; Sterer, N.; Liron, T.; Kohavi, D.; Gabet, Y. Scaling of titanium implants entrains inflammation-induced osteolysis. *Sci. Rep.* **2017**, *7*, 39612. [CrossRef]

11

Dysfunction of Salivary Glands, Disturbances in Salivary Antioxidants and Increased Oxidative Damage in Saliva of Overweight and Obese Adolescents

Anna Zalewska [1,*], Agnieszka Kossakowska [1], Katarzyna Taranta-Janusz [2], Sara Zięba [3], Katarzyna Fejfer [4], Małgorzata Salamonowicz [4], Paula Kostecka-Sochoń [4], Anna Wasilewska [2] and Mateusz Maciejczyk [5,*]

1 Experimental Dentistry Laboratory, Medical University of Bialystok, 15-222 Bialystok, Poland; a_kossak@op.pl
2 Department of Pediatrics and Nephrology, Medical University of Bialystok, 15-222 Bialystok, Poland; katarzyna.taranta@wp.pl (K.T.-J.); annwasil@interia.pl (A.W.)
3 Students Scientific Club "Biochemistry of Civilization Diseases" at the Department of Hygiene, Epidemiology and Ergonomics, Medical University of Bialystok, 15-222 Bialystok, Poland; sarap.zieba@gmail.com
4 Conservative Dentistry Department, Medical University of Bialystok, 15-222 Bialystok, Poland; katarzyna.fejfer@gmail.com (K.F.); wrobmalg@gmail.com (M.S.); p.kosta@wp.pl (P.K.-S.)
5 Department of Hygiene, Epidemiology and Ergonomics, Medical University of Bialystok, 15-222 Bialystok, Poland
* Correspondence: azalewska426@gmail.com (A.Z.); mat.maciejczyk@gmail.com (M.M.)

Abstract: Obesity is inseparably connected with oxidative stress. This process may disturb the functioning of the oral cavity, although the effect of oxidative stress on salivary gland function and changes in the qualitative composition of saliva are still unknown. Our study is the first to evaluate salivary redox homeostasis in 40 overweight and obese adolescents and in the age- and gender-matched control group. We demonstrated strengthening of the antioxidant barrier (↑superoxide dismutase, ↑catalase, ↑peroxidase, ↑uric acid, ↑total antioxidant capacity (TAC)) with a simultaneous decrease in reduced glutathione concentration in saliva (non-stimulated/stimulated) in overweight and obese teenagers compared to the controls. The concentration of the products of oxidative damage to proteins (advanced glycation end products), lipids (malondialdehyde, 4-hydroxynonenal) and DNA (8-hydroxydeoxyguanosine) as well as total oxidative status were significantly higher in both non-stimulated and stimulated saliva as well as plasma of overweight and obese adolescents. Importantly, we observed more severe salivary and plasma redox alterations in obese adolescents compared to overweight individuals. In the study group, we also noted a drop in stimulated salivary secretion and a decrease in total protein content. Interestingly, dysfunction of parotid glands in overweight and obese teenagers intensified with the increase of BMI. We also showed that the measurement of salivary catalase and TAC could be used to assess the central antioxidant status of overweight and obese adolescents.

Keywords: oxidative stress; antioxidants; saliva; salivary biomarkers; obesity

---

1. Introduction

Overweight/obesity is a social problem worldwide, characterized by an increase in body weight that results in excessive accumulation of fat [1]. In recent years, we have observed a steady growth in the frequency of overweight and obesity, observed not only among adults, but also children and adolescents [2]. This results from various genetic, environmental and economic (easy access to cheap and highly calorific food) factors as well as evolutionary conditioning (sedentary lifestyle, low physical activity, low energy expenditure) [1,3]. According to the latest WHO report, nearly 41 million children under 5 years of age are overweight or obese [4]. Interestingly, studies have shown that about 40% of overweight children will continue to gain weight during the puberty period, and about 80% of these obese teenagers will remain obese as adults [5]. Although obesity rates are higher in developed countries, more overweight or obese children live in developing countries, and this trend also applies to European countries.

It has been shown that obesity is associated with an increase in oxidative stress (OS). OS is a condition characterized by disturbed balance between the amount of reactive oxygen species (ROS) produced by the body and activity/concentration of antioxidants responsible for neutralizing ROS [6]. ROS are chemically reactive molecules which, when unbalanced, lead to oxidative modifications of proteins, lipids, carbohydrates and nucleic acids, resulting in obesity-related complications.

It should be emphasized that obesity has been recognized as a major underlying factor in the pathogenesis of serious OS-related health problems, such as hyperlipidemia [7], insulin resistance [8], hypertension [9], type 2 diabetes [10], cardiovascular diseases [7] and certain types of cancer [11]. Overweight/obesity has been shown to adversely affect the condition of the oral cavity, including salivary gland function [12–14]. The pathogenesis of salivary gland lesions in the course of obesity is not fully understood, although the influence of OS is emphasized. It has been demonstrated that adult morbid obesity is associated with disorders of antioxidant systems [15,16] and oxidative damage to salivary proteins, lipids, and DNA [17], while bariatric treatment generally lowers the levels of salivary oxidative damage. However, it does not rescue antioxidant capacity of non-stimulated and stimulated saliva [16,17].

Recently, more and more attention has been paid to the use of saliva in laboratory medical diagnostics, particularly in connection with pediatric diseases, as the collection of saliva samples is non-invasive and thus acceptable to children. It has been shown that proteins and other substances are transported to saliva from blood via the passive process of diffusion, ultrafiltration and active transport. The concentrations of numerous substances in saliva can be correlated with their concentrations in blood plasma, allowing for the use of saliva as an alternative diagnostic material. Moreover, the use of oxidative stress biomarkers is proposed in diagnosing patients with obesity due to the observed changes in enzymatic and non-enzymatic antioxidant levels as well as accumulation of protein and lipid oxidation products in plasma and saliva of obese patients [16,17].

There have been numerous studies on OS in saliva and blood of overweight and obese adults [15–18], whereas no research has been conducted to evaluate salivary redox markers and their usefulness in diagnosing adolescents with excessive body weight. Therefore, the aim of our work is to evaluate antioxidant systems as well as oxidative modifications of proteins and lipids in non-stimulated and stimulated saliva of overweight and obese adolescents.

2. Materials and Methods

2.1. Patients

The study was approved by the Ethics Committee at the Medical University of Bialystok, Poland (permission number R-I-002/43/2018). After explaining the purpose and methodology of the study to patients and their parents, written informed content was obtained from each parent/legal guardian.

Our study included adolescents aged 11–18: overweight with BMI z-score ≤ + 1 + 2 < SD (*n* = 20, 10 teenagers) and obese with BMI z-score ≥ + 2 SD (*n* = 20, 10 teenagers).

The control group consisted of adolescents (*n* = 40, 20 teenagers) with normal body weight (BMI z-score < –1 + 1 <, matched by age and gender to the study group.

The adolescents included in the study group were recruited in the Department of Pediatrics and Nephrology of the Medical University of Bialystok, during routine follow-up visits, after performing a dental and biochemical blood test and meeting the conditions for inclusion/exclusion to the study.

The adolescents included in the control group were recruited during dental follow-up visits in the Children's Outpatient Dentistry Clinic (Specialist Dental Centre of the Medical University of Bialystok), initially based on BMI index and a health survey. Then, after obtaining the written consent of participants and their legal guardians, biochemical blood tests were performed. If the participants met the conditions for inclusion/exclusion in the study, they were finally included in the control group.

Patients from the study and control group were qualified by the same experienced pediatrician (K.T.J.) as well as a pediatric dentist (A.Z.). The control group consisted of patients of the Children's Outpatient Dentistry Clinic because, in the Pediatrics and Nephrology Clinic, there were only a few healthy controls that met the inclusion criteria for the study.

Clinical data of the subjects are presented in Table 1.

Table 1. Clinical characteristics of patients and healthy controls.

	C $n = 40$	OWT $n = 20$	OB $n = 20$
Age (years)	16 ± 2.0	16 ± 1.9	15.8 ± 2.2
Sex (male/female) n	20/20	10/10	10/10
Weight (kg)	55 ± 3.1	65 ± 10 *	90 ± 21 *
Height (cm)	167 ± 4.5	163 ± 12	162 ± 14
BMI (kg/m^2)	20 ± 1.5	28 ± 1.5 *	34 ± 2.7 *
cc BMI	50 ± 2.5	97 ± 1.2	99 ± 0.83
SDS BMI	0.5 ± 0.2	2.5 ± 0.28	3.9 ± 0.81
Systolic BP (mmHg)	109 ± 1.0	110 ± 1.2	111 ± 1.0
Diastolic BP (mmHg)	58 ± 4.2	73 ± 10	76 ± 9.8
WBC (thousand/μL)	5.8 ± 1.3	6.7 ± 2.2	6.7 ± 1.1
Hgb (g/dL)	13.9 ± 1.1	14 ± 1.2	14 ± 1.0
Hct (%)	42.0 ± 2.3	41 ± 3.3	42 ± 3.2
PLT (thousand/μL)	278 ± 46	294 ± 71	263 ± 48
sCre (mg/dL)	0.63 ± 0.1	0.64 ± 0.19	0.79 ± 0.56
Urea (mg/dL)	15.4 ± 3.6	24 ± 9.7 *	27 ± 13 *
HDL (mg/dL)	47 ± 2.2	52 ± 1.4	43 ± 8.1
LDL (mg/dL)	70 ± 5.2	87 ± 24	106 ± 21 *
Total cholesterol (mg/dL)	120 ± 9	132 ± 30	161 ± 39 *
TG (mg/dL)	68 ± 8	102 ± 75 *	139 ± 75 *
Glucose (mg/dL)	86 ± 5.3	86 ± 9.9	91 ± 5.4
eGFR (mL/min/1.73 m^2)	132 ± 10	120 ± 42	122 ± 43
IL-6 (pg/mL)	1.7 ± 0.71	2.3 ± 0.74	3 ± 1.13

Body weight, height and head and chest circumferences were measured by standard methods. BMI was calculated as weight (kg) divided by the square of height (m^2). BMI z-scores that reflect the standard deviation score (SD) for age- and gender-appropriate BMI distribution, were calculated according to the LMS method [19], using reference values from the WHO study [20]. Based on the international norms from the World Health Organization for age- (with an accuracy of 1 month) and gender-specific BMI, BMI cut-offs for children over 5 years of age were the following: overweight–BMI z-score $\leq +1+2 <$ SD; obesity–BMI z-score $\geq +2$ SD [21].

The inclusion criteria were: adolescents of both sexes (in the case of girls, those who had had menarche) with full permanent dentition. On the day of material collection, the teenage girls were in the first phase of their menstrual cycle.

Patients with deciduous and mixed dentition, with gingivitis (gingival index, GI > 0.5) and pathological changes in the oral cavity mucosa were excluded from the study. Negative general medical history was a necessary factor to qualify for the experiment. The questionnaire completed by the patients included: infectious, autoimmune and metabolic diseases (type 2 diabetes) as well as hypertension, insulin resistance and diseases of respiratory, cardiovascular, digestive, genitourinary and coagulation systems. The exclusion criteria also covered inappropriate behavior and/or refusal to cooperate with the examiner. At least 3 months before the study, patients and the healthy controls had not taken any oral non-steroidal anti-inflammatory drugs, glucocorticosteroids, vitamins, other supplements, or antibiotics. The participants were non-smokers and did not drink alcohol more frequently than once a month.

2.2. Blood Collection

Blood was collected on an empty stomach, during routine examinations in the case of adolescents from the control group, and for the study groups: during admission to the Pediatric and Nephrology Clinic of the Medical University of Bialystok. Blood was collected in the amount of 10 mL using an S-Monovette® EDTA K3 tube (Sarstedt, Nümbrecht, Germany). After collection, the blood was centrifuged (3000 g, 10 min, 4 °C). No hemolysis was observed in any of the obtained plasma samples. Blood cell mass was rinsed 3 times with 0.9% NaCl, and then underwent osmotic lysis using 50 mM cold phosphate buffer (pH 7.4) 1:9 (v/v) [17]. To prevent sample oxidation, 0.5 M BHT (Sigma-Aldrich, Saint Louis, MO, USA; 10 µl/ml blood) was added to the plasma and red blood cell lysate [17]. Plasma and blood lysate were frozen (–82 °C). The samples were stored deep-frozen for no longer than 6 months.

2.3. Saliva Collection

Non-stimulated and stimulated saliva was collected by the spitting method between 7 and 8 a.m., one day after admission to the Pediatrics and Nephrology Clinic of the UMB or during a routine dental check-up. The time since the last meal, tooth-brushing and taking medications was at least 10 h. Samples were collected in a separate room to ensure comfort for the subjects. After rinsing the mouth with water, participants spat out non-stimulated saliva accumulated at the bottom of the oral cavity for 15 min. Stimulated saliva was collected after a 5-min break. Stimulation was performed by dropping 20 µl of 2% citric acid on the tongue every 20 s for 5 min. Both types of saliva were collected in test tubes placed on ice. To prevent sample oxidation, 0.5 M BHT (Sigma-Aldrich, Saint Louis, MO, USA; 10 µl/ml blood) was added to the saliva. After collecting the samples, the volume of saliva was measured in a calibrated pipette with accuracy of 100 µL and saliva flow rate was estimated. Saliva samples were centrifuged (3000 g, 20 min, 4 °C, MPW 351, MPW Med. Instruments, Warsaw, Poland) and then frozen (–82 °C). Frozen samples were stored for no longer than 6 months.

In each of the obtained saliva samples, the concentration of transferrin was determined by the ELISA test to identify samples contaminated with blood. Transferrin was not detected in any of the saliva samples (data not shown).

2.4. Dental Examination

Immediately after saliva collection, dental examination was performed by the selected dentists (K. F., M. S., P. K.-S.) in artificial light, using a mirror, an explorer and a periodontal probe (WHO, 621) in accordance with the WHO criteria. The dental examination included the evaluation of DMFT (decayed, missing, filled teeth) and GI (gingival index). The interrater reliability for DMFT was $r = 0.92$, and for GI was $r = 0.94$.

2.5. Biochemical Determination

The performed assays included: antioxidant enzymes (salivary peroxidase (Px), EC 1.11.1.7, catalase (CAT), EC 1.11.1.6 and superoxide dismutase (SOD), EC 1.15.1.1), non-enzymatic antioxidants (reduced glutathione (GSH), uric acid (UA) and albumin), redox status (total oxidant status (TOS), total antioxidant capacity (TAC) and oxidative stress index (OSI)), advanced glycation end products (AGE), malondialdehyde (MDA), 4-NHE-protein adduct (4-HNE) and 8-hydroxy-D-guanosine (8-OHdG). All results were standardized to mg of total protein. The total protein content was determined using the bicinchoninic acid (BCA) method and bovine serum albumin (BSA) as a standard (Thermo Scientific PIERCE BCA Protein Assay (Rockford, IL, USA).

In the saliva samples, we analyzed all redox biomarkers. In erythrocytes, antioxidant enzymes were assayed, while in the blood plasma we evaluated non-enzymatic antioxidants, redox status and oxidative damage products as well as interleukin-6 (IL-6) concentration. All assays were performed in duplicate samples (TOS in triplicate samples), and the absorbance/fluorescence of the samples was measured with an Infinite M200 PRO Multimode Microplate Reader (Tecan).

2.6. *Antioxidant Enzymes*

The activity of salivary peroxidase (Px, E.C. 1.11.1.7) was determined colorimetrically according to Mansson-Rahemtulla et al. [22] based on the reduction of 5,5′-dithiobis-(2-nitrobenzoic acid) (DTNB) to thionitrobenzoic acid, which then reacted with thiocyanate anions (SCN^-) formed as a result of potassium thiocyanate (KSCN) oxidation by Px. The absorbance was measured at a 412 nm wavelength. The activity of catalase (CAT, E.C. 1.11.1.6) was determined by the colorimetric method described by Aebi [23], based on the measurement of the hydrogen peroxide (H_2O_2) decomposition rate in phosphate buffer at pH 7.0. The absorbance was measured at 240 nm wavelength. One unit of CAT activity was defined as the amount of the enzyme that decomposes 1 mM H_2O_2 for 1 min. The activity of superoxide dismutase-1 (SOD, E.C. 1.15.1.1) was determined colorimetrically according to Misra and Fridovich [24] based on the measurement of cytoplasmic activity of the SOD subunit in the reaction of inhibiting the oxidation of epinephrine to adrenochrome at a 320 nm wavelength. It was assumed that one unit of SOD activity inhibits epinephrine oxidation in 50%.

2.7. *Non-Enzymatic Antioxidants*

The concentration of reduced glutathione (GSH) was determined colorimetrically based on DTNB reduction to 2-nitro-5-mercaptobenzoic acid under the influence of GSH contained in the assayed samples [25]. Absorbance changes were measured at 412 nm wavelength. Uric acid (UA) concentration was determined by the colorimetric method using a set of ready-made reagents (QuantiChrom TM Uric Acid Assay Kit DIUA-250, BioAssay System Harward, CA, USA). The method is based on the reaction of 2,4,6-tripyridyl-s-triazine with iron (3+) ions in the presence of UA contained in the samples. Changes in the absorbance of the resulting complex were measured at a 590 nm wavelength.

2.8. *Redox Status*

Total antioxidant capacity (TAC) was determined colorimetrically as described by Erel [26], based on the measurement of the ability to neutralize the radical cation ABTS $^{\cdot+}$ [2,2-azino-bis-(3-ethylbenzothiazoline-6-sulfonate)] under the influence of antioxidants contained in the tested samples. Changes in the absorbance of ABTS $^{\cdot+}$ solution were measured at a 660 nm wavelength. Total oxidant status (TOS) was determined using the colorimetric method described by Erel [27], based on the oxidation of iron (2+) ions to iron (3+) ions in the presence of oxidants contained in the sample, followed by the detection of Fe^{3+} ions by xylene orange. TOS concentration was calculated from the standard curve for hydrogen peroxide and presented in nM H_2O_2 equivalent/mg total protein. TOS determination was performed in triplicate samples. The oxidative stress index (OSI) was presented as the quotient of TOS to TAC and expressed in % [28,29].

2.9. *Products of Oxidative Damage to Proteins and Lipids*

The content of protein advanced glycation end products (AGE) was determined fluorimetrically by the method described by Kalousová et al. [30] based on the measurement of fluorescence of furyl-furanyl-imidazole (FFI), carboxymethyl lysine (CML), pyraline and pentosidine at the excitation wavelength 350 nm and emission wavelength 440 nm. To determine the AGE content, the samples were diluted in PBS buffer (0.02 M, pH 7.0) in a volume ratio of 1:5, and mixed thoroughly [31]. AGE content was determined in duplicate samples and expressed in fluorescence arbitrary units AFU/mg total protein. The concentration of malondialdehyde (MDA) was determined colorimetrically using thiobarbituric acid (TBA) [32]. The MDA reaction with TBA produces a colored adduct with the maximum absorption at 535 nm wavelength. The concentrations of 4-HNE and 8-OHdG were assessed by ELISA with commercial sets (Cell Biolabs, Inc. San Diego, CA, USA; USCN Life Science, Wuhan, China, respectively), following the manufacturer's instructions included in the package.

2.10. Statistical Analysis

Statistical analysis of the results was performed using GraphPad Prism 8 and Microsoft Excel 16.16.12 for MacOS. The D'Agostino–Pearson test and Shapiro–Wilk test were used to assess the distribution of the results. Individual groups were compared using the analysis of variance (ANOVA) followed by Tukey's honest significant difference test (Tukey's HSD test). The multiplicity adjusted p value was also calculated. Correlations between redox biomarkers were assessed based on the Pearson correlation coefficient. The results were presented as mean and standard deviation (SD) using tables or graphs. Diagnostic usefulness of the redox biomarkers was evaluated by means of receiver operating characteristic (ROC) analysis. Statistical significance was assumed at $p \leq 0.05$.

The number of subjects was determined based on our previous experiment, assuming that the power of the test would equal 0.9.

3. Results

3.1. General Characteristics

Stimulated secretion was significantly lower in the group of overweight and obese adolescents compared to the controls (↓40%, $p < 0.0001$; ↓51%, $p < 0.0001$, respectively). Teenagers with obesity secreted considerably less saliva after stimulation than their overweight peers (18%, $p = 0.004$). The secretion of non-stimulated saliva did not differ significantly between the study groups as well as in comparison with the control group (Table 2).

Table 2. Salivary flow rate, total protein and stomatological findings.

	C $n = 40$	O $n = 20$	OB $n = 20$
NWS (mL/min)	0.42 ± 0.05	0.39 ± 0.11	0.41 ± 0.11
SWS (mL/min)	1.5 ± 0.1	0.9 ± 0.2 *	0.74 ± 0.18 *#
TP NWS (μg/mL)	1291 ± 227	1167 ± 299	1139 ± 245
TP SWS (μg/mL)	986 ± 327	658 ± 208 *	598 ± 197 *
DMFT	6 ± 2	8 ± 3	8 ± 2
GI	0.1 ± 0.1	0.1 ± 0.15	0.1 ± 0.12

NWS- non-stimulated salivary flow rate, SWS- stimulated salivary flow rate, TP- total protein, C- control, OWT- overweight, OB- obese, DMFT= decay, missing, filling teeth, PBI- papilla bleeding index, GI- gingival index, * $p < 0.05$ vs. C; # $p < 0.05$ vs. OWT.

Total protein concentration in stimulated saliva of overweight and obese adolescents was significantly lower than in the control group (↓33%, $p = 0.0001$; 40%, $p < 0.0001$, respectively). Protein concentration in non-stimulated saliva did not differ significantly between the study groups and compared to the control group (Table 2).

Scatter plots for BMI and NWS/SWS flow rate are presented in Figure 1.

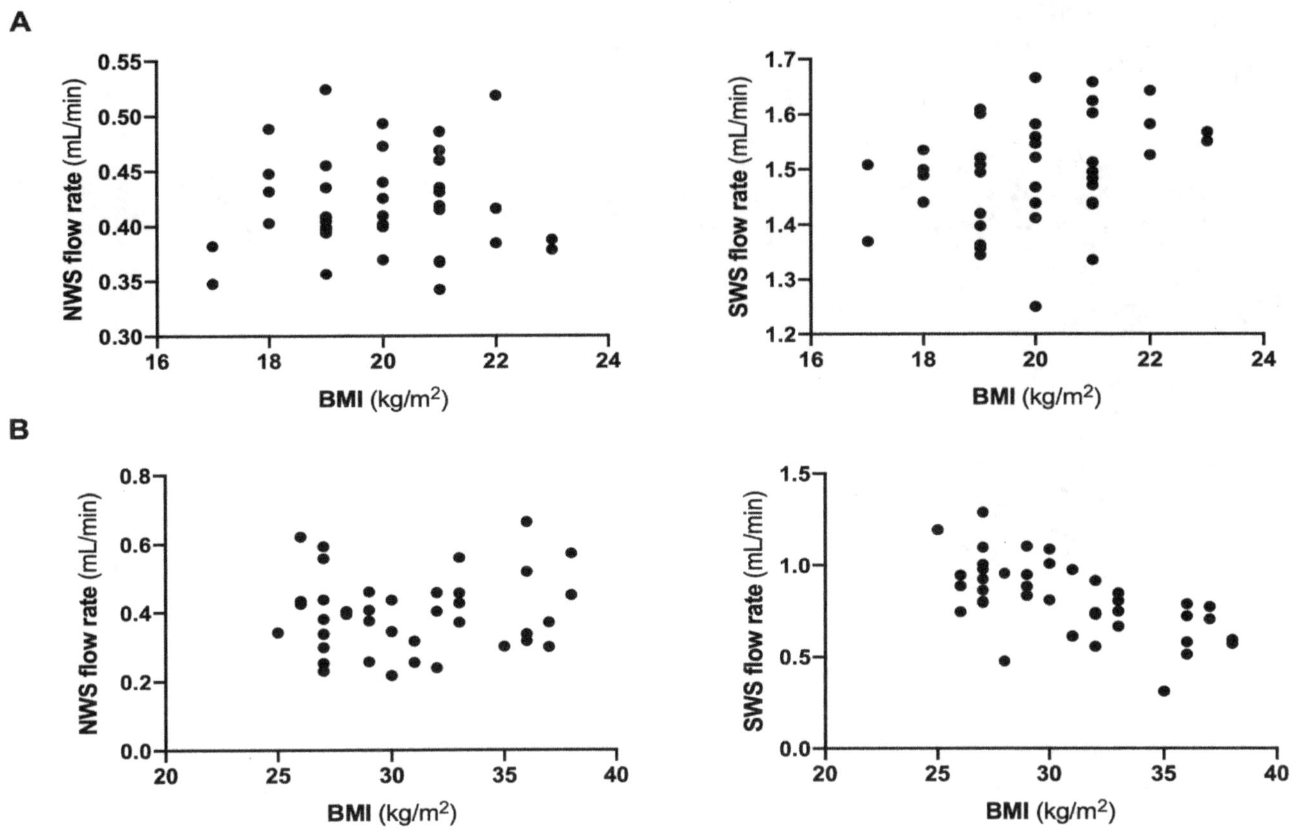

Figure 1. Scatter plots for BMI and non-stimulated and stimulated salivary flow rate in healthy children (**A**) as well as overweight and obese adolescents (**B**). BMI- body mass index; NWS- non-stimulated whole saliva; SWS- stimulated whole saliva.

There were no significant differences in the dental indexes DMFT and GI between the controls and the groups of overweight and obese adolescents (Table 2).

3.2. *Enzymatic Antioxidants*

The activity of SOD in non-stimulated and stimulated saliva of overweight adolescents was significantly higher than in the control group of adolescents with normal weight (↑60%, $p < 0.001$; ↑48%, $p = 0.002$, respectively). Similar significant differences were observed in the group of obese adolescents, in whom SOD activity in non-stimulated and stimulated saliva was significantly higher than in the control group (↑125%, $p < 0.001$; ↑78%, $p < 0.001$, respectively). There were no differences in salivary SOD activity between overweight and obese subjects. SOD activity in erythrocytes of both overweight (↓59%, $p < 0.001$) and obese (↓58%, $p < 0.001$) adolescents was considerably lower than in erythrocytes of teenagers with normal body weight, and did not differ between the study groups.

The activity of CAT in non-stimulated saliva of obese adolescents was significantly higher compared to the controls (↑75%, $p < 0.001$) and overweight adolescents (↑75%, $p < 0.001$).

The activity of CAT in stimulated saliva of overweight (↑62%, $p < 0.001$) and obese (↑90%, $p < 0.001$) adolescents was significantly higher than in the control group. CAT activity in erythrocytes of obese teenagers was considerably lower than in the control group (↓49%, $p < 0.001$) and in overweight adolescents (↓38%, $p = 0.02$).

The activity of Px in non-stimulated saliva did not differ between the study groups and the controls. Px activity in stimulated saliva and erythrocytes of overweight (↑78%, $p < 0.001$; ↑153%, $p < 0.001$, respectively) and obese (↑57%, $p < 0.001$; ↑153%, $p < 0.001$, respectively) adolescents was significantly higher than in saliva and erythrocytes of the control group (Figure 2).

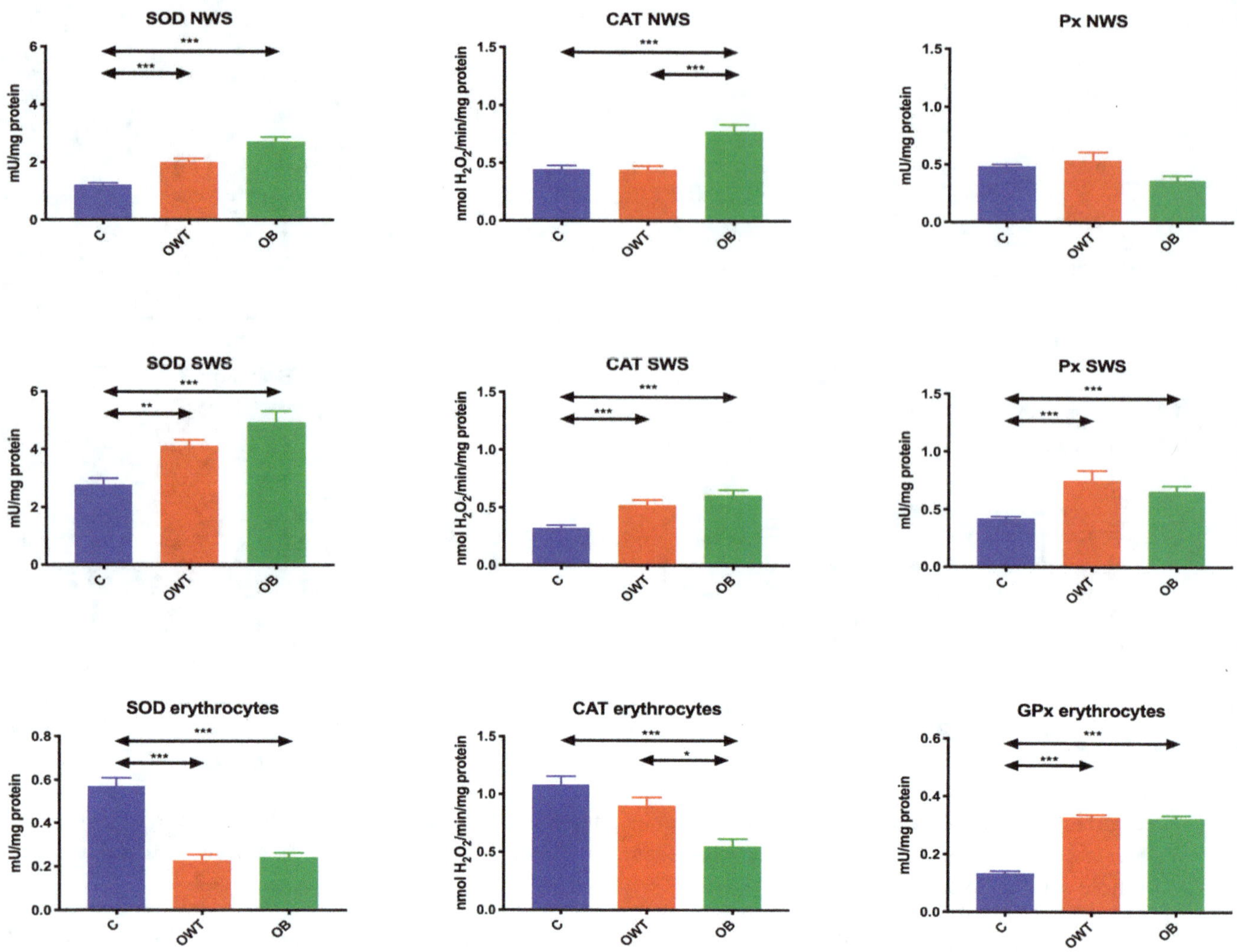

Figure 2. Enzymatic antioxidants in overweight and obese adolescents as well as healthy controls. C- control, CAT- catalase, NWS- non-stimulated whole saliva, OB- obese, OWT- overweight, Px- salivary peroxidase, SOD- superoxide dismutase, SWS- stimulated whole saliva. Differences statistically significant at: * $p < 0.05$, ** $p < 0.005$, *** $p < 0.0005$.

3.3. Non-Enzymatic Antioxidants

The concentration of GSH in non-stimulated and stimulated saliva of overweight (↓47%, $p < 0.001$; ↓26%, $p = 0.005$, respectively) and obese (↓65%, $p < 0.001$; ↓54%, $p < 0.001$, respectively) adolescents was significantly lower than in the control group. However, the GSH concentration in overweight adolescents was significantly higher only in stimulated saliva compared to obese subjects (↑38%, $p < 0.001$). Plasma GSH concentration in obese adolescents was significantly lower than in the control group (↓29%, $p < 0.006$).

The concentration of UA in non-stimulated saliva of obese adolescents was significantly higher than in the controls (↑37%, $p < 0.001$). UA concentration in stimulated saliva of overweight and obese adolescents was considerably higher than in the control group (↑157%, $p < 0.001$; ↑198%, $p < 0.001$, respectively). Plasma UA concentration in overweight and obese adolescents was significantly elevated compared to their peers with normal body weight (↑43%, $p < 0.001$; ↑45%, $p < 0.001$, respectively) (Figure 3).

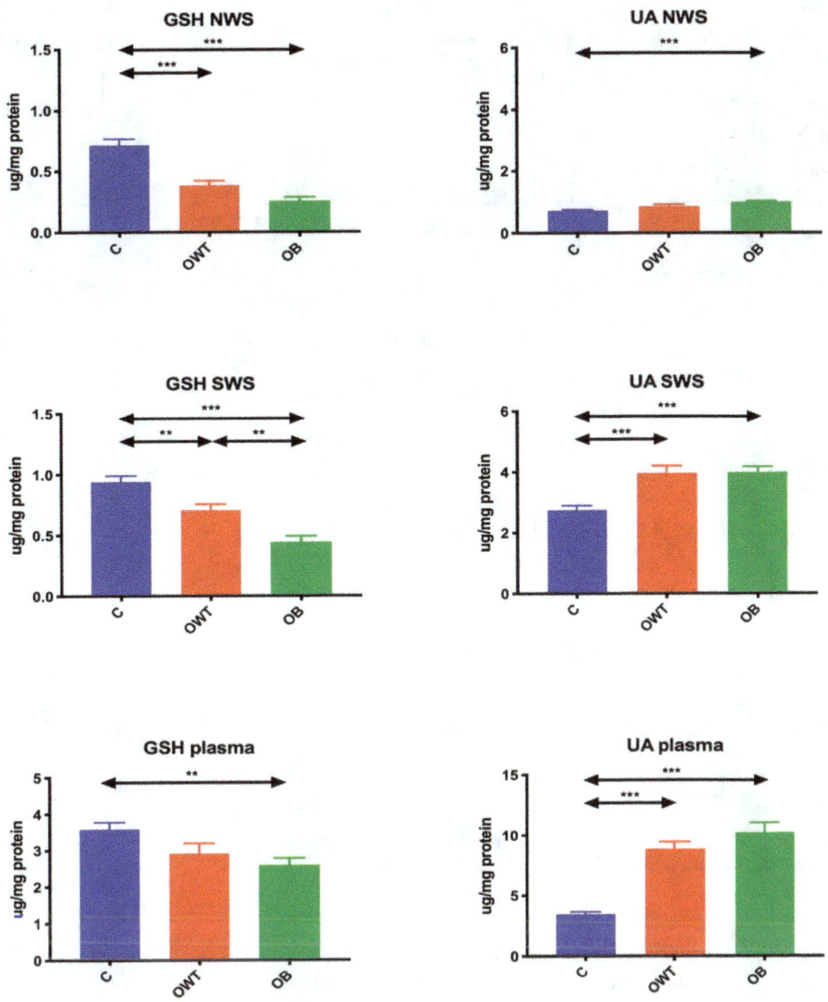

Figure 3. Non-enzymatic antioxidants in overweight and obese adolescents as well as healthy controls. C- control, GSH- reduced glutathione, NWS- non-stimulated whole saliva, OB- obese, OWT- overweight, SWS- stimulated whole saliva, UA- uric acid. Differences statistically significant at: ** $p < 0.005$, *** $p < 0.0005$.

3.4. Redox Status

In overweight and obese adolescents, TAC in non-stimulated (↑110%, $p < 0.001$; ↑122%, $p < 0.001$, respectively) and stimulated (↑62%, $p < 0.001$; ↑56%, $p < 0.001$, respectively) saliva as well as plasma (↑61%, $p < 0.001$; ↑75%, $p < 0.001$, respectively) was considerably higher than in the control group.

TOS in non-stimulated (↑113%, $p < 0.001$; ↑288%, $p < 0.001$, respectively) and stimulated (↑115%, $p < 0.001$; ↑170%, $p < 0.001$, respectively) saliva as well as plasma (↑103%, $p < 0.001$; ↑97%, $p \leq 0.001$, respectively) of overweight and obese adolescents was significantly raised compared to the control group. TOS in non-stimulated (↑129%, $p < 0.001$) and stimulated (↑25%, $p = 0.001$) saliva of obese teenagers was considerably higher than in their overweight peers.

OSI in non-stimulated and stimulated saliva as well as plasma in obese adolescents was significantly higher than in the controls (↑153%, $p < 0.001$; ↑105%, $p = 0.001$; ↑48%, $p = 0.01$, respectively) (Figure 4).

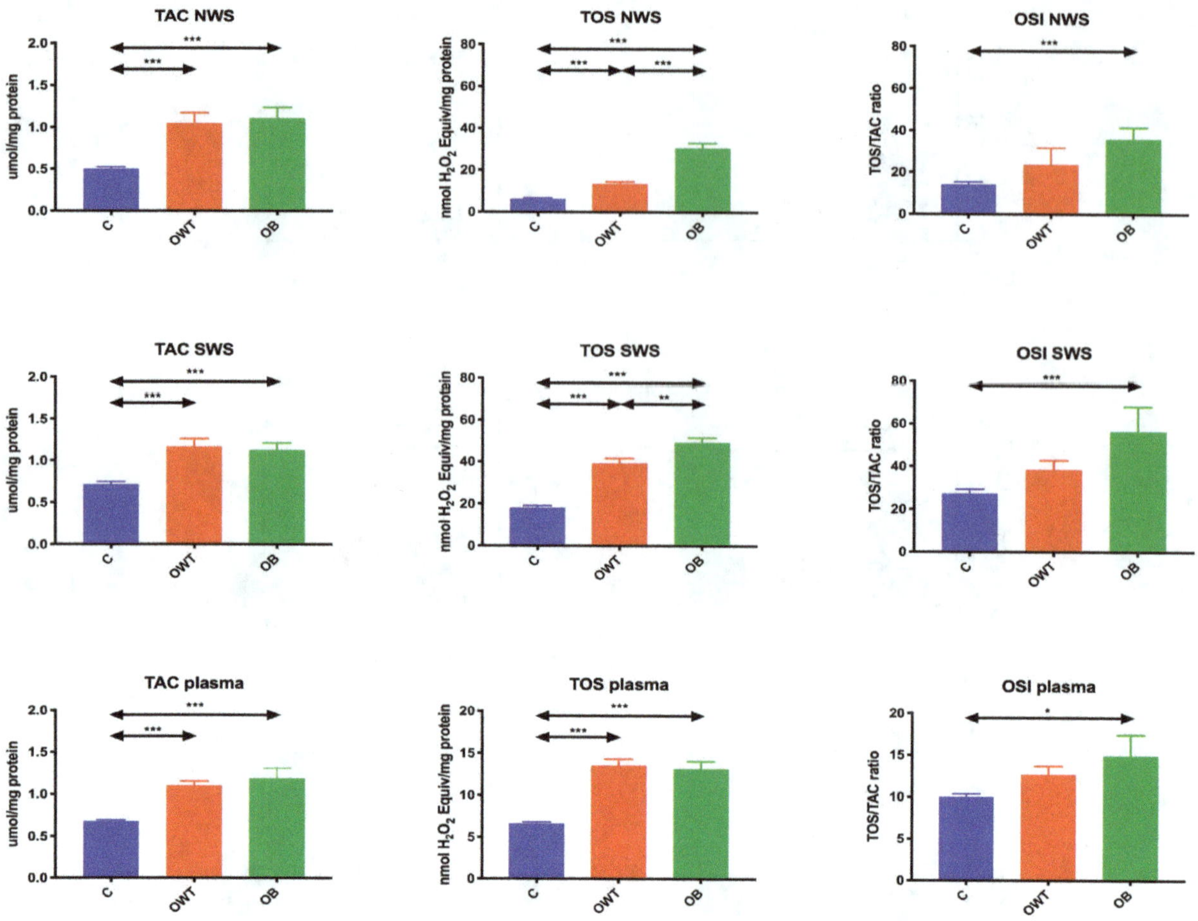

Figure 4. Redox status in overweight and obese adolescents as well as healthy controls. C- control, NWS- non-stimulated whole saliva, OB- obese, OSI- oxidative stress index, OWT- overweight, SWS- stimulated whole saliva, TAC- total antioxidant capacity, TOS- total oxidative status. Differences statistically significant at: * $p < 0.05$, ** $p < 0.005$, *** $p < 0.0005$.

3.5. Oxidation Products

AGEs in non-stimulated and stimulated saliva as well as plasma of both overweight (↑281%, $p < 0.001$; ↑209%, $p < 0.001$; ↑203%, $p < 0.001$, respectively) and obese (↑347%, $p < 0.001$; ↑423%, $p < 0.001$; ↑244%, $p < 0.001$, respectively) adolescents were significantly higher compared to the saliva of the control group. Only AGEs in stimulated saliva of obese adolescents were considerably higher than in overweight adolescents (↑69%, $p < 0.001$).

MDA in non-stimulated and stimulated saliva as well as plasma in both overweight (↑43%, $p < 0.001$; ↑63%, $p = 0.001$; ↑41%, $p < 0.001$, respectively) and obese (↑43%, $p < 0.001$; ↑79%, $p < 0.001$; ↑55%, $p < 0.001$, respectively) teenagers were significantly higher than in saliva of control group adolescents.

The concentration of 4-HNE was notably higher in non-simulated and stimulated saliva as well as plasma of overweight (33% $p = 0.01$; 50% $p < 0.001$; 41% $p = 0.003$) and obese adolescents (84% $p < 0.001$; 95% $p < 0.001$; 104% $p < 0.001$) compared to the control group. The concentration of 4-HNE in non-simulated and stimulated saliva as well as plasma of obese adolescents was considerably higher than in overweight adolescents (37% $p < 0.001$; 50% $p < 0.001$; 43% $p < 0.001$). Similarly, the concentration of 8-OHdG in non-stimulated and stimulated saliva as well as plasma of both overweight (53% $p < 0.001$; 25% $p = 0.04$; 62% $p < 0.001$) and obese adolescents (121% $p < 0.001$; 73% $p < 0.001$; 118% $p < 0.001$) was significantly higher than in saliva and plasma of the controls. The 8-OHdG concentration in non-stimulated and stimulated saliva as well as plasma of obese teenagers was considerably higher than in their overweight peers (43% $p = 0.001$, 38% $p = 0.007$; 34% $p < 0.001$) (Figure 5).

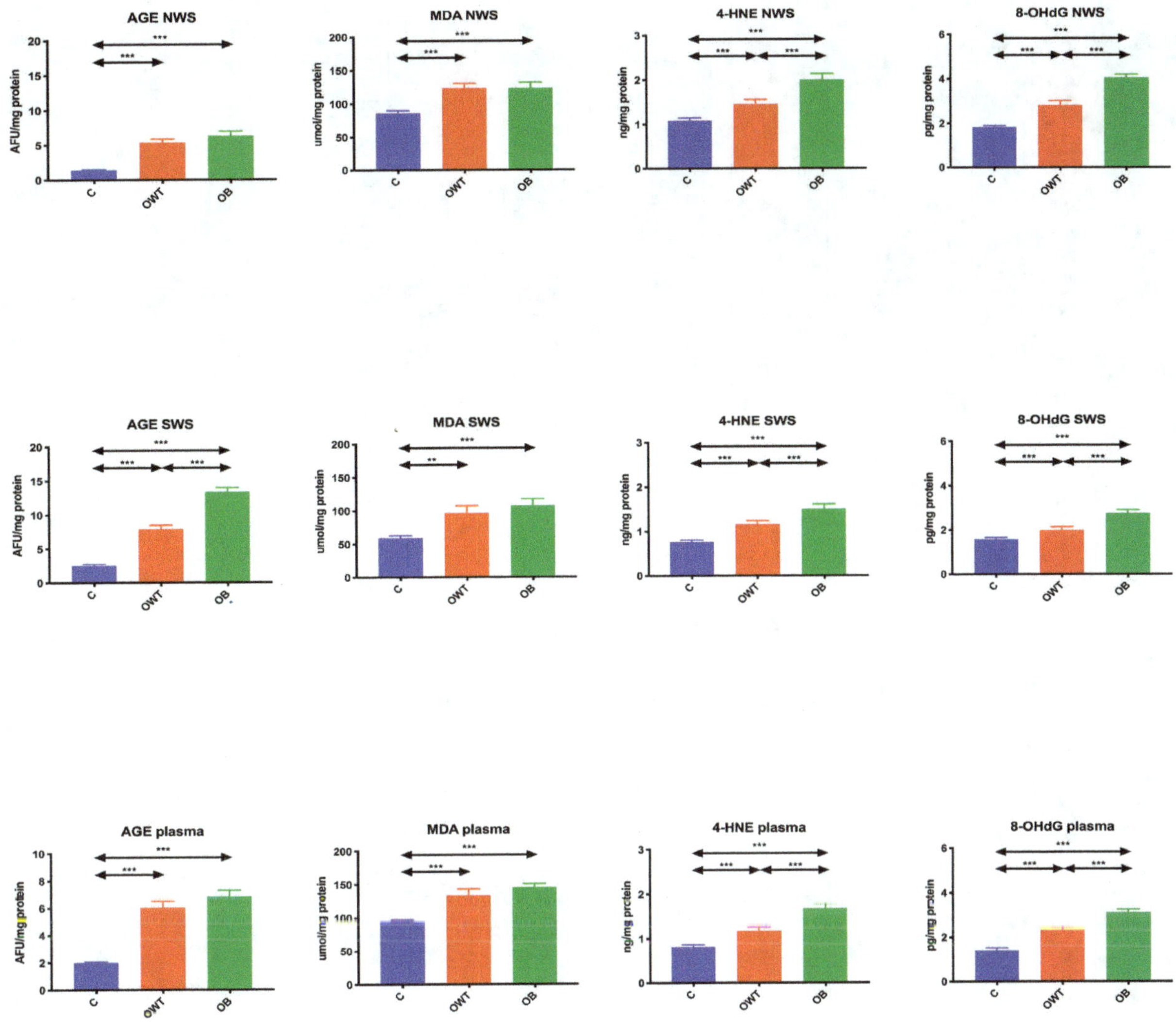

Figure 5. Protein, lipid, and DNA oxidation products in overweight and obese adolescents as well as healthy controls. AGE- advanced glycation end products, C- control, MDA- malondialdehyde, NWS- non-stimulated whole saliva, OB- obese, OWT- overweight, SWS- stimulated whole saliva, 4-HNE- 4-hydroxynoneal protein adduct, 8-OHdG- 8-hydroxy-D-guanosine. Differences statistically significant at: ** $p < 0.005$, *** $p < 0.0005$.

3.6. ROC Analysis

The diagnostic utility of salivary redox parameters to differentiate children who are overweight from those who are obese is presented in Table 3. For this purpose, ROC curves were generated, and then the area under the curve (AUC) was calculated. Optimal cut-off values were determined for each parameter that ensured high sensitivity with high specificity. The maximum AUC value, from 0 to 1, is a parameter that determines the discriminatory power of the test.

Particular attention should be paid to SOD, CAT, TOS and OSI in NWS, GSH and AGE in SWS, and CAT in erythrocytes—the AUC of which is close to 1.0, which differentiates overweight adolescents from obese ones (Figure 6).

Table 3. Receiver operating characteristic (ROC) analysis to differentiate between overweight and obese children.

Parameter	NWS						SWS						Plasma/Erythrocytes					
	AUC	95% Confidence Interval	*p* Value	Cut-Off	Sensitivity (%)	Specificity (%)	AUC	95% Confidence Interval	*p* Value	Cut-Off	Sensitivity (%)	Specificity (%)	AUC	95% Confidence Interval	*p* Value	Cut-Off	Sensitivity (%)	Specificity (%)
Antioxidants																		
SOD (mU/mg protein)	0.7775	0.6222–0.9328	0.0027	>2.469	53.13	63.96	0.615	0.4360–0.7940	0.2134	>4.536	29.93	43.29	0.5325	0.3490–0.7160	0.7251	>0.2348	38.66	38.66
CAT (nmol H_2O_2/min/mg protein)	0.8875	0.7711–1.000	<0.0001	>0.5747	63.96	69.90	0.6675	0.4954–0.8396	0.0699	>0.5692	43.29	48.10	0.795	0.6515–0.9385	0.0014	<0.6559	53.13	53.13
Px/GPx (mU/mg protein)	0.6575	0.4818–0.8332	0.0884	<0.4494	43.29	38.66	0.5525	0.3675–0.7375	0.57	<0.6815	38.66	34.21	0.5	0.3167–0.6833	>0.9999	>0.3117	34.21	29.93
GSH (μg/mg protein)	0.7	0.5359–0.8641	0.0305	<0.3304	53.1	43.29	0.7925	0.6531–0.9319	0.0016	<0.5908	53.13	48.10	0.5875	0.4058–0.7692	0.3438	<2.823	43.29	34.21
UA (ng/mg protein)	0.67	0.5018–0.8382	0.0659	>0.8843	48.10	34.21	0.5075	0.3247–0.6903	0.9353	>3.912	29.93	29.93	0.6125	0.4345–0.7905	0.2235	>9.354	38.66	43.29
Redox Status																		
TAC (Trolox μmol/mg protein)	0.52	0.3370–0.7030	0.8287	>1.018	34.21	29.93	0.5175	0.3348–0.7002	0.8498	>1.202	29.93	38.66	0.5425	0.3511–0.7339	0.6456	>1.143	34.21	38.66
TOS (nmol H_2O_2 Equiv./mg protein)	0.9325	0.8344–1.000	<0.0001	>20.77	90	100	0.7425	0.5847–0.9003	0.0087	>45.71	70	80	0.55	0.3685–0.7315	0.5885	<14.48	34.21	29.93
OSI (TOS/TAC ratio)	0.7875	0.6377–0.9373	0.0019	>20.12	80	75	0.655	0.4836–0.8264	0.0935	>38.18	65	60	0.5525	0.3664–0.7386	0.57	<12.63	43.29	34.21
Oxidative Damage																		
AGE (AFU/mg protein)	0.5825	0.3937–0.7713	0.372	>6.116	38.66	48.10	0.9325	0.8547–1.000	<0.0001	>10.24	69.90	69.90	0.6175	0.4395–0.7955	0.2036	>6.360	38.66	38.66
MDA (μmol/mg protein)	0.5325	0.3480–0.7170	0.7251	>127.4	38.66	38.66	0.565	0.3828–0.7472	0.4819	>98.43	43.29	34.21	0.6625	0.4817–0.8433	0.0787	>143.0	53.13	48.10
4-HNE (ng/mg protein)	0.7625	0.6138–0.9112	0.0045	>1.787	65	70	0.705	0.5400–0.8700	0.0265	>1.268	70	70	0.81	0.6730–0.9470	0.0008	>1.386	75	80
8-OHdG (pg/mg protein)	0.8625	0.7452–0.9798	<0.0001	<3.440	80	80	0.795	0.6501–0.9399	0.0014	<2.226	75	80	0.8075	0.6761–0.9389	0.0009	>2.690	65	70

AGE- advanced glycation end products, CAT- catalase, GSH- reduced glutathione, MDA- malondialdehyde, NWS- non-stimulated whole saliva, OSI- oxidative stress index, Px- salivary peroxidase, SOD- superoxide dismutase, SWS- stimulated whole saliva, TAC- total antioxidant capacity, TOS- total oxidative status, UA- uric acid, 4-HNE- 4-hydroxynoneal protein adduct, 8-OHdG- 8-hydroxy-D-guanosine.

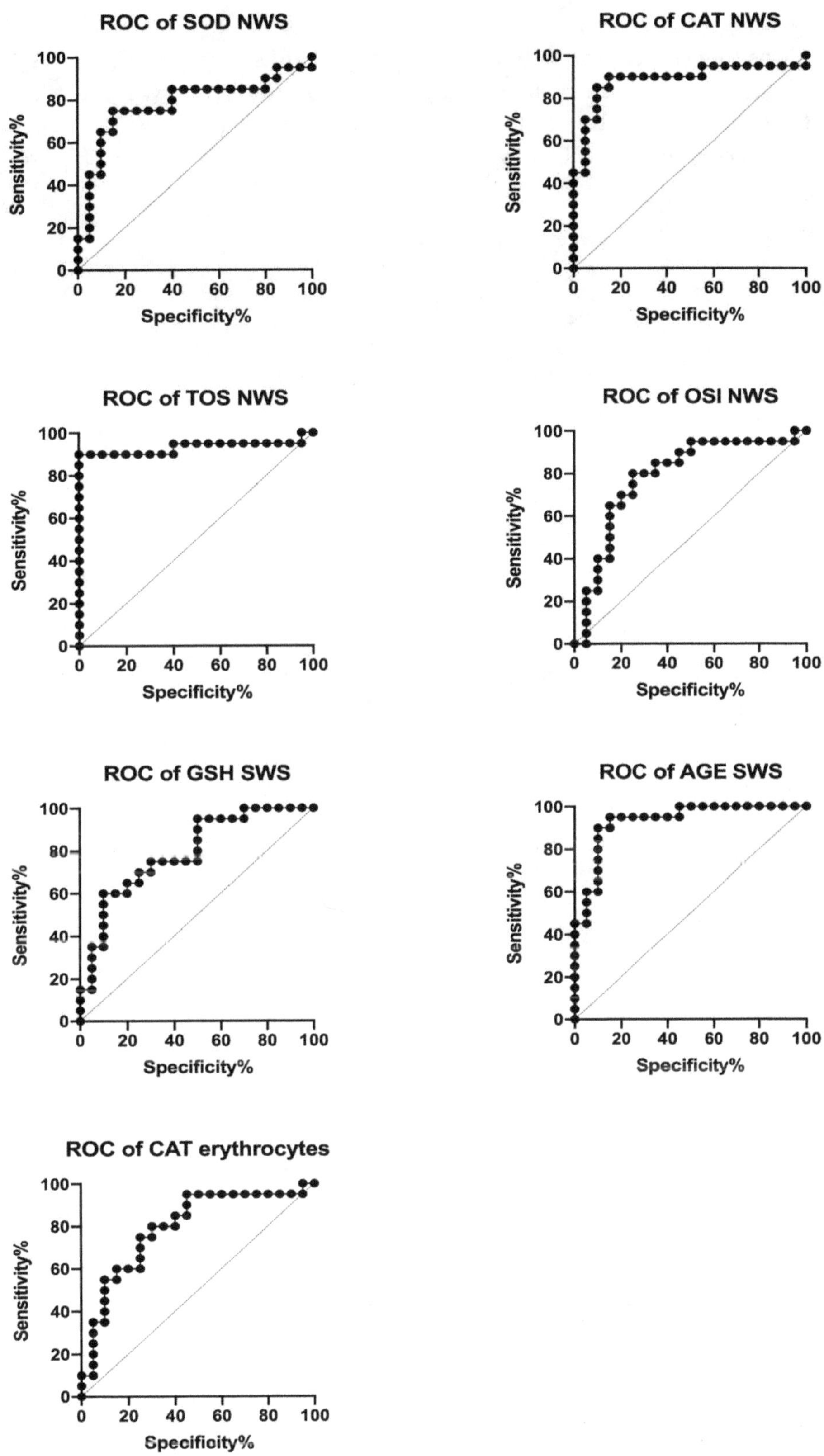

Figure 6. Area under the curve (AUC) of selected redox biomarkers in overweight and obese children. AGE- advanced glycation end products, CAT- catalase, GSH- reduced glutathione, NWS- non-stimulated whole saliva, OSI- oxidative stress index, SOD- superoxide dismutase, SWS- stimulated whole saliva, TOS- total oxidative status, UA- uric acid, 4-HNE- 4-hydroxynoneal protein adduct,.

3.7. Correlations

We showed a positive correlation between erythrocyte and salivary CAT and TAC in overweight and obese adolescents. We also demonstrated a positive correlation between UA content in plasma and non-stimulated/stimulated saliva of the study group patients (Figure 7B). However, we did not observe a saliva–blood correlation of UA in healthy children and adolescents (Figure 7A).

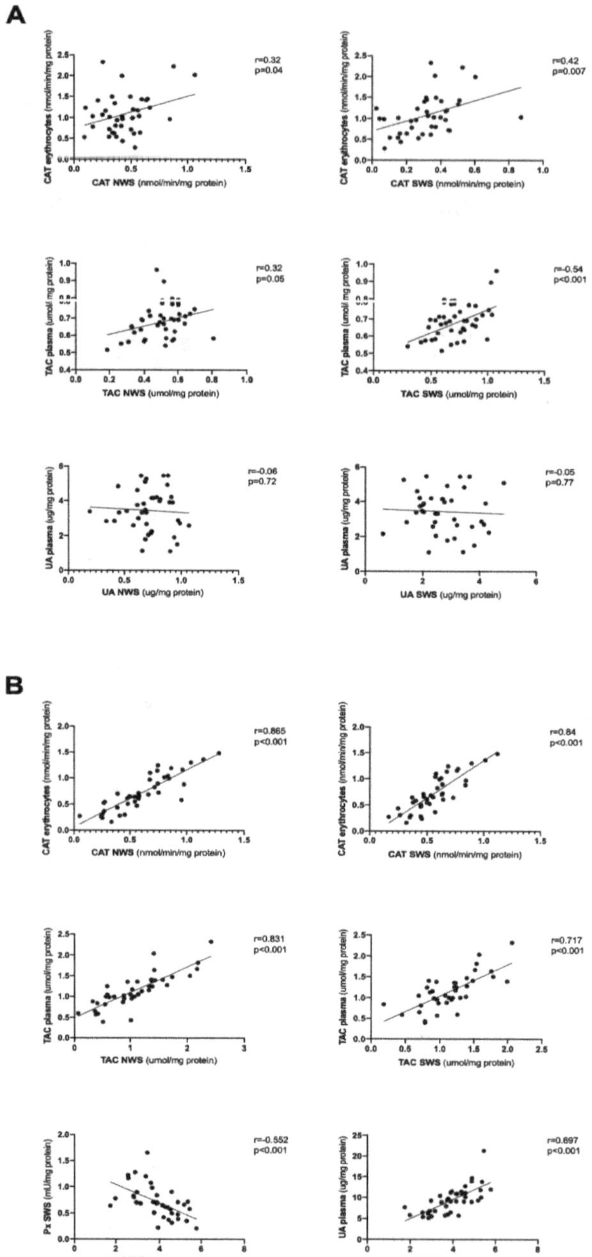

Figure 7. Saliva–blood correlations of the analyzed redox biomarkers in healthy controls (**A**) as well as overweight and obese adolescents (**B**). CAT- catalase, NWS- non-stimulated whole saliva, SWS- stimulated whole saliva, TAC- total antioxidant capacity, UA- uric acid.

Correlations between BMI and salivary redox biomarkers and presented in Figures 8 and 9. Interestingly, BMI correlates with most salivary antioxidants and oxidative damage products but only in the study group.

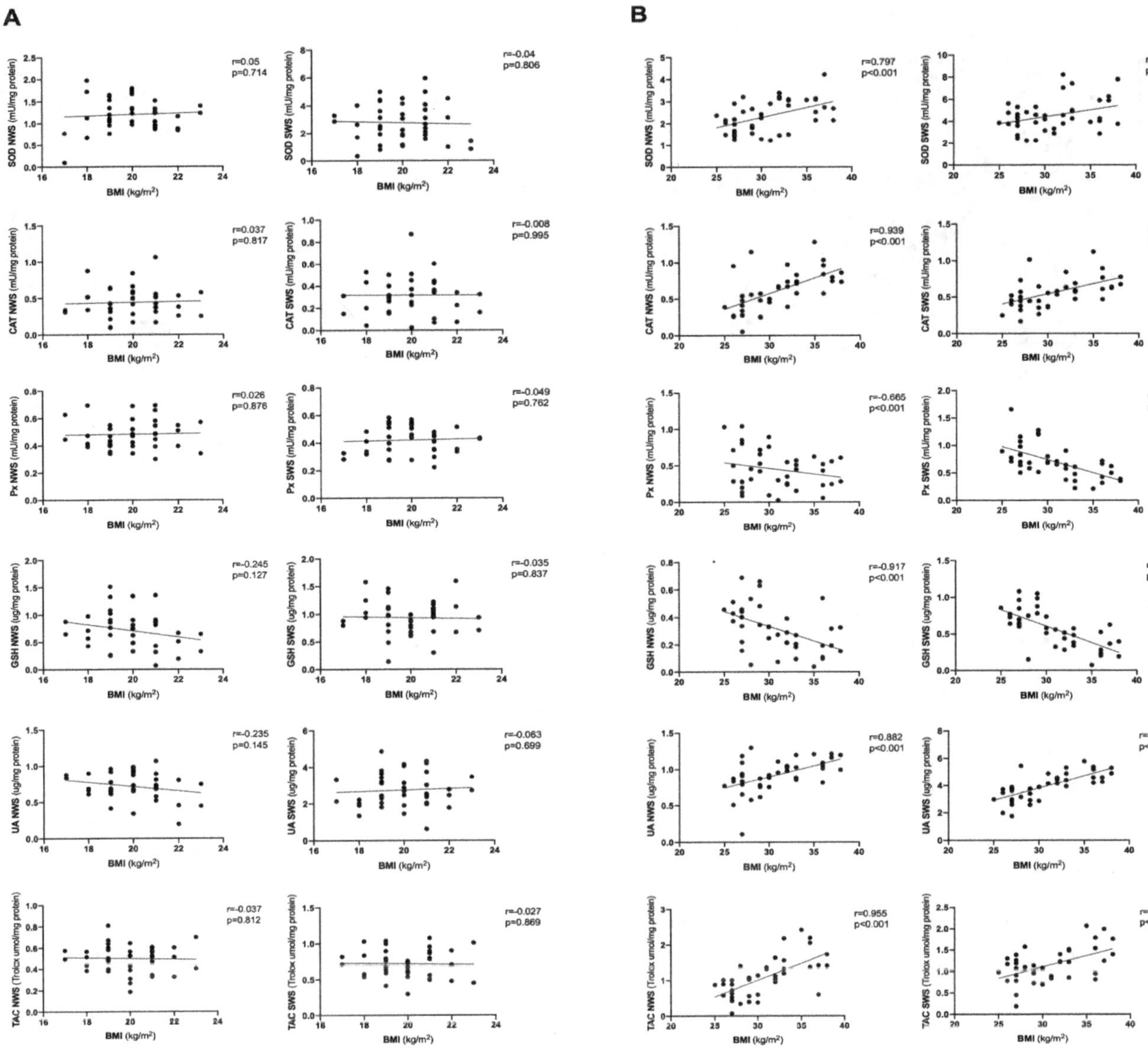

Figure 8. Correlations between BMI and salivary antioxidants in healthy children (**A**) as well as overweight and obese adolescents (**B**). BMI- body mass index, CAT- catalase, GSH- reduced glutathione, NWS- non-stimulated whole saliva, Px- salivary peroxidase, SOD- superoxide dismutase, SWS- stimulated whole saliva, TAC- total antioxidant capacity, UA- uric acid.

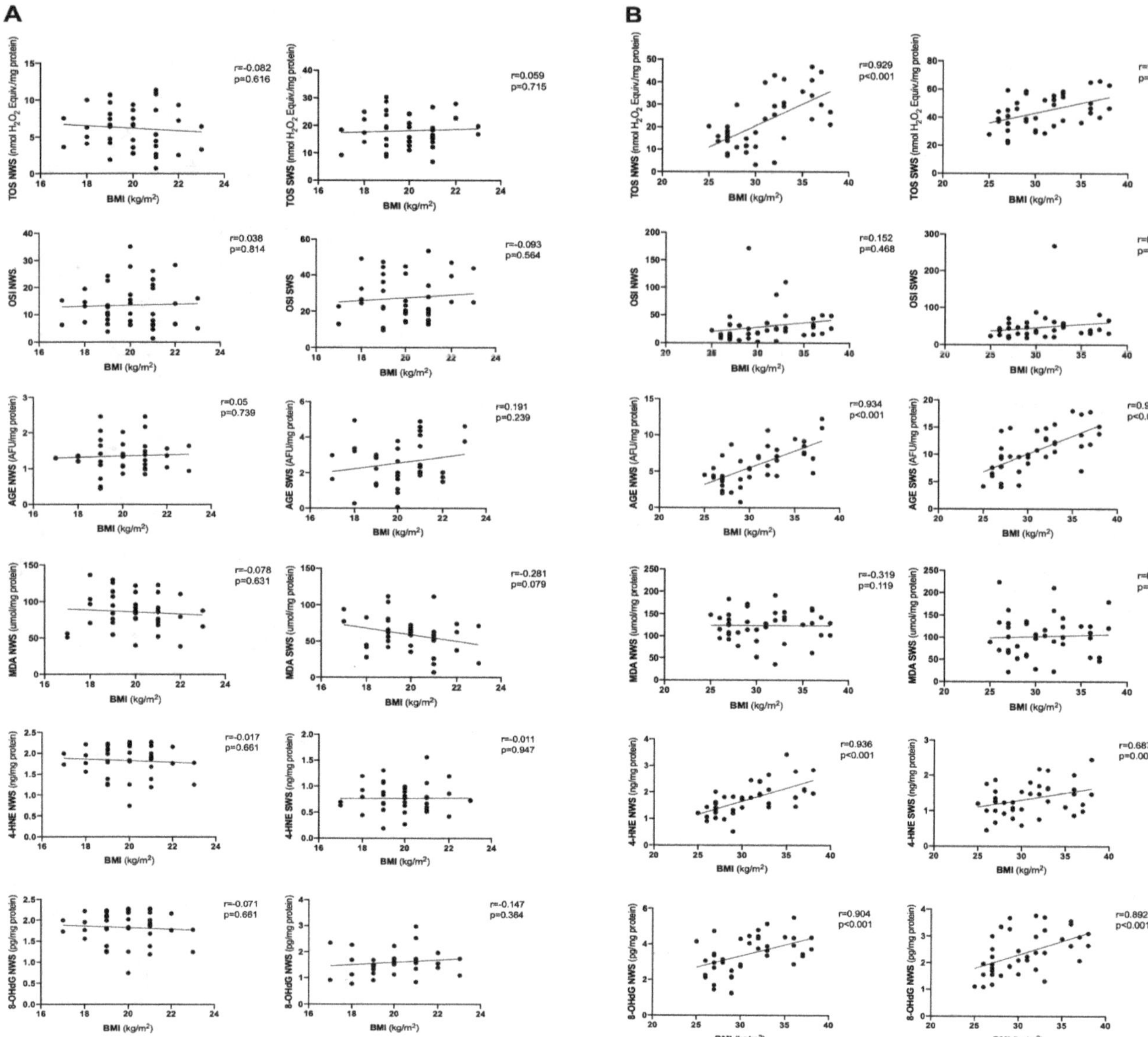

Figure 9. Correlations between BMI and salivary oxidative damage in healthy children (**A**) as well as overweight and obese adolescents (**B**). BMI- body mass index, AGE- advanced glycation end products, MDA- malondialdehyde, NWS- non-stimulated whole saliva, OSI- oxidative stress index, SWS- stimulated whole saliva, TOS- total oxidative status, 4-HNE- 4-hydroxynoneal protein adduct, 8-OHdG- 8-hydroxy-D-guanosine.

4. Discussion

This publication is the first to analyze redox balance in the saliva of overweight and obese adolescents. Generally, we demonstrated disturbances in the activity/concentration of antioxidants as well as oxidative stress in non-stimulated and stimulated saliva of both examined groups compared to their peers with normal body weight, with a higher intensity of oxidative modifications in the saliva of obese adolescents.

Excessive body weight is characterized by chronic (low-grade) inflammation with permanently elevated OS. It has been demonstrated that adipose tissue induces the synthesis of proinflammatory cytokines, such as TNFα, IL-1 and IL-6, which increase the generation of ROS and nitrogen radicals by macrophages and monocytes. ROS production promotes inflammation and expression of molecules as well as growth factors by redox-sensitive transcription factors, mainly NF-κB and the NADPH oxidase pathway [33,34]. The inefficiency of antioxidant systems, observed in the plasma of obese individuals [16], entails oxidative damage to cellular components and development of obesity-related complications.

It has been shown that obesity results in the dysfunction of salivary glands as well as changes in salivary flow and composition [15–17,35]. As saliva is essential for maintaining appropriate functions of the body, such as swallowing, chewing, carbohydrate digestion, healing of the oral mucosa and tooth enamel remineralization, it is not surprising that excessive body weight increases the risk of gingivitis [36], periodontitis [37], caries [38,39] and inflammatory changes in the oral cavity mucosa [40]. Recently, a significant influence of OS has been increasingly emphasized in explaining the pathogenesis of salivary gland lesions in the course of overweight/obesity in adults [16,17,41]. To the best of our knowledge, there have been no studies evaluating redox balance in the oral cavity of overweight and obese adolescents.

The study by Brown et al. [42] demonstrated that failure of antioxidant systems is related to the duration of obesity. Considering that our study covered adolescents aged 11 to 18 with relatively short overweight/obesity history (4/4.3 years, respectively, data not shown), it is not surprising that salivary and plasma TAC (the sum of both enzymatic and non-enzymatic antioxidants) as well as the content of enzymatic antioxidants were elevated in both non-stimulated and stimulated saliva of overweight and obese adolescents. Therefore, the higher activity of enzymatic antioxidants may be an expression of a highly effective antioxidant barrier that has not been exhausted in oxidative stress conditions. On the other hand, a significant increase in salivary TAC and enzymatic antioxidants as well as, generally, plasma biomarkers (despite the decline in SOD activity, which we explain further) can be considered as a positive adaptative response to the increased ROS generation (↑TOS in plasma as well as non-stimulated and stimulated saliva of both study groups). It was demonstrated that decreased activity of antioxidant enzymes in erythrocytes, accompanying increased plasma TAC, is likely to result from cell damage due to an inflammatory process and leakage of enzymes into the extracellular space [43]. On the other hand, it may result from the use of enzymes in the process of ROS control, or from inactivation of enzymes by free radicals [44].

Interestingly, we found a significant positive correlation between erythrocyte and salivary CAT and TAC in overweight and obese adolescents, which suggests that these salivary parameters could assess the general antioxidant status of overweight and obese adolescents.

Uric acid constitutes 40% of the antioxidant potential of saliva [45]; however, it has been found that at high concentrations it can induce and intensify oxidative damage [46]. Obesity has been demonstrated to increase UA concentration by reducing its renal secretion and accumulating metabolites for UA production [47], which was confirmed by our study. We observed an increase in uric acid concentration both in plasma and stimulated saliva of overweight and obese adolescents as well as in non-stimulated saliva of the latter. The negative correlation between the concentrations of UA and protein in non-stimulated saliva of overweight and obese adolescents, as well as the negative correlation between UA content and Px activity in stimulated saliva, suggest that in both groups UA shifts salivary redox balance towards oxidation and does not oxidize hydroxyl or peroxyl radicals, preventing OS. Moreover, we demonstrated a positive correlation between UA levels in plasma and stimulated saliva of overweight and obese subjects. Considering that plasma UA is a strong predictor of future development of type 2 diabetes [48], measurements of salivary UA may be useful in assessing the risk of this disease.

Although changes in the activity/concentration of antioxidants or ROS concentration may suggest redox imbalance, they are not sufficient to determine the existence and extent of OS. The most reliable determinants of oxidative stress are increased concentrations of oxidative damage products [49,50]. There are numerous markers of oxidative damage to biomolecules; in our study, we assessed 4-HNE protein adducts, MDA, AGE and 8-OHdG. These are only few selected markers, which should be taken into account when interpreting the presented results. The use of other OS indicators could change our observations and conclusions.

Our research showed, however, that the overproduction of free radicals exceeds the capabilities of antioxidant systems of the examined adolescents at the central level as well as in both salivary glands, which was observed as increased concentration of oxidative modification products in plasma and non-stimulated as well as stimulated saliva. It should be noted that intensified oxidative modifications reveal a certain tendency (AGE and MDA in plasma and non-stimulated saliva; MDA in stimulated saliva) or are significantly higher (4-HNE, 8-OHdG in plasma and stimulated and non-stimulated saliva, and AGE in stimulated saliva) in obese adolescents compared to their overweight peers. The obtained results prove that oxidative damage occurred in the salivary glands of overweight adolescents, and was more severe in obese subjects. We noted a significant increase of TOS in non-stimulated and stimulated saliva in obese adolescents compared to the overweight group, but observed no such dependence for TAC and antioxidant enzymes (except CAT in non-stimulated saliva). In our opinion, this is a worrying phenomenon and may be evidence of the beginning of subclinical inefficiency of antioxidant mechanisms, leading to the boost of oxidative damage to the salivary glands of obese adolescents.

We demonstrated that in both non-stimulated and stimulated saliva of overweight and obese patients, GSH levels were significantly decreased and considerably lower in the stimulated saliva of patients with obesity compared to overweight ones. Our results suggest that, GSH is the first to be used up, and perhaps forms the first line of defense against free radicals, which can be easily explained. The main function of GSH is maintaining thiol groups of proteins in a reduced state, which is often necessary for preserving the functional activity of these proteins. It has been shown that the most probable primary object of ROS attack is proteins, and, according to this theory, fatty and nucleic acids are protected by proteins and therefore undergo oxidation at a later stage [51]. A mediator of biomolecule damage in cells is the hydroxyl radical ($OH^{\cdot}$) [52]. It was shown that the percentage share of primary substrates of the $OH^{\cdot}$ reaction is 75% proteins, 21% lipids, and 4% DNA, which is related to the specificity of the mechanism of $OH^{\cdot}$ radical production in the Fenton reaction [52].

It is worth mentioning that the stimulation of saliva secretion activates parotid glands, while at rest the main source of saliva is the submandibular glands. Therefore, it was assumed that any disturbances in secretion/composition of non-stimulated saliva reflects disturbances of the submandibular gland function, and disturbed secretion/composition of stimulated saliva indicates disturbed activity of parotid glands [53].

The ability of salivary glands of overweight and obese adolescents to secrete saliva at rest was similar to the results of their peers of normal weight. Protein secretion by submandibular glands of the examined adolescents also did not differ from the control group of normal weight. In relation to the stimulated salivary flow, overweight and obese subjects showed reduced salivary secretion compared to the control group, which is consistent with the results of Modéer et al. [38]. Moreover, the dysfunction of parotid glands intensified with the increase in BMI, as obese adolescents produce significantly less stimulated saliva than their overweight peers, and in 8 obese individuals we recorded the salivary flow value of 0.7 mL/min, which is classified as hyposalivation. Modéer et al. [38] claimed that BMI SDS may be a potential factor to exclude subjects with reduced flow of stimulated saliva. Protein concentration in SWS of overweight and obese adolescents was also reduced compared to the controls. The decrease in stimulated saliva secretion and protein concentration is most probably caused by steatosis of the parotid (but not submandibular) glands observed in obese patients, which decreases the number of secretory units (acini and ducts) [54,55]. It can also be assumed that obesity-related inflammatory milieu (up-regulation of proinflammatory cytokines, ROS), similarly to Sjögren's syndrome [56], activates metalloproteinases, thus disrupting the stromal tissue. This phenomenon may disturb the neurotransmission between the residual neural network and residual secretory units, as well as inhibit the response of follicular cells [57,58].

Our study showed reduced salivary production and enhanced oxidative stress in overweight and obese teenagers. However, in obese children, alterations in salivary gland function are more severe than those who are overweight. This is also reflected in the redox status of saliva (greater disturbances in the antioxidant barrier) as well as higher severity of oxidative damage in children with obesity vs. overweight.

5. Conclusions

Obese and overweight adolescents present impaired systemic and salivary oxidative status in contrast to their normal weight peers.

Both parotid and submandibular salivary glands lose the ability to maintain redox balance at the level observed in the control group, which was shown by an increased level of oxidized biomolecules. However, redox equilibrium in our study was more disturbed in the saliva and plasma of obese adolescents compared to overweight subjects.

Excess of adipose tissue and deficiency of GSH are the main factors responsible for oxidative damage to the salivary glands.

Dysfunction of parotid glands in relation to salivary secretion deepens with the increase of BMI. Dysfunction of mechanisms responsible for protein synthesis/secretion observed at the overweight stage does not worsen with the increase of body weight in adolescents.

Determinations of salivary CAT and TAC could be used to assess the central antioxidant status of overweight and obese adolescents.

Author Contributions: Conceptualization, A.Z., M.M.; Data curation, A.Z. and M.M.;A.K., S.Z., Formal analysis, A.Z. and M.M. A.K., S.Z.; Funding acquisition, A.Z.; Investigation, A.Z. and M.M.; Methodology, A.Z., M.M., Material collection: A.K., K.F., M.S., P.K-S., Supervision, A.Z., K.T-J., A.W.; Validation, A.Z. and M.M.; Visualization, A.Z. and M.M.; Writing—original draft, A.Z. and M.M.; Writing—review and editing, A.Z. and M.M. All authors have read and agreed to the published version of the manuscript.

References

1. Marseglia, L.; Manti, S.; D'Angelo, G.; Nicotera, A.; Parisi, E.; Di Rosa, G.; Gitto, E.; Arrigo, T. Oxidative stress in obesity: A critical component in human diseases. *Int. J. Mol. Sci.* **2014**, *16*, 378–400. [CrossRef]
2. Rowicka, G.; Dylag, H.; Ambroszkiewicz, J.; Riahi, A.; Weker, H.; Chelchowska, M. Total Oxidant and Antioxidant Status in Prepubertal Children with Obesity. *Oxid. Med. Cell. Longev.* **2017**. [CrossRef] [PubMed]
3. Matczuk, J.; Zalewska, A.; Łukaszuk, B.; Knaś, M.; Maciejczyk, M.; Grabowska, M.; Ziembicka, D.M.; Waszkiel, D.; Chabowski, A.; Żendzian-Piotrowska, M.; et al. Insulin resistance and obesity affect lipid profile in the salivary glands. *J. Diabetes Res.* **2016**. [CrossRef] [PubMed]
4. WHO. Global Database on Body Mass Index. Available online: http://www.who.int/bmi (accessed on 16 January 2020).
5. Freedman, D.S.; Khan, L.K.; Serdula, M.K.; Dietz, W.H.; Srinivasan, S.R.; Berenson, G.S. The relation of childhood BMI to adult adiposity: The Bogalusa Heart Study. *Pediatrics* **2005**, *115*, 22–27. [CrossRef] [PubMed]
6. Knaś, M.; Maciejczyk, M.; Waszkiel, D.; Zalewska, A. Oxidative stress and salivary antioxidants. *Dent. Med. Probl.* **2013**, *50*, 461–466.
7. Holven, K.B.; Ulven, S.M.; Bogsrud, M.P. Hyperlipidemia and cardiovascular disease with focus on familial hypercholesterolemia. *Curr. Opin. Lipidol.* **2017**, *28*, 445–447. [CrossRef]
8. Kurek, K.; Miklosz, A.; Lukaszuk, B.; Chabowski, A.; Gorski, J.; Zendzian-Piotrowska, M. Inhibition of Ceramide De Novo Synthesis Ameliorates Diet Induced Skeletal Muscles Insulin Resistance. *J. Diabetes Res.* **2015**. [CrossRef]
9. Outon, S.; Galceran, I.; Pascual, J.; Oliveras, A. Central blood pressure in morbid obesity and after bariatric surgery. *Nefrologia* **2019**. [CrossRef]
10. Greig, F.; Hyman, S.; Wallach, E.; Hildebrandt, T.; Rapaport, R. Which obese youth are at increased risk for type 2 diabetes? Latent class analysis and comparison with diabetic youth. *Pediatr. Diabetes* **2012**, *13*, 181–188. [CrossRef]
11. Sanchez, A.; Furberg, H.; Kuo, F.; Vuong, L.; Ged, Y.; Patil, S.; Ostrovnaya, I.; Petruzella, S.; Reising, A.; Patel, P.; et al. Transcriptomic signatures related to the obesity paradox in patients with clear cell renal cell carcinoma: A cohort study. *Lancet Oncol.* **2019**. [CrossRef]

12. Gerdin, E.W.; Angbratt, M.; Aronsson, K.; Eriksson, E.; Johansson, I. Dental caries and body mass index by socio-economic status in Swedish children. *Commun. Dent. Oral. Epidemiol.* **2008**, *36*, 459–465. [CrossRef] [PubMed]
13. Willerhausen, B.; Blettner, M.; Kasaj, A.; Hohenfellner, K. Association between body mass index and dental health in 1,290 children of elementary schools in a German city. *Clin. Oral. Invesitg.* **2007**, *11*, 195–200. [CrossRef]
14. Zeigler, C.C.; Persson, G.R.; Wondimu, B.; Marcus, C.; Sobko, T.; Modèer, T. Microbiota in the oral subgingival biofilm is associated with obesity in adolescence. *Obesity* **2012**, *20*, 157–164. [CrossRef] [PubMed]
15. Chielle, E.O.; Casarin, J.N. Evaluation of salivary oxidative parameters in overweight and obese young adults. *Arch. Epidemiol. Metab.* **2017**, *61*, 152–159. [CrossRef] [PubMed]
16. Knaś, M.; Maciejczyk, M.; Sawicka, K.; Hady Razak, H.; Niczyporuk, M.; Ładny, J.R.; Matczuk, J.; Waszkiel, D.; Żendzian-Piotrowska, M.; Zalewska, A. Impact of morbid obesity and bariatric surgery on antioxidant/oxidant balance of the unstimulated and stimulated saliva. *J. Oral. Pathol. Med.* **2016**, *45*, 455–464. [CrossRef]
17. Fejfer, K.; Buczko, P.; Niczyporuk, M.; Ładny, J.R.; Hady, R.H.; Knaś, M.; Waszkiel, D.; Klimiuk, A.; Zalewska, A.; Maciejczyk, M. Oxidative Modicication of biomolecules in the nonstiumulated and stimulated saliva of patients with morbid obesity treated with bariatric surgery. *BioMed Res. Int.* **2017**. [CrossRef]
18. Narotzki, B.; Reznick, A.Z.; Mitki, T.; Aizenbud, D.; Levy, Y. Enhanced cardiovascular risk and altered oxidative status in elders with moderate excessive body fat. *Rejuvenation Res.* **2014**, *17*, 334–340. [CrossRef]
19. Cole, T.J.; Green, P.J. Smoothing reference centile curves: The LMS method and penalized likelihood. *Stat. Med.* **1992**, *11*, 1305–1319. [CrossRef]
20. WHO. *WHO Child Growth Standards: Length/Height-for-Age, Weight-for-Age, Weight-for-Length, Weight-for-Height and Body Mass Index-Forage: Methods and Development*; WHO: Genewa, Switzerland, 2006.
21. De Onis, M.; Lobstein, T. Defining obesity risk status in the general childhood population: Which cut-offs should we use? *Int. J. Pediatr. Obese.* **2010**, *5*, 458–460. [CrossRef]
22. Mansson-Rahemtulla, B.; Baldone, D.C.; Pruitt, K.M.; Rahemtulla, F. Specific assays for peroxidases in human saliva. *Arch. Oral. Biol.* **1986**, *31*, 661–668. [CrossRef]
23. Aebi, H. Catalase in vitro. *Methods Enzymol.* **1984**, *105*, 121–126. [PubMed]
24. Misra, H.P.; Fridovich, I. The role of superoxide anion in the autoxidation of epinephrine and a simple assay for superoxide dismutase. *J. Biol. Chem.* **1972**, *247*, 3170–3175. [PubMed]
25. Griffith, O.W. Determination of glutathione and glutathione disulfide using glutathione reductase and 2-vinylpyridine. *Anal. Biochem.* **1980**, *106*, 207–212. [CrossRef]
26. Erel, O. A novel automated direct measurement method for total antioxidant capacity using a new generation, more stable ABTS radical cation. *Clin. Biochem.* **2004**, *37*, 227–285. [CrossRef] [PubMed]
27. Erel, O. A new automated colorimetric method for measuring total oxidant status. *Clin. Biochem.* **2005**, *38*, 1103–1111. [CrossRef]
28. Kołodziej, U.; Maciejczyk, M.; Niklińska, W.; Waszkiel, D.; Żendzian-Piotrowska, M.; Żukowski, P.; Zalewska, A. Chronic high-protein diet induces oxidative stress and alters the salivary gland function in rats. *Arch. Oral. Biol.* **2017**, *84*, 6–12. [CrossRef]
29. Abuelo, A.; Hernandez, J.; Benedito, J.L.; Castillo, C. Oxidative stress index (OSI) as a new tool to assess redox status in dairy cattle during transition period. *Animal* **2013**, *7*, 1374–1378. [CrossRef]
30. Kalousová, M.; Skrha, J.; Zima, T. Advanced glycation end-products and advanced oxidation protein products in patients with diabetes mellitus. *Physiol. Res.* **2002**, *51*, 597–604.
31. Maciejczyk, M.; Zalewska, A.; Ladny, J.R. Salivary Antioxidant Barrier, Redox Status, and Oxidative Damage to Proteins and Lipids in Healthy Children, Adults, and the Elderly. *Oxid. Med. Cell. Longev.* **2019**. [CrossRef]
32. Buege, J.A.; Aust, S.D. Microsomal lipid peroxidation. *Methods Enzymol.* **1978**, *52*, 302–310.
33. Farhangi, M.A.; Mesgari-Abbasi, M.; Hajiluian, G.; Nameni, G.; Shahabi, P. Adipose Tissue Inflammation and Oxidative Stress: The Ameliorative Effects of Vitamin D. *Inflammation* **2017**, *40*, 1688–1697. [CrossRef] [PubMed]
34. Alcala, M.; Calderon-Dominguez, M.; Bustos, E.; Ramos, P.; Casals, N.; Serra, D.; Viana, M.; Herrero, L. Increased inflammation, oxidative stress and mitochondrial respiration in brown adipose tissue from obese mice. *Sci. Rep.* **2017**. [CrossRef] [PubMed]
35. Pannunzio, E.; Silverio Amancio, O.M.; de Souza Vitalle, M.S.; Nesadal de Souza, D.; Medeiros Mendes, F.;

Nicolau, J. Analysis of the stimulated whole saliva in overweight and obese children. *Rev. Assoc. Med. Bras.* **2010** *56*, 32–36. [CrossRef] [PubMed]

36. Zhao, B.; Jin, C.; Li, L.; Wang, Y. Increased Expression of TNF-alpha Occurs Before the Development of Periodontitis Among Obese Chinese Children: A Potential Marker for Prediction and Prevention of Periodontitis. *Oral. Health Prev. Dent.* **2016**, *14*, 71–75. [CrossRef]
37. Scorzetti, L.; Marcattili, D.; Pasini, M.; Mattei, A.; Marchetti, E.; Marzo, G. Association between obesity and periodontal disease in children. *Eur. J. Pediatr. Dent.* **2013**, *14*, 181–184.
38. Modeer, T.; Blomberg, C.C.; Wondimu, B.; Julihn, A.; Marcus, C. Association between obesity, flow rate of whole saliva, and dental caries in adolescents. *Obesity* **2010**, *18*, 2367–2373. [CrossRef]
39. Fadel, H.T.; Pliaki, A.; Gronowitz, E.; Mårild, S.; Ramberg, P.; Dahlèn, G.; Yucel-Lindberg, T.; Heijl, L.; Birkhed, D. Clinical and biological indicators of dental caries and periodontal disease in adolescents with or without obesity. *Clin. Oral. Investig.* **2014**, *18*, 359–368. [CrossRef]
40. Patrascu, V.; Giurca, C.; Ciurea, R.N.; Georgescu, C.C.; Ciurea, M.E. Ulcerated necrobiosis lipoidica to a teenager with diabetes mellitus and obesity. *Rom. J. Morphol. Embryol.* **2014**, *55*, 171–176.
41. Dursun, E.; Akalin, F.A.; Genc, T.; Cinar, N.; Erel, O.; Yildiz, B.O. Oxidative stress and periodontal disease in obesity. *Medicine* **2016**, *95*, e3136. [CrossRef]
42. Brown, L.A.; Kerr, C.J.; Whiting, P.; Finer, N.; McEneny, J.; Ashton, T. Oxidant stress in healthy normal-weight, overweight, and obese individuals. *Obesity* **2009**, *17*, 460–466. [CrossRef]
43. Goth, L.; Lenkey, A.; Bigler, W.N. Blood catalase deficiency and diabetes in Hungary. *Diabetes Care* **2001**, *24*, 1839–1840. [CrossRef] [PubMed]
44. Zalewska, A.; Knaś, M.; Waszkiewicz, N.; Klimiuk, A.; Litwin, K.; Sierakowski, S.; Waszkiel, D. Salivary antioxidants in patients with systemic sclerosis. *J. Oral. Pathol. Med.* **2014**, *43*, 61–68. [CrossRef] [PubMed]
45. Zalewska, A.; Knaś, M.; Żendzian-Piotrowska, M.; Waszkiewicz, N.; Szulimowska, J.; Prokopiuk, S.; Waszkiel, D.; Car, H. Antioxidant profile of salivary glands in high fat diet- induced insulin resistance rats. *Oral. Dis.* **2014**, *20*, 560–566. [CrossRef] [PubMed]
46. Al-Rawi, N.H. Oxidative stress, antioxidant status and lipid profile in the saliva of type 2 diabetics. *Diabetes Vasc. Dis. Res.* **2011**, *8*, 22–28. [CrossRef]
47. Yuan, H.; Yang, X.; Shi, X.; Tian, R.; Zhao, Z. Association of serum uric acid with different levels of glucose and related factors. *Chin. Med. J.* **2011**, *124*, 1443–1448. [PubMed]
48. Wang, Z.N.; Li, P.; Jiang, R.H.; Li, L.; Li, X.; Li, L.; Liu, C.; Tian, C.L. The association between serum uric acid and metabolic syndrome among adolescents in northeast China. *Int. J. Clin. Exp. Med.* **2015**, *8*, 21122–21129.
49. Lushchak, V.I. Free radicals, reactive oxygen species, oxidative stress and its classification. *Chem. Biol. Interact.* **2014**, *224*, 164–175. [CrossRef]
50. Lushchak, V.I. Classification of oxidative stress based on its intensity. *Exp. Clin. Sci.* **2014**, *13*, 922–937.
51. Adamczyk-Sowa, M.; Bieszczad-Bedrejczuk, E.; Galiniak, S.; Rozmilowska, I.; Czyzewski, D.; Bartosz, G.; Sadowska-Bartosz, I. Oxidative modifications of blood serum proteins in myasthenia gravis. *J. Neuroimmunol.* **2017**, *305*, 145–153. [CrossRef]
52. Gębicki, J.M.; Bartosz, G. Rola białek jako przekaźników uszkodzeń indukowanych przez reaktywne formy tlenu in vivo. *Postepy Biochem.* **2010**, *56*, 115–123.
53. Choromańska, M.; Klimiuk, A.; Kostecka-Sochoń, P.; Wilczyńska, K.; Kwiatkowski, M.; Okuniewska, N.; Waszkiewicz, N.; Zalewska, A.; Maciejczyk, M. Antioxidant defence, oxidative stress and oxidative damage in saliva, plasma and erythrocytes of dementia patients. Can salivary AGE be a marker of dementia? *Int. J. Mol. Sci.* **2017**, *18*, 2205. [CrossRef] [PubMed]
54. Bozzato, A.; Burger, P.; Zenk, J.; Ulter, W.; Iro, H. Salivary gland biometry in female patients with eating disorders. *Eur. Arch. Oto-Rhino-Laryngol.* **2008**, *265*, 1095–1102. [CrossRef]
55. Heo, M.S.; Lee, S.C.; Lee, S.S.; Choi, H.M.; Choi, S.C.; Park, T.W. Quantitative analysis of normal major salivary glands using computed tomography. *Oral Surg. Oral Med. Oral Pathol. Oral Radiol. Endodontol.* **2001**, *92*, 240–244. [CrossRef] [PubMed]
56. Sekiguchi, M.; Iwasaki, T.; Kitano, M.; Kuno, H.; Hashimoto, N.; Kawahito, Y.; Azuma, M.; Hla, T.; Sano, H. Role of sphingosine 1-phosphate in the pathogenesis of Sjögren's syndrome. *J. Immunol.* **2008**, *180*, 1921–1928. [CrossRef]
57. Uemura, T.; Suzuki, T.; Saiki, R.; Dohmae, N.; Ito, S.; Takahashi, H.; Toida, T.; Kashiwagi, K.; Igarashi, K.

Activation of MMP-9 activity by acrolein in saliva from patients with primary Sjögren's syndrome and its mechanism. *Int. J. Biochem. Cell Biol.* **2017**, *88*, 84–91. [CrossRef] [PubMed]
58. Norheim, K.B.; Jonsson, G.; Harboe, E.; Hanasand, M.; Goransson, L.; Omdal, R. Oxidative stress, as measured by protein oxidation, is increased in primary Sjögren's syndrome. *Free Radic. Res.* **2012**, *46*, 141–146. [CrossRef] [PubMed]

12

Saliva and Oral Diseases

Emanuela Martina [†], Anna Campanati [*,†], Federico Diotallevi and Annamaria Offidani

Dermatology Clinic, Department of Clinical and Molecular Sciences, Polytechnic Marche University, via Conca 71, 60126 Ancona, Italy; ema.martina@gmail.com (E.M.); federico.diotallevi@hotmail.it (F.D.); a.offidani@ospedaliriuniti.marche.it (A.O.)

* Correspondence: anna.campanati@gmail.com

† These authors contributed equally to the manuscript.

Abstract: Saliva is a fascinating biological fluid which has all the features of a perfect diagnostic tool. In fact, its collection is rapid, simple, and noninvasive. Thanks to several transport mechanisms and its intimate contact with crevicular fluid, saliva contains hundreds of proteins deriving from plasma. Advances in analytical techniques have opened a new era—called "salivaomics"—that investigates the salivary proteome, transcriptome, microRNAs, metabolome, and microbiome. In recent years, researchers have tried to find salivary biomarkers for oral and systemic diseases with various protocols and technologies. The review aspires to provide an overall perspective of salivary biomarkers concerning oral diseases such as lichen planus, oral cancer, blistering diseases, and psoriasis. Saliva has proved to be a promising substrate for the early detection of oral diseases and the evaluation of therapeutic response. However, the wide variation in sampling, processing, and measuring of salivary elements still represents a limit for the application in clinical practice.

Keywords: biomarkers; saliva; oral cancer; oral lichen planus; psoriasis; oral diseases

---

1. Introduction

Saliva is a biological fluid secreted by major and minor salivary glands. The major salivary glands are the parotid, submandibular, and sublingual glands. Minor salivary glands are widely disseminated throughout the entire oral cavity. Saliva provides lubrication; facilitates mastication, digestion, and taste; it has antimicrobial properties; and serves as buffer for acidic food. Moreover, saliva inhibits the demineralization of teeth and protects from caries [1]. The physiological secretion generates 0.75–1.5 L per day, with a decrease during the night [2]. Saliva contains 99% water and proteins for the remaining 1% (mucins, enzymes, immunoglobulins), electrolytes, lipids, and inorganic substances [3].

There are many advantages to employing saliva as a substrate for diagnostic analysis. Its sampling is fast, inexpensive, non-invasive, and well tolerated by children and people with disabilities; moreover, it is a safe procedure for healthcare providers [4]. Many serum substances enter saliva through passive diffusion, active transport, or extracellular ultrafiltration [5]. Obviously, compared with blood, levels of several analytes are lower, which was an obstacle until a few years ago [6]. Nowadays, highly sensitive molecular methods are available and can be used in the detection of many elements in saliva, despite their dimensions and concentrations [7].

In recent decades, enormous progress has been made in early diagnosis and screening for many diseases, especially for neoplastic conditions. However, some of these methods are invasive or expensive, and for certain conditions, accurate tests are still not available. This is the case for oral cancer, the sixth most common cancer worldwide, frequently diagnosed at an advanced stage with a 5 year survival rate of 50% [8].

In accordance with Biomarkers Definitions Working Group 2011, a biomarker is a characteristic that can be objectively measured and evaluated as indicator of normal biological or pathogenic processes, or as an indicator of pharmacologic response to therapeutic interventions [9]. The detection of salivary biomarkers and their use in clinical practice in the near future is one of the most ambitious aims of contemporary researchers.

2. Materials and Methods

The review was conducted in accordance with the PRISMA (Preferred Reporting Items for Systematic Reviews and Meta-Analyses) checklist. A search in the PubMed database was carried out using the keywords "saliva", "salivary", "biomarkers", "oral diseases", "oral lichen planus", "oral cancer", and associations between terms. We selected only articles written in English. The papers were selected first by analyzing titles and abstracts, in order to choose a correct match with our topic; full-text articles were then studied and included in the revision.

3. Sampling and Processing Techniques

Many factors can alter the composition and total amount of saliva. The time of day, hydration, body position, drugs intake, smoking, psychological stimuli, food assumption, and other factors related to systemic conditions can change the characteristics of saliva in a single subject [10]. A sample of saliva can be collected at rest or after stimulation. This procedure consists of offering a gum or swab to chew, or specific taste stimuli such as citric acid [11]. The stimulation changes not only the volume, but also the composition of saliva; it has been demonstrated that parasympathetic stimulation produces a high flow rate, but sympathetic stimulation produces a small flow richer in proteins and peptides [12]. Consequently, proteome profile and proportion are changeable as a reaction to neural activation [13].

As regards clinical trials, saliva is usually collected at rest ("unstimulated saliva") after at least 1 h of fasting, without drinking or smoking; the patient must be comfortably seated, avoid oro-facial movements for 5 min, and, just before the sampling, has to rinse their mouth with deionized water [11].

Saliva specimens can be collected from whole saliva or from a single gland (for example, the parotid gland). This procedure, which uses a different method, can be uncomfortable for patients and therefore is rarely used [14]. It should be specified that whole saliva has a higher proportion of non-salivary materials such as food debris, bacteria, desquamated epithelial cells, and leukocytes [15].

The gold standard method is to drain saliva using special devices (Salivette®, Sarstedt, Nümbrecht, Germany; Quantisal®, Immunalysis, Pomona, CA, USA; Orapette®, Trinity Biotech, Dublin, Ireland and SCS® Greiner Bio-One, Kremsmünster, Austria) [16].

Controversies are evident in the literature regarding centrifugation and speed, addition of PIC (protease inhibitor cocktail), and storage temperature. Most authors recommended the use of a protease inhibitor mixture in order to stabilize the substrate; moreover, the samples collected must be immediately stored in ice containers and, after processing, stored at −80 °C [17]. All these steps are necessary for bacterial growth inhibition and the minimal impairment of salivary proteins.

4. "Salivaomics"

The term "salivaomics" was coined in 2008 to emphasize the various "omics" found in saliva: genome, transcriptome, proteome, metabolome, and microbiome [18]. Salivaomics has been widely studied in recent years thanks to the advent of more advanced analytical techniques. Nearly 70% of the genome in saliva is human; the remaining 30% belongs to the oral microbiota [19]. The DNA contained in saliva is approximately 24 μg (range 0.2–52 μg), which is almost 10 times lower than in blood, but genotyping techniques require as little as 5 ng/mL of DNA to work effectively [20]. Polymerase chain reaction (PCR) and sequencing arrays can be applied to saliva samples. The analysis of salivary DNA aims especially to detect aberrant DNA methylation, which is the first epigenetic mark of neoplastic alterations [21].

4.1. *Transcriptomes*

mRNA and microRNA secreted from cells can be easily detected in saliva. Reverse transcriptase polymerase chain reaction and microarray are the most commonly used analyses. Zhang et al. first developed a technique to permit stabilization and to process salivary RNA [22]. The great potential of transcriptome study in the early detection of cancer and other diseases has been reported [23–25]. More recently, noncoding RNAs (ncRNAs) or microRNAs (miRNA) have been the subject of many studies because of their role in oncogenesis and their great stability in biological fluids, including saliva [26]. MicroRNAs are encoded by genes but are not translated into proteins; it is now generally accepted that these small nucleotides are involved in cell differentiation, proliferation, and survival. Moreover, many studies have already demonstrated the dysregulation of miRNAs in cancer tissues [27,28]. Surprisingly, salivary microRNAs are more stable than mRNAs, which makes this biological fluid a suitable substrate for transcriptome analysis.

4.2. *Metabolome*

The endogenous metabolites are nucleic acids, vitamins, lipids, organic acids, carbohydrates, thiols, and amino acids. The study of the salivary metabolome can provide an overview of the general health status or modification during systemic diseases [29]. In 2010, Sugimoto et al. first used salivary metabolome analysis with capillary electrophoresis and mass spectrometry to detect differences between healthy controls and patients with solid cancer [30]. The authors identified three metabolites that were oral-cancer-specific and eight metabolites that were pancreatic-cancer-specific. Nuclear magnetic resonance (NMR) spectroscopy can detect and measure metabolites in a solution with minimal sample preparation. This quantitative technique is based on the magnetic properties of atomic nuclei [31]. Each compound has a characteristic resonance frequency that makes it easy to distinguish. Moreover, the area under a signal peak is proportional to the concentration of the metabolite [32]. Liquid chromatography–mass spectrometry (LC-MS) is considered the gold standard in metabolomics. In fact, it is able to analyze an enormous range of analytes with a greater sensitivity than NMR [33]. This technique provides very high chromatographic resolution and its results are easily interpretable using libraries of molecular fragmentation patterns [34].

4.3. *Proteome*

The term "proteome" encompasses all proteins in the oral cavity. Saliva contains more than 2000 proteins with a multitude of biological activities [35] and one quarter of salivary proteins are detectable in plasma. The greatest obstacle to salivary proteome analysis is its rapid degradation, which occurs just minutes after sample collection. For this reason, the majority of researchers combine the saliva with protease inhibitor cocktails (PIC) before storage and analysis, as suggested by Xiao et al. [36]. Proteomics takes advantage of NMR spectroscopy and gas and liquid chromatography–mass spectrometry (GC-MS and LC-MS), described above. In this research field, two-dimensional polyacrylamide gel electrophoresis (2D-PAGE) and capillary electrophoresis with electrochemical detection are essential tools [37]. 2D-PAGE, which precedes the advent of 2D-difference gel electrophoresis (2D-DIGE), fractionates proteins on the basis of their isoelectric points in the first dimension and apparent molecular weight in the second [38]. An amphoteric carrier or an ampholyte is added to a gel and subjected to electrophoresis under a continuously regulated temperature. The acrylamide gel is placed in a glass tube and proteins are separated via an isoelectric gradient; it is easy to understand why this method is poorly accurate with multiple samples. 2D-DIGE dramatically improved 2D-PAGE thanks to the possibility of labeling each sample with distinct fluorescent dyes and then reading them using a laser scanner. Immunoassay is one of the most commonly used analytical techniques to detect the expression of an antibody or an antigen in a test sample. Enzyme-linked immunosorbent assay (ELISA) has been used for a variety of applications including diagnostic tools and quality controls [39]. The four basic setups are direct, indirect, sandwich, and competitive ELISAs. Direct ELISA is the simplest format, requiring an antigen and an enzyme-conjugated antibody specific to the antigen [40]. The ELISA method is a sensitive and specific test that rapidly produces results and for these advantages has found a wide field of applications in clinical practice (e.g., in viral serology tests).

4.4. Microbiome

The study of microbiota has probably been the largest topic in scientific literature in recent years. In fact, next-generation sequencing has allowed the identification of thousands of phylotypes of microorganism throughout the entire human body, and research is ongoing. About 19,000 microorganisms have been identified in saliva [41]. Oral dysbiosis can lead to periodontal disease [42], caries [43], and some evidence exists supporting an association with cancer and systemic diseases [44,45]. Nowadays, molecular biology methods such as 16S ribosomal RNA (rRNA) gene sequencing, polymerase chain reaction (PCR), and other related PCR-based methods are very popular thanks to their high sensitivity and reproducibility. However, these techniques are no longer employed in routine diagnostics due to their costs. Alternative approaches include electromigration techniques (two-dimensional gel electrophoresis, capillary zone electrophoresis) and MS methods, such as matrix-assisted laser desorption ionization time-of-flight mode (MALDI-TOF MS). MALDI-TOF MS is a fast and accurate method based on the ionization of intact microorganism cells with short laser pulses and the subsequent acceleration of the particles in a vacuum by way of an electric field. Each microorganism has a specific spectrum profile [46].

Histopathology, in some cases with direct immunofluorescence, remains the gold standard for the diagnosis of oral disease. In fact, it is often necessary to perform a biopsy to confirm the diagnosis of bullous diseases (together with DIF) [47], Sjögren's syndrome [48], and for all lesions suspected for malignancy [49].

5. Fields of Application

In this article, we have summarized the latest findings on the use of saliva as a diagnostic tool in oral inflammatory diseases. In particular, we chose the most epidemiologically relevant conditions or where the oral cavity is a typical location of a systemic disease. In fact, mouth disorders can often precede the onset of systemic symptoms (e.g., in bullous pemphigus), and early diagnosis of oral disease can change the prognosis of these patients. In this scenario, the study of salivary biomarkers is a promising tool for early diagnosis and screening in susceptible populations (e.g., in smokers).

5.1. Oral Lichen Planus

Oral lichen planus (OLP) is one of the most common chronic inflammatory condition of the oral mucosa, with 0.5%–2% prevalence in adults and a slight predominance in women [50]. OLP affects oral mucosa symmetrically, with a predilection for oral mucosa. Clinically, it is possible to distinguish different aspects: reticular (the most prevalent form), erythematous, ulcerative or erosive, plaque-like, bullous, or papular [51,52]. The histopathology of OLP is typical, with a prominent lymphocyte infiltrate at the interface of epithelium, acanthosis, and degeneration of the basal cell layer [53]. Direct immunofluorescence (DIF) permits deposition of Immunoglobulin M as colloid bodies and C3 in granular and linear patterns in the basement membrane zone to be detected [54]. Although the exact pathogenesis of OLP is mostly unknown, it is believed that autoreactive T cells play a crucial role in the disease. Several risks/triggers factors have been described, such as stress, HCV and viral infections, and drugs [55]. OLP has been classified as a premalignant lesion for its risk of malignant transformation (0.04–1.74 per year) in squamous cell carcinoma (OSCC) [56]. Patients affected by OLP suffer from burning and itching sensations up to a severe pain in the erosive form; the disease has a huge negative impact on quality of life due to impairment in daily activities such as eating or oral hygiene [57]. Published articles focused on salivary biomarkers in OLP are quite recent and concern the diagnosis of OLP, but in particular the early detection of malignant transformation.

In 2018, Sineepat et al. enrolled five OLP patients and five healthy controls using a proteomic approach on saliva with two-dimensional gel electrophoresis followed by mass spectrometry. The authors detected three proteins that showed a potential role in OLP patients (cystatin SA, chain C of human complement component C3c, and chain B of fibrinogen fragment D) and tested with ELISA. All the analytical techniques confirmed with statistical significance that fibrinogen fragment D and complement component C3c were increased and cystatin SA was decreased in OLP patients compared with healthy subjects [58]. Fibrinogen fragments D and C3c play a central role in inflammation, whereas cystatin SA belongs to the cystatin superfamily, a group of cysteine protease inhibitors with antimicrobial activity. In fact, fibrinogen expression and C3 deposition are typical findings in OLP using IFD [54].

A different and more complex panel of proteins was reported by another study, published in 2017 [59]. The study was conducted on 10 patients, investigating with mass spectrometry 108 proteins differentially expressed in OLP subjects in comparison to healthy controls. The first finding was the absence of proteins essential to lubrication and viscoelasticity, supporting the xerostomia symptom frequently reported by patients. The authors interestingly tried to link protein expression in saliva with histological findings in OLP, discussing the known functions of each peptide. In particular, S100A8 and S100A9 (also called MRP8 and MRP14) are calcium- and zinc-binding proteins with a role in inflammation and cytokine production via IL-17. S100A8 can also induce apoptosis via attraction to skin of $CD8^+$ cells and natural killer (NK) cells [60]. Another player in the scene of T-cell proliferation and differentiation is AZGP1 (zinc-alpha-2-glycoprotein), which is an adipocytokine [61]. The study also confirmed the crucial role of oxidative stress in OLP; reactive oxygen species (ROS) induce apoptosis and dysfunction in keratinocytes and, moreover, ROS can be further produced from $TCD4^+$ lymphocytes infiltrating in OLP in a vicious circle.

Oxidative stress in OLP was previously discussed in 2016 in a case–control study enrolling 62 patients and 30 healthy individuals [62]. The authors demonstrated significant differences between patients and the control group concerning the average concentration of total antioxidant capacity (TAC, determined using the Benzie and Strain method [26]), glutathione (GSH, measured spectrophotometrically), and thiobarbituric-acid-reactive substances (TBARS, determined using the Aust method), which are a product of lipid peroxidation [63]. In patients suffering from OLP, as expected, TAC and GSH had lower values, while TBARS was higher than in healthy controls. More interestingly, patients with an erosive form of lichen had more marked values, demonstrating severe oxidative stress and a great concordance with clinical features. These findings could support the oral or topical use of antioxidants [64].

Many authors have suggested salivary cortisol as a biomarker in OLP [65–70]. Cortisol is considered a biological marker of stress and anxiety, the variation of which can alter cytokine profiles [71]. OLP has a double connection with stress: anxiety and stressful events are considered a trigger for OLP onset but, at the same time, oral lichen itself represent a source of stress for patients. In this intricate scenario, the evaluation of salivary cortisol seems to mimic the ancestral question "Which came first, the chicken or the egg?" In fact, data from the literature are controversial, and cortisol is probably not suitable as a biomarker in OLP. As previously discussed, OLP is a T-cell-driven disease; however, it is still unclear if the inflammation is due to Th1 or Th2 expression. In fact, in OLP, there are numerous cytokines expressed both from recruited lymphocytes and from affected keratinocytes, in a mechanism of self-amplification [72]. The evaluation of specific interleukin in saliva is certainly a good trace to detect biomarkers in OLP and, moreover, to design tailored therapies. Nowadays, more consistent results concern IL-6 and IL-8. Interleukin-6 is involved in B- and T cell differentiation and is able to inactivate p53 with tumor progression of some cancers [73]. Mozaffari et al. revealed in a meta-analysis that IL-6 levels in saliva and serum of OLP patients were significantly higher than in healthy controls, with higher values in saliva than in serum [74]. For this reason, saliva seemed to be more useful than serum for the detection of IL-6. Interleukin-8 is an important mediator of host response to injury and inflammation; it can activate neutrophils, basophils, and T cells [75]. The group of Mozaffari conducted a meta-analysis on this topic [76]. The most interesting finding was that IL-8 plays a key role in the transformation from reticular to erosive form of lichen, probably due to the loss of efficacy in the repairing mechanisms of keratinocytes [77]. IL-8 also revealed a potential application in therapeutic monitoring, as demonstrated via its decrease in saliva after dexamethasone administration [78].

5.2. Oral Cancer

Oral cancer is the sixth most common cancer worldwide [79] with a higher incidence in India, because of the chewing of areca nut/betel quid [80]. The mortality rate after 5 years from diagnosis is still 50% [79]. Well-known risk factors include tobacco consumption, alcohol abuse, and human papilloma virus infections [81]. The onset of an oral cancer is frequently asymptomatic, but most oral carcinomas develop from premalignant conditions such as leukoplakia and oral lichen planus [82,83]. Nowadays, the gold standard for diagnosis is tissue biopsy, an invasive technique that requires specific training and creates public health costs [84]. It is therefore easy to understand the need for an early detection method for pre-cancer and cancer by validating salivary biomarkers. Above, we discussed the great diagnostic potential of miRNA both in saliva and serum. In 2018, a well-designed study enrolled 30 patients with OLP, 15 patients with OSCC and 15 healthy donors [85]. Saliva samples were analyzed by quantitative RT-PCR for miR-21, miR-125a, miR31, and miR200a. Results showed that miRNA-21 and -125a were, respectively, higher and lower in OSCC patients and in OLP with dysplasia compared to healthy controls with statistical significance. miR-21 has been widely studied in oral, head, and neck cancer and has been postulated that it might have a role in inhibition of tumor suppression and apoptosis [86]. In contrast, miR-125a may act as a tumor suppressor, downregulating target oncogens [87]. Based on these data, the authors suggested a negative prognostic role of decreased salivary miR-125a levels in association with increased salivary miR-21 levels in OLP patients. Ishikawa et al. recently suggested a metabolomics approach to distinguish OLP from OSCC [88]; the authors detected higher levels of 12 salivary metabolites in OSCC patients compared with OLP patients. More specifically, the combination of indole-3-acetate and ethanolamine phosphate showed the best statistical accuracy. The aim of Mikkonen's research was to investigate the potential of nuclear magnetic resonance (NMR) spectroscopy for detecting the salivary metabolic changes associated with head and neck squamous cell carcinoma (HNSCC). The Authors found two metabolites, fucose and 1,2-propanediol, to be significantly upregulated, whereas proline was significantly downregulated in patients affected by HNSCC. The combination of four salivary metabolites (fucose, glycine, methanol, and proline) together provided maximum discrimination among HNSCC patients and healthy controls [31]. The role of fucosylation of glycoproteins in the development of cancer has been studied in recent years [89]. Ample evidence exists to prove that in normal tissues, fucosylation levels are relatively low, but this rapidly increases during carcinogenesis [90]. Aberrant glycosylation in cancer development is also an investigation area in oral diseases; in particular, researchers have focused attention on sialic acid (N-acetyl neuraminic acid), which is an important terminal sugar in cell membrane glycoproteins and glycolipids. Previous studies have shown elevated levels of salivary sialic acid in various carcinomas, including oral pre-cancer and OC [91–93].

The fascinating study of the microbiome has a wide field of application in the oral cavity. An extensive work has just been published regarding the alterations of salivary microbial community in oropharyngeal and hypopharyngeal carcinoma patients. In fact, the microbiome is considered a potential modulator of cancer metabolism [94]. The authors found 13 phylotypes of microorganism as potential diagnostic biomarkers in oral cancer. The role of the microbiome in malignant change in the oral cavity is still controversial because of the lack of large cohort studies. Healy et al. considered the implication of risk factors such as smoking or alcohol consumption in promoting epithelial dysplasia and production of carcinogenic agents [95]. Acetaldehyde (ACH) and N-nitrosamine compounds are potential genotoxic agents that are increased in the saliva of smokers; these compounds can be produced in vitro by microbial cultures [96,97]. In vitro studies have demonstrated the leading role of *Neisseria* species and *Candida* species in ACH production [98,99]. However, one study revealed the reduction of *Neisseria* species in the oral cavity of smokers, with a theoretical improvement of ACH levels [100]. Current theories hypothesize that the presence of these organisms could accelerate the progression of dysplasia towards OSCC in association with predisposing factors such as diet, age, or smoking/alcohol consumption habits in a multifactorial vision.

5.3. Blistering Diseases

Bullous pemphigoid (BP) and pemphigus vulgaris (PV) are acquired bullous diseases affecting the mucosa and/or skin. In both diseases, autoantibodies react with adhesion cell mechanisms or with the basement layer, resulting in blistering. Blisters are intraepithelial/intraepidermal in PV, whereas in BP they are subepithelial/subepidermal [101]. The diagnosis is first clinical, then confirmed with histopathology and direct immunofluorescence (IFD). In BP, bullae involving the skin and oral lesions are rare; in contrast, PV frequently begins with oral blistering or oral lesions following cutaneous involvement. IFD reveals IgG and C3 (BP180) deposition on the basement membrane in BP, while in PV it shows intercellular IgG antibody deposition to desmoglein (Dsg) 1 and/or desmoglein 3, which are trans-membrane desmosomal proteins [102]. In recent years, the use of ELISA to detect autoantibodies in the serum of BP and PV patients has entered clinical practice for diagnosis and therapeutic monitoring [101]. Starting from this technique, some authors have proposed the use of saliva as substrate for the research of BP180 and Dsg1 and 3. In 2006, Andreadis et al. first applied ELISA in both the serum and saliva of PV and BP patients, finding a great concordance in serum and saliva levels of Dsg1 and 3, while the BP180 determination on saliva failed [103]. Similar results emerged from Ali's study [104] on Dsg1 and 3. The potential of salivary testing in PV prognosis and mucosal severity has been investigated in two studies. Hallaji et al. included 50 patients with histologically confirmed PV and performed ELISA for Dsg1 and 3 on serum and saliva samples [105]. There was statistically significant concordance between serum and salivary levels of Dsg; more interestingly, there was a significant relationship between salivary anti-Dsg1 antibody and mucosal severity. The authors explained these data with the loss of integrity in mucosa and the largest transition of antibodies in saliva. The study of De et al. perfectly reproduced this finding and the authors perfectly agreed with the explanation concerning higher Dsg1 levels in severe disease [106]. In contrast to the previously discussed research, one Italian study was designed to assess the use of a BIOCHIP approach compared with ELISA in PV [107]. In fact, the authors considered saliva an unsuitable substrate for autoantibody detection because of the discordance between techniques found when using saliva samples.

5.4. Sjögren's Syndrome

Sjögren's syndrome (SS) is a systemic autoimmune disease characterized by the inflammation and consecutive destruction of exocrine glands, as well as salivary and lacrimal glands, with the occurrence of a lymphoepithelial sialadenitis [108]. The majority of patients are women of menopausal age; oral manifestations are frequently present at the onset of disease, but some patients develop a systemic disease with the involvement of joints, the gastrointestinal tract, the central nervous system, and with an increased risk of lymphoma [109]. Patients suffering from SS typically complain about xerostomia and its impact on their quality of life [110]. Current research on salivary biomarkers in SS is pursuing a non-invasive diagnostic test, a therapeutic monitoring marker, and, moreover, an early detection of lymphoma onset. One of the current diagnostic approaches is the detection of anti-Ro/SSA and/or anti-La/SSB in serum; studies from different groups have demonstrated the presence of these autoantibodies in the saliva of SS patients [111,112]. The determination of salivary autoantibodies seemed to be effective in discriminating SS patients from patients affected by systemic lupus erythematosus (SLE) [113]. A few studies have investigated cytokine profiles in SS saliva; data from these studies showed significantly higher levels of Th1, Th2, and Th17, in accordance with serum findings [114,115]. The proteomic approach in SS comprises proteins, enzymes, calcium-binding proteins, and immune-related molecules. Summarizing, data from the literature report high levels of inflammatory-phase proteins in saliva that can provide a great indication of gland status [116]. Lee et al.

recently published the results of determination of soluble sialic-acid-binding immunoglobulin-like lectin (siglec)-5 in saliva and sera by ELISA [117]. The level of salivary siglec-5 was significantly higher in the saliva from SS patients, which reflects the severity of hyposalivation. Several novel miRNAs have been described in SS [118]. Pauley et al. demonstrated that the expression of miR-146a was significantly increased in SS patients [119]. In Alevizos' research, another two miRNAs, miR-768-3p and miR-574, were associated with minor salivary gland inflammation in 15 patients with SS [120]. The pathogenesis of autoimmune diseases is a very complex interaction of many factors; epigenetic modifications are now considered crucial to the control of gene expression associated with these diseases [121,122]. Thabet et al. proposed that the dysfunction of salivary gland epithelial cells in SS might be partially linked to epigenetic modifications. Their analysis showed that blood global DNA methylation was reduced in SS patients and the expression of the gene DNMT1, which encodes DNA methyltransferase 1, was decreased compared to healthy controls. In contrast, the expression of the gene Gadd45a, which encodes the growth arrest and DNA-damage-inducible protein GADD45 alpha (GADD45a), was increased [123]. Probably the most interesting field in saliva and SS is the early diagnosis and prevention of MALT-type lymphoma [124]. The neoplasm has an insidious onset, almost asymptomatic, with a fast progression and dissemination. Cui et al. described a triad of markers (anti-cofillin-1, anti-alpha-enolase, and anti-Rho GDP-dissociation inhibitor 2) overexpressed in patients with SS who developed MALT lymphoma compared with SS patients and healthy individuals [125]. Sharma et al. recently examined the role of the microbiome in SS compared to healthy controls [126]. The analysis, performed with DNA isolation and 16rRNA sequencing, revealed four genera (Bifidobacterium, Dialister, Lactobacillus, and Leptotrichia) that were different between the two groups. The results were consistent with previous studies, revealing a role of Actinobacteria and Firmicutes phila [127,128]. More interestingly, Sharma et al. identified a difference in alpha diversity in patients treated with steroids, suggesting the potential role of microbiome analysis in therapeutic response.

5.5. Psoriasis

Psoriasis is now classified as an immune-mediated inflammatory disease (IMID) of the skin. It is being recognized that patients with psoriasis are at higher risk of developing systemic co-morbidities, e.g., metabolic syndrome and cardiovascular diseases [129,130].

Oral involvement in course of psoriasis is still debated. Recently, it has been hypothesized that gingivitis and periodontitis share the same underlying inflammatory pathogenic process as psoriasis. Thus, in our previous study, psoriatic patients were investigated for oral mucosa lesion prevalence as well as gum disease. Results displayed an increased association between gingivitis/periodontitis and psoriasis, which may suggest common underlying pathogenic risk factors [131].

Furthermore, salivary secretions, collected from patients with active psoriasis and healthy control subjects, were investigated for expression of interleukin (IL)-1b, IL-6, transforming growth factor (TGF)-β1, IL-8, tumor necrosis factor (TNF)-α, interferon (IFN)-χ, IL-17A, IL-4, IL-10, monocyte chemoattractant protein (MCP)-1, microphage inflammatory protein (MIP)-1a, and MIP-1b using a Multi-Analyte ELISArray Kit (Qiagen, Venlo, the Netherlands). Patients with active psoriasis had significantly higher salivary IL1β, TNF-α, TGF-β, and MCP-1 levels than healthy controls [132].

Thus, saliva can be a valid non-invasive tool for monitoring inflammation in psoriasis [133].

6. Conclusions

In the era of precision medicine, salivaomics approaches seem to be a promising field of research. Despite encouraging results reported in this review, there is a large variability in study designs, protocols, sampling collections, and techniques. Moreover, the study of new molecules with new technologies requires a well-established range of values without random decisions. Future studies should standardize accurate methodologies in order to validate new salivary biomarkers in clinical practice.

Author Contributions: E.M. was responsible for the literature revision and drafting; A.C. was responsible for final drafting and revision; F.D. contributed to article analysis; A.O. gave her final revision. All authors have read and agree to the published version of the manuscript.

References

1. Qin, R.; Steel, A.; Fazel, N. Oral mucosa biology and salivary biomarkers. *Clin. Dermatol.* **2017**, *35*, 477–483. [CrossRef] [PubMed]
2. Holmberg, K.V.; Hoffman, M.P. Anatomy, Biogenesis and Regeneration in Salivary Glands. *Monogr. Oral Sci.* **2014**, *24*, 1–13. [PubMed]
3. Mese, H.; Matsuo, R. Salivary secretion, taste and hyposalivation. *J. Oral Rehabil.* **2007**, *34*, 711–723. [CrossRef] [PubMed]
4. Kaczor-Urbanowicz, K.E.; Martin Carreras-Presas, C.; Aro, K.; Tu, M.; Garcia-Godoy, F.; Wong, D.T.W. Saliva diagnostics—Current views and directions. *Exp. Biol. Med.* **2017**, *242*, 459–472. [CrossRef]
5. Pfaffe, T.; Cooper-White, J.; Beyerlein, P.; Kostner, K.; Punyadeera, C. Diagnostic potential of saliva: Current state and future applications. *Clin. Chem.* **2011**, *57*, 675–687. [CrossRef]
6. Javaid, M.A.; Ahmed, A.S.; Durand, R.; Tran, S.D. Saliva as a diagnostic tool for oral and systemic diseases. *J. Oral Biol. Craniofacial Res.* **2016**, *6*, 67–76. [CrossRef]
7. Iguiniz, M.; Heinisch, S. Two-dimensional liquid chromatography in pharmaceutical analysis. Instrumental aspects, trends and applications. *J. Pharm. Biomed. Anal.* **2017**, *145*, 482–503. [CrossRef]
8. Petti, S. Pooled estimate of world leukoplakia prevalence: A systematic review. *Oral Oncol.* **2003**, *39*, 770–780. [CrossRef]
9. Delli, K.; Villa, A.; Farah, C.S.; Celentano, A.; Ojeda, D.; Peterson, D.; Jensen, S.B.; Glurich, I.; Vissink, A. World Workshop on Oral Medicine VII: Biomarkers predicting lymphoma in the salivary glands of patients with Sjögren's syndrome—A systematic review. *Oral Dis.* **2019**, *25*, 49–63. [CrossRef]
10. Siqueira, W.L.; Dawes, C. The salivary proteome: Challenges and perspectives. *PROTEOMICS Clin. Appl.* **2011**, *5*, 575–579. [CrossRef]
11. Navazesh, M. Methods for Collecting Saliva. *Ann. N. Y. Acad. Sci.* **1993**, *694*, 72–77. [CrossRef] [PubMed]
12. Lorenzo-Pouso, A.I.; Pérez-Sayáns, M.; Bravo, S.B.; López-Jornet, P.; García-Vence, M.; Alonso-Sampedro, M.; Carballo, J.; García-García, A.; Zalewska, A. Protein-Based Salivary Profiles as Novel Biomarkers for Oral Diseases. *Dis. Markers* **2018**, *2018*, 6141845. [CrossRef] [PubMed]
13. Proctor, G.B.; Carpenter, G.H. Salivary Secretion: Mechanism and Neural Regulation. In *Monographs in Oral Science*; KARGER: Basel, Switzerland, 2014; Volume 24, pp. 14–29. ISBN 0077-0892.
14. Henson, B.S.; Wong, D.T. Collection, Storage, and Processing of Saliva Samples for Downstream Molecular Applications. In *Oral Biology. Methods in Molecular Biology (Methods and Protocols)*; Humana Press: Totowa, NJ, USA, 2010; Volume 666H.
15. Kaufman, E.; Lamster, I.B. The diagnostic applications of saliva—A review. *Crit. Rev. Oral Biol. Med.* **2002**, *13*, 197–212. [CrossRef] [PubMed]
16. Khurshid, Z.; Zohaib, S.; Najeeb, S.; Zafar, M.S.; Slowey, P.D.; Almas, K. Human Saliva Collection Devices for Proteomics: An Update. *Int. J. Mol. Sci.* **2016**, *17*, 846. [CrossRef]
17. Schipper, R.; Loof, A.; de Groot, J.; Harthoorn, L.; Dransfield, E.; van Heerde, W. SELDI-TOF-MS of saliva: Methodology and pre-treatment effects. *J. Chromatogr. B* **2007**, *847*, 45–53. [CrossRef]
18. Ai, J.; Smith, B.; Wong, D.T. Saliva Ontology: An ontology-based framework for a Salivaomics Knowledge Base. *BMC Bioinform.* **2010**, *11*, 302. [CrossRef]
19. Rylander-Rudqvist, T.; Håkansson, N.; Tybring, G.; Wolk, A. Quality and Quantity of Saliva DNA Obtained from the Self-administrated Oragene Method—A Pilot Study on the Cohort of Swedish Men. *Cancer Epidemiol. Biomark. Prev.* **2006**, *15*, 1742–1745. [CrossRef]
20. Abraham, J.E.; Maranian, M.J.; Spiteri, I.; Russell, R.; Ingle, S.; Luccarini, C.; Earl, H.M.; Pharoah, P.P.D.; Dunning, A.M.; Caldas, C. Saliva samples are a viable alternative to blood samples as a source of DNA for high throughput genotyping. *BMC Med. Genom.* **2012**, *5*, 19. [CrossRef]
21. Gaździcka, J.; Gołąbek, K.; Strzelczyk, J.K.; Ostrowska, Z. Epigenetic Modifications in Head and Neck Cancer. *Biochem. Genet.* **2019**. [CrossRef]
22. Lee, Y.-H.; Zhou, H.; Reiss, J.K.; Yan, X.; Zhang, L.; Chia, D.; Wong, D.T.W. Direct Saliva Transcriptome Analysis. *Clin. Chem.* **2011**, *57*, 1295–1302. [CrossRef]

23. Tutar, Y. Editorial (Thematic Issue: "miRNA and Cancer; Computational and Experimental Approaches"). *Curr. Pharm. Biotechnol.* **2014**, *15*, 429. [CrossRef] [PubMed]
24. Kaczor-Urbanowicz, K.E.; Martín Carreras-Presas, C.; Kaczor, T.; Tu, M.; Wei, F.; Garcia-Godoy, F.; Wong, D.T.W. Emerging technologies for salivaomics in cancer detection. *J. Cell. Mol. Med.* **2017**, *21*, 640–647. [CrossRef] [PubMed]
25. Prattichizzo, F.; Giuliani, A.; Recchioni, R.; Bonafè, M.; Marcheselli, F.; De Carolis, S.; Campanati, A.; Giuliodori, K.; Rippo, M.R.; Brugè, F.; et al. Anti-TNF-α treatment modulates SASP and SASP-related microRNAs in endothelial cells and in circulating angiogenic cells. *Oncotarget* **2016**, *7*, 11945–11958. [CrossRef] [PubMed]
26. Majem, B.; Rigau, M.; Reventós, J.; Wong, D.T. Non-coding RNAs in saliva: Emerging biomarkers for molecular diagnostics. *Int. J. Mol. Sci.* **2015**, *16*, 8676–8698. [CrossRef]
27. Bartel, D.P. MicroRNAs: Target recognition and regulatory functions. *Cell* **2009**, *136*, 215–233. [CrossRef]
28. Adams, B.D.; Kasinski, A.L.; Slack, F.J. Aberrant regulation and function of microRNAs in cancer. *Curr. Biol.* **2014**, *24*, R762–R776. [CrossRef]
29. Bessonneau, V.; Bojko, B.; Pawliszyn, J. Analysis of human saliva metabolome by direct immersion solid-phase microextraction LC and benchtop orbitrap MS. *Bioanalysis* **2013**, *5*, 783–792. [CrossRef]
30. Sugimoto, M.; Wong, D.T.; Hirayama, A.; Soga, T.; Tomita, M. Capillary electrophoresis mass spectrometry-based saliva metabolomics identified oral, breast and pancreatic cancer-specific profiles. *Metabolomics* **2010**, *6*, 78–95. [CrossRef]
31. Mikkonen, J.J.W.; Singh, S.P.; Akhi, R.; Salo, T.; Lappalainen, R.; González-Arriagada, W.A.; Lopes, M.A.; Kullaa, A.M.; Myllymaa, S. Potential role of nuclear magnetic resonance spectroscopy to identify salivary metabolite alterations in patients with head and neck cancer. *Oncol. Lett.* **2018**, *16*, 6795–6800. [CrossRef]
32. Emwas, A.-H.M. The Strengths and Weaknesses of NMR Spectroscopy and Mass Spectrometry with Particular Focus on Metabolomics Research. In *Metabonomics: Methods and Protocols*; Bjerrum, J.T., Ed.; Springer: New York, NY, USA, 2015; pp. 161–193. ISBN 978-1-4939-2377-9.
33. McBride, E.M.; Lawrence, R.J.; McGee, K.; Mach, P.M.; Demond, P.S.; Busch, M.W.; Ramsay, J.W.; Hussey, E.K.; Glaros, T.; Dhummakupt, E.S. Rapid liquid chromatography tandem mass spectrometry method for targeted quantitation of human performance metabolites in saliva. *J. Chromatogr. A* **2019**, *1601*, 205–213. [CrossRef]
34. Beale, D.J.; Jones, O.A.H.; Karpe, A.V.; Dayalan, S.; Oh, D.Y.; Kouremenos, K.A.; Ahmed, W.; Palombo, E.A. A review of analytical techniques and their application in disease diagnosis in breathomics and salivaomics research. *Int. J. Mol. Sci.* **2017**, *18*, 24. [CrossRef] [PubMed]
35. Esteves, C.V.; de Campos, W.G.; de Souza, M.M.; Lourenço, S.V.; Siqueira, W.L.; Lemos-Júnior, C.A. Diagnostic potential of saliva proteome analysis: A review and guide to clinical practice. *Braz. Oral Res.* **2019**, *33*. [CrossRef] [PubMed]
36. Xiao, H.; Wong, D.T.W. Method development for proteome stabilization in human saliva. *Anal. Chim. Acta* **2012**, *722*, 63–69. [CrossRef] [PubMed]
37. Mishra, S.; Saadat, D.; Kwon, O.; Lee, Y.; Choi, W.S.; Kim, J.H.; Yeo, W.H. Recent advances in salivary cancer diagnostics enabled by biosensors and bioelectronics. *Biosens. Bioelectron.* **2016**, *81*, 181–197. [CrossRef]
38. Kondo, T. Cancer biomarker development and two-dimensional difference gel electrophoresis (2D-DIGE). *Biochim. Biophys. Acta Proteins Proteom.* **2019**, *1867*, 2–8. [CrossRef]
39. Zhang, Y.; Li, X.; Di, Y.P. Fast and Efficient Measurement of Clinical and Biological Samples Using Immunoassay-Based Multiplexing Systems. In *Molecular Toxicology Protocols*; Keohavong, P., Singh, K.P., Gao, W., Eds.; Springer: New York, NY, USA, 2020; pp. 129–147. ISBN 978-1-0716-0223-2.
40. Lin, A. V Direct ELISA. In *ELISA: Methods and Protocols*; Hnasko, R., Ed.; Springer: New York, NY, USA, 2015; pp. 61–67. ISBN 978-1-4939-2742-5.
41. Zaura, E.; Brandt, B.W.; Prodan, A.; Teixeira de Mattos, M.J.; Imangaliyev, S.; Kool, J.; Buijs, M.J.; Jagers, F.L.; Hennequin-Hoenderdos, N.L.; Slot, D.E.; et al. On the ecosystemic network of saliva in healthy young adults. *ISME J.* **2017**, *11*, 1218–1231. [CrossRef]
42. Ge, X.; Rodriguez, R.; Trinh, M.; Gunsolley, J.; Xu, P. Oral microbiome of deep and shallow dental pockets in chronic periodontitis. *PLoS ONE* **2013**, *8*, e65520. [CrossRef]
43. Burne, R.A.; Zeng, L.; Ahn, S.J.; Palmer, S.R.; Liu, Y.; Lefebure, T.; Stanhope, M.J.; Nascimento, M.M. Progress dissecting the oral microbiome in caries and health. *Adv. Dent. Res.* **2012** *24*, 77–80. [CrossRef]

44. Schwabe, R.F.; Jobin, C. The microbiome and cancer. *Nat. Rev. Cancer* **2013**, *13*, 800–812. [CrossRef]
45. Torres, P.J.; Fletcher, E.M.; Gibbons, S.M.; Bouvet, M.; Doran, K.S.; Kelley, S.T. Characterization of the salivary microbiome in patients with pancreatic cancer. *PeerJ* **2015**, *3*, e1373. [CrossRef]
46. Buszewski, B.; Rogowska, A.; Pomastowski, P.; Złoch, M.; Railean-Plugaru, V. Identification of microorganisms by modern analytical techniques. *J. AOAC Int.* **2017**, *100*, 1607–1623. [CrossRef]
47. Rashid, H.; Lamberts, A.; Diercks, G.F.H.; Pas, H.H.; Meijer, J.M.; Bolling, M.C.; Horváth, B. Oral Lesions in Autoimmune Bullous Diseases: An Overview of Clinical Characteristics and Diagnostic Algorithm. *Am. J. Clin. Dermatol.* **2019**, *20*, 847–861. [CrossRef] [PubMed]
48. Jonsson, R.; Brokstad, K.A.; Jonsson, M.V.; Delaleu, N.; Skarstein, K. Current concepts on Sjögren's syndrome–classification criteria and biomarkers. *Eur. J. Oral Sci.* **2018**, *126*, 37–48. [CrossRef] [PubMed]
49. Warnakulasuriya, S. Oral potentially malignant disorders: A comprehensive review on clinical aspects and management. *Oral Oncol.* **2020**, *102*, 104550. [CrossRef] [PubMed]
50. McCartan, B.E.; Healy, C.M. The reported prevalence of oral lichen planus: A review and critique. *J. Oral Pathol. Med.* **2008**, *37*, 447–453. [CrossRef] [PubMed]
51. Thorn, J.J.; Holmstrup, P.; Rindum, J.P.J. Course of various clinical forms of oral lichen planus. A prospective follow-up study of 611 patients. *J. Oral Pathol.* **1988**, *17*, 213–218. [CrossRef] [PubMed]
52. Campanati, A.; Brandozzi, G.; Giangiacomi, M.; Simonetti, O.; Marconi, B.; Offidani, A.M. Lichen striatus in adults and pimecrolimus: Open, off-label clinical study. *Int. J. Dermatol.* **2008**, *47*, 732–736. [CrossRef]
53. Cheng, Y.-S.L.; Gould, A.; Kurago, Z.; Fantasia, J.; Muller, S. Diagnosis of oral lichen planus: A position paper of the American Academy of Oral and Maxillofacial Pathology. *Oral Surg. Oral Med. Oral Pathol. Oral Radiol.* **2016**, *122*, 332–354. [CrossRef]
54. Buajeeb, W.; Okuma, N.; Thanakun, S.; Laothumthut, T. Direct Immunofluorescence in Oral Lichen Planus. *J. Clin. Diagn. Res.* **2015**, *9*, ZC34–ZC37. [CrossRef]
55. Lodi, G.; Scully, C.; Carrozzo, M.; Griffiths, M.; Sugerman, P.B.; Thongprasom, K. Current controversies in oral lichen planus: Report of an international consensus meeting. Part 1. Viral infections and etiopathogenesis. *Oral Surg. Oral Med. Oral Pathol. Oral Radiol.* **2005**, *100*, 40–51. [CrossRef]
56. Van der Meij, E.H.; Schepman, K.-P.; van der Waal, I. The possible premalignant character of oral lichen planus and oral lichenoid lesions: A prospective study. *Oral Surg. Oral Med. Oral Pathol. Oral Radiol.* **2003**, *96*, 164–171. [CrossRef]
57. Radwan-Oczko, M.; Zwyrtek, E.; Owczarek, J.E.; Szcześniak, D. Psychopathological profile and quality of life of patients with oral lichen planus. *J. Appl. Oral Sci.* **2018**, *26*, e20170146. [CrossRef] [PubMed]
58. Talungchit, S.; Buajeeb, W.; Lerdtripop, C.; Surarit, R.; Chairatvit, K.; Roytrakul, S.; Kobayashi, H.; Izumi, Y.; Khovidhunkit, S.-o.P. Putative salivary protein biomarkers for the diagnosis of oral lichen planus: A case-control study. *BMC Oral Health* **2018**, *18*, 42. [CrossRef] [PubMed]
59. Souza, M.M.; Florezi, G.P.; Nico, M.M.S.; de Paula, F.; Paula, F.M.; Lourenço, S.V. Salivary proteomics in lichen planus: A relationship with pathogenesis? *Oral Dis.* **2018**, *24*, 784–792. [CrossRef]
60. De Carvalho, G.C.; Domingues, R.; de Sousa Nogueira, M.A.; Branco, A.C.C.; Manfrere, K.C.G.; Pereira, N.V.; Aoki, V.; Sotto, M.N.; da Silva Duarte, A.J.; Sato, M.N. Up-regulation of Proinflammatory Genes and Cytokines Induced by S100A8 in CD8 + T Cells in Lichen Planus. *Acta Derm. Venereol.* **2016**, *96*, 485–489. [CrossRef]
61. Severo, J.S.; Morais, J.B.S.; Beserra, J.B.; dos Santos, L.R.; de Sousa Melo, S.R.; de Sousa, G.S.; de Matos Neto, E.M.; Henriques, G.S.; do Nascimento Marreiro, D. Role of Zinc in Zinc-α2-Glycoprotein Metabolism in Obesity: A Review of Literature. *Biol. Trace Elem. Res.* **2020**, *193*, 81–88. [CrossRef]
62. Darczuk, D.; Krzysciak, W.; Vyhouskaya, P.; Kesek, B.; Galecka-Wanatowicz, D.; Lipska, W.; Kaczmarzyk, T.; Gluch-Lutwin, M.; Mordyl, B.; Chomyszyn-Gajewska, M. Salivary oxidative status in patients with oral lichen planus. *J. Physiol. Pharmacol.* **2016**, *67*, 885–894.
63. Abdolsamadi, H.; Rafieian, N.; Goodarzi, M.T.; Feradmal, J.; Davoodi, P.; Jazayeri, M.; Taghavi, Z.; Hoseyni, S.-M.; Ahmadi-Motamayel, F. Levels of salivary antioxidant vitamins and lipid peroxidation in patients with oral lichen planus and healthy individuals. *Chonnam Med. J.* **2014**, *50*, 58–62. [CrossRef]
64. Rivarola de Gutierrez, E.; Di Fabio, A.; Salomón, S.; Lanfranchi, H. Topical treatment of oral lichen planus with anthocyanins. *Med. Oral Patol. Oral Cir. Bucal* **2014**, *19*, e459–e466. [CrossRef]

65. Skrinjar, I.; Vidranski, V.; Brzak, B.L.; Juras, D.V.; Rogulj, A.A.; Brailo, V.; Boras, V.V. Salivary cortisol levels in patients with oral lichen planus—A pilot case-control study. *Dent. J.* **2019**, *7*, 59. [CrossRef]
66. Mansourian, A.; Najafi, S.; Nojoumi, N.; Parhami, P.M.M. Salivary Cortisol and Salivary Flow Rate in Clinical Types of Oral Lichen Planus. *Skinmed* **2018**, *16*, 19–22. [PubMed]
67. Lopez-Jornet, P.; Zavattaro, E.; Mozaffari, H.R.; Ramezani, M.; Sadeghi, M. Evaluation of the salivary level of cortisol in patients with oral lichen planus: A meta-analysis. *Medicina* **2019**, *55*, 213. [CrossRef] [PubMed]
68. Nadendla, L.K.; Meduri, V.; Paramkusam, G.; Pachava, K.R. Association of salivary cortisol and anxiety levels in lichen planus patients. *J. Clin. Diagn. Res.* **2014**, *8*, ZC01. [CrossRef] [PubMed]
69. Rödström, P.-O.; Jontell, M.; Hakeberg, M.; Berggren, U.; Lindstedt, G. Erosive oral lichen planus and salivary cortisol. *J. Oral Pathol. Med.* **2001**, *30*, 257–263. [CrossRef] [PubMed]
70. Koray, M.; Dülger, O.; Ak, G.; Horasanli, S.; Üçok, A.; Tanyeri, H.; Badur, S. The evaluation of anxiety and salivary cortisol levels in patients with oral lichen planus. *Oral Dis.* **2003**, *9*, 298–301. [CrossRef]
71. Stojanovich, L. Stress and autoimmunity. *Autoimmun. Rev.* **2010**, *9*, A271–A276. [CrossRef] [PubMed]
72. Wei, W.; Sun, Q.; Deng, Y.; Wang, Y.; Du, G.; Song, C.; Li, C.; Zhu, M.; Chen, G.; Tang, G. Mixed and inhomogeneous expression profile of Th1/Th2 related cytokines detected by cytometric bead array in the saliva of patients with oral lichen planus. *Oral Surg. Oral Med. Oral Pathol. Oral Radiol.* **2018**, *126*, 142–151. [CrossRef]
73. Hodge, D.R.; Peng, B.; Cherry, J.C.; Hurt, E.M.; Fox, S.D.; Kelley, J.A.; Munroe, D.J.; Farrar, W.L. Interleukin 6 Supports the Maintenance of p53 Tumor Suppressor Gene Promoter Methylation. *Cancer Res.* **2005**, *65*, 4673–4682. [CrossRef]
74. Mozaffari, H.R.; Sharifi, R.; Sadeghi, M. Interleukin-6 levels in the serum and saliva of patients with oral lichen planus compared with healthy controls: A meta-analysis study. *Cent. Eur. J. Immunol.* **2018**, *43*, 103–108. [CrossRef]
75. Baggiolini, M.; Clark-Lewis, I. Interleukin-8, a chemotactic and inflammatory cytokine. *FEBS Lett.* **1992**, *307*, 97–101. [CrossRef]
76. Mozaffari, H.R.; Sharifi, R.; Mirbahari, S.; Montazerian, S.; Sadeghi, M.; Rostami, S. A systematic review and meta-analysis study of salivary and serum interleukin-8 levels in oral lichen planus. *Postep. Dermatol. Alergol.* **2018**, *35*, 599–604. [CrossRef] [PubMed]
77. Rhodus, N.L.; Cheng, B.; Myers, S.; Miller, L.; Ho, V.; Ondrey, F. The feasibility of monitoring NF-κB associated cytokines: TNF-α, IL-1α, IL-6, and IL-8 in whole saliva for the malignant transformation of oral lichen planus. *Mol. Carcinog.* **2005**, *44*, 77–82. [CrossRef] [PubMed]
78. Rhodus, N.L.; Cheng, B.; Bowles, W.; Myers, S.; Miller, L.; Ondrey, F. Proinflammatory cytokine levels in saliva before and after treatment of (erosive) oral lichen planus with dexamethasone. *Oral Dis.* **2006**, *12*, 112–116. [CrossRef] [PubMed]
79. Warnakulasuriya, S. Global epidemiology of oral and oropharyngeal cancer. *Oral Oncol.* **2009**, *45*, 309–316. [CrossRef] [PubMed]
80. Mehrtash, H.; Duncan, K.; Parascandola, M.; David, A.; Gritz, E.R.; Gupta, P.C.; Mehrotra, R.; Amer Nordin, A.S.; Pearlman, P.C.; Warnakulasuriya, S.; et al. Defining a global research and policy agenda for betel quid and areca nut. *Lancet Oncol.* **2017**, *18*, e767–e775. [CrossRef]
81. Yete, S.; D'Souza, W.; Saranath, D. High-Risk Human Papillomavirus in Oral Cancer: Clinical Implications. *Oncology* **2018**, *94*, 133–141. [CrossRef]
82. Scheifele, C.; Reichart, P.A. Is there a natural limit of the transformation rate of oral leukoplakia? *Oral Oncol.* **2003**, *39*, 470–475. [CrossRef]
83. Offidani, A.; Simonetti, O.; Bernardini, M.L.; Alpagut, A.; Cellini, A.; Bossi, G. General Practitioners' Accuracy in Diagnosing Skin Cancers. *Dermatology* **2002**, *205*, 127–130. [CrossRef]
84. Mignogna, M.D.; Fedele, S.; Russo, L.L.; Ruoppo, E.; Muzio, L.L. Oral and pharyngeal cancer: Lack of prevention and early detection by health care providers. *Eur. J. Cancer Prev.* **2001**, *10*, 381–383. [CrossRef]
85. Mehdipour, M.; Shahidi, M.; Manifar, S.; Jafari, S.; Mashhadi Abbas, F.; Barati, M.; Mortazavi, H.; Shirkhoda, M.; Farzanegan, A.; Elmi Rankohi, Z. Diagnostic and prognostic relevance of salivary microRNA-21, -125a, -31 and -200a levels in patients with oral lichen planus—A short report. *Cell. Oncol.* **2018**, *41*, 329–334. [CrossRef]
86. Park, N.J.; Zhou, H.; Elashoff, D.; Henson, B.S.; Kastratovic, D.A.; Abemayor, E.; Wong, D.T. Salivary

microRNA: Discovery, characterization, and clinical utility for oral cancer detection. *Clin. Cancer Res.* **2009**, *15*, 5473–5477. [CrossRef]
87. Sun, Y.-M.; Lin, K.-Y.; Chen, Y.-Q. Diverse functions of miR-125 family in different cell contexts. *J. Hematol. Oncol.* **2013**, *6*, 6. [CrossRef] [PubMed]
88. Ishikawa, S.; Sugimoto, M.; Edamatsu, K.; Sugano, A.; Kitabatake, K.; Iino, M. Discrimination of oral squamous cell carcinoma from oral lichen planus by salivary metabolomics. *Oral Dis.* **2020**, *26*, 35–42. [CrossRef] [PubMed]
89. Ma, B.; Simala-Grant, J.L.; Taylor, D.E. Fucosylation in prokaryotes and eukaryotes. *Glycobiology* **2006**, *16*, 158R–184R. [CrossRef] [PubMed]
90. Miyoshi, E.; Moriwaki, K.; Nakagawa, T. Biological Function of Fucosylation in Cancer Biology. *J. Biochem.* **2008**, *143*, 725–729. [CrossRef] [PubMed]
91. Sanjay, P.; Hallikeri, K.; Shivashankara, A. Evaluation of salivary sialic acid, total protein, and total sugar in oral cancer: A preliminary report. *Indian J. Dent. Res.* **2008**, *19*, 288–291. [PubMed]
92. Dhakar, N.; Astekar, M.; Jain, M.; Saawarn, S.; Saawarn, N. Total sialic acid, total protein and total sugar levels in serum and saliva of oral squamous cell carcinoma patients: A case control study. *Dent. Res. J.* **2013**, *10*, 343–347.
93. Dadhich, M.; Prabhu, V.; Pai, V.; D'Souza, J.; Harish, S.; Jose, M. Serum and salivary sialic acid as a biomarker in oral potentially malignant disorders and oral cancer. *Indian J. Cancer* **2014**, *51*, 214–218.
94. Panda, M.; Rai, A.K.; Rahman, T.; Das, A.; Das, R.; Sarma, A.; Kataki, A.C.; Chattopadhyay, I. Alterations of salivary microbial community associated with oropharyngeal and hypopharyngeal squamous cell carcinoma patients. *Arch. Microbiol.* **2019**. [CrossRef]
95. Healy, C.M.; Moran, G.P. The microbiome and oral cancer: More questions than answers. *Oral Oncol.* **2019**, *89*, 30–33. [CrossRef]
96. Marttila, E.; Uittamo, J.; Rusanen, P.; Lindqvist, C.; Salaspuro, M.; Rautemaa, R. Acetaldehyde production and microbial colonization in oral squamous cell carcinoma and oral lichenoid disease. *Oral Surg. Oral Med. Oral Pathol. Oral Radiol.* **2013**, *116*, 61–68. [CrossRef]
97. Marttila, E.; Uittamo, J.; Rusanen, P.; Lindqvist, C.; Salaspuro, M.; Rautemaa, R. Site-specific acetaldehyde production and microbial colonization in relation to oral squamous cell carcinoma and oral lichenoid disease. *Oral Surg. Oral Med. Oral Pathol. Oral Radiol.* **2015**, *119*, 697–699. [CrossRef] [PubMed]
98. Alnuaimi, A.D.; Ramdzan, A.N.; Wiesenfeld, D.; O'Brien-Simpson, N.M.; Kolev, S.D.; Reynolds, E.C.; McCullough, M.J. Candida virulence and ethanol-derived acetaldehyde production in oral cancer and non-cancer subjects. *Oral Dis.* **2016**, *22*, 805–814. [CrossRef] [PubMed]
99. Moritani, K.; Takeshita, T.; Shibata, Y.; Ninomiya, T.; Kiyohara, Y.; Yamashita, Y. Acetaldehyde production by major oral microbes. *Oral Dis.* **2015**, *21*, 748–754. [CrossRef] [PubMed]
100. Wu, J.; Peters, B.A.; Dominianni, C.; Zhang, Y.; Pei, Z.; Yang, L.; Ma, Y.; Purdue, M.P.; Jacobs, E.J.; Gapstur, S.M.; et al. Cigarette smoking and the oral microbiome in a large study of American adults. *ISME J.* **2016**, *10*, 2435–2446. [CrossRef] [PubMed]
101. Corbaux, C.; Joly, P. Bullous Diseases. In *Current Problems in Dermatology*; KARGER: Basel, Switzerland, 2017; Volume 53, pp. 64–69. ISBN 1421-5721.
102. Murrell, D.F.; Peña, S.; Joly, P.; Marinovic, B.; Hashimoto, T.; Diaz, L.A.; Sinha, A.A.; Payne, A.S.; Daneshpazhooh, M.; Eming, R.; et al. Diagnosis and Management of Pemphigus: Recommendations by an International Panel of Experts. *J. Am. Acad. Dermatol.* **2019**. [CrossRef] [PubMed]
103. Andreadis, D.; Lorenzini, G.; Drakoulakos, D.; Belazi, M.; Mihailidou, E.; Velkos, G.; Mourellou-Tsatsou, O.; Antoniades, D. Detection of pemphigus desmoglein 1 and desmoglein 3 autoantibodies and pemphigoid BP180 autoantibodies in saliva and comparison with serum values. *Eur. J. Oral Sci.* **2006**, *114*, 374–380. [CrossRef]
104. Ali, S.; Kelly, C.; Challacombe, S.J.; Donaldson, A.N.A.; Bhogal, B.S.; Setterfield, J.F. Serum and salivary IgG and IgA antibodies to desmoglein 3 in mucosal pemphigus vulgaris. *Br. J. Dermatol.* **2016**, *175*, 113–121. [CrossRef]
105. Hallaji, Z.; Mortazavi, H.; Lajevardi, V.; Tamizifar, B.; Amirzargar, A.; Daneshpazhooh, M.; Chams-Davatchi, C. Serum and salivary desmoglein 1 and 3 enzyme-linked immunosorbent assay in pemphigus vulgaris: Correlation with phenotype and severity. *J. Eur. Acad. Dermatology Venereol.* **2010**, *24*, 275–280. [CrossRef]

106. De, D.; Khullar, G.; Handa, S.; Joshi, N.; Saikia, B.; Minz, R.W. Correlation between salivary and serum anti-desmoglein 1 and 3 antibody titres using ELISA and between anti-desmoglein levels and disease severity in pemphigus vulgaris. *Clin. Exp. Dermatol.* **2017**, *42*, 648–650. [CrossRef]
107. Russo, I.; Saponeri, A.; Michelotto, A.; Alaibac, M. Salivary samples for the diagnosis of Pemphigus vulgaris using the BIOCHIP approach: A pilot study. *In Vivo* **2017**, *31*, 97–100. [CrossRef] [PubMed]
108. Brito-Zerón, P.; Baldini, C.; Bootsma, H.; Bowman, S.J.; Jonsson, R.; Mariette, X.; Sivils, K.; Theander, E.; Tzioufas, A.; Ramos-Casals, M. Sjögren syndrome. *Nat. Rev. Dis. Prim.* **2016**, *2*, 16047. [CrossRef] [PubMed]
109. Pasoto, S.G.; Adriano de Oliveira Martins, V.; Bonfa, E. Sjögren's syndrome and systemic lupus erythematosus: Links and risks. *Open Access Rheumatol. Res. Rev.* **2019**, *11*, 33–45.
110. Fernández-Martínez, G.; Zamora-Legoff, V.; Hernández Molina, G. Oral health-related quality of life in primary Sjögren's syndrome. *Reumatol. Clínica (Engl. Ed.)* **2019**. [CrossRef]
111. Ben-Chetrit, E.; Fischel, R.; Rubinow, A. Anti-SSA/Ro and anti-SSB/La antibodies in serum and saliva of patients with Sjogren's syndrome. *Clin Rheumatol.* **1993**, *12*, 471–474. [CrossRef] [PubMed]
112. Ching, K.H.; Burbelo, P.D.; Gonzalez-Begne, M.; Roberts, M.E.P.; Coca, A.; Sanz, I.; Iadarola, M.J. Salivary anti-Ro60 and anti-Ro52 antibody profiles to diagnose Sjogren's Syndrome. *J. Dent. Res.* **2011**, *90*, 445–449. [CrossRef]
113. Hu, S.; Vissink, A.; Arellano, M.; Roozendaal, C.; Zhou, H.; Kallenberg, C.G.M.; Wong, D.T. Identification of autoantibody biomarkers for primary Sjögren's syndrome using protein microarrays. *Proteomics* **2011**, *11*, 1499–1507. [CrossRef]
114. Ohyama, K.; Moriyama, M.; Hayashida, J.-N.; Tanaka, A.; Maehara, T.; Ieda, S.; Furukawa, S.; Ohta, M.; Imabayashi, Y.; Nakamura, S. Saliva as a potential tool for diagnosis of dry mouth including Sjögren's syndrome. *Oral Dis.* **2015**, *21*, 224–231. [CrossRef]
115. Kang, E.H.; Lee, Y.J.; Hyon, J.Y.; Yun, P.Y.; Song, Y.W. Salivary cytokine profiles in primary Sjögren's syndrome differ from those in non-Sjögren sicca in terms of TNF-α levels and Th-1/Th-2 ratios. *Clin. Exp. Rheumatol.* **2011**, *29*, 970–976.
116. Katsiougiannis, S.; Wong, D.T.W. The Proteomics of Saliva in Sjögren's Syndrome. *Rheum. Dis. Clin. N. Am.* **2016**, *42*, 449–456. [CrossRef]
117. Lee, J.; Lee, J.; Baek, S.; Koh, J.H.; Kim, J.-W.; Kim, S.-Y.; Chung, S.-H.; Choi, S.S.; Cho, M.-L.; Kwok, S.-K.; et al. Soluble siglec-5 is a novel salivary biomarker for primary Sjogren's syndrome. *J. Autoimmun.* **2019**, *100*, 114–119. [CrossRef]
118. Tandon, M.; Gallo, A.; Jang, S.-I.; Illei, G.G.; Alevizos, I. Deep sequencing of short RNAs reveals novel microRNAs in minor salivary glands of patients with Sjögren's syndrome. *Oral Dis.* **2012**, *18*, 127–131. [CrossRef] [PubMed]
119. Pauley, K.M.; Stewart, C.M.; Gauna, A.E.; Dupre, L.C.; Kuklani, R.; Chan, A.L.; Pauley, B.A.; Reeves, W.H.; Chan, E.K.L.; Cha, S. Altered miR-146a expression in Sjögren's syndrome and its functional role in innate immunity. *Eur. J. Immunol.* **2011**, *41*, 2029–2039. [CrossRef] [PubMed]
120. Alevizos, I.; Alexander, S.; Turner, R.J.; Illei, G.G. MicroRNA expression profiles as biomarkers of minor salivary gland inflammation and dysfunction in Sjögren's syndrome. *Arthritis Rheum.* **2011**, *63*, 535–544. [CrossRef] [PubMed]
121. Ibáñez-Cabellos, J.S.; Seco-Cervera, M.; Osca-Verdegal, R.; Pallardó, F.V.; García-Giménez, J.L. Epigenetic Regulation in the Pathogenesis of Sjögren Syndrome and Rheumatoid Arthritis. *Front. Genet.* **2019**, *10*, 1104. [CrossRef]
122. Konsta, O.D.; Thabet, Y.; Le Dantec, C.; Brooks, W.H.; Tzioufas, A.G.; Pers, J.O.; Renaudineau, Y. The contribution of epigenetics in Sjogren's Syndrome. *Front. Genet.* **2014**, *5*, 71. [CrossRef] [PubMed]
123. Thabet, Y.; Le Dantec, C.; Ghedira, I.; Devauchelle, V.; Cornec, D.; Pers, J.-O.; Renaudineau, Y. Epigenetic dysregulation in salivary glands from patients with primary Sjögren's syndrome may be ascribed to infiltrating B cells. *J. Autoimmun.* **2013**, *41*, 175–181. [CrossRef]
124. Baldini, C.; Giusti, L.; Ciregia, F.; Da Valle, Y.; Giacomelli, C.; Donadio, E.; Ferro, F.; Galimberti, S.; Donati, V.; Bazzichi, L.; et al. Correspondence between salivary proteomic pattern and clinical course in primary Sjögren syndrome and non-Hodgkin's lymphoma: A case report. *J. Transl. Med.* **2011**, *9*, 188. [CrossRef]
125. Cui, L.; Elzakra, N.; Xu, S.; Xiao, G.G.; Yang, Y.; Hu, S. Investigation of three potential autoantibodies in Sjogren's syndrome and associated MALT lymphoma. *Oncotarget* **2017**, *8*, 30039–30049.

126. Sharma, D.; Sandhya, P.; Vellarikkal, S.K.; Surin, A.K.; Jayarajan, R.; Verma, A.; Kumar, A.; Ravi, R.; Danda, D.; Sivasubbu, S.; et al. Saliva microbiome in primary Sjögren's syndrome reveals distinct set of disease-associated microbes. *Oral Dis.* **2019**. [CrossRef]
127. Siddiqui, H.; Chen, T.; Aliko, A.; Mydel, P.M.; Jonsson, R.; Olsen, I. Microbiological and bioinformatics analysis of primary Sjögren's syndrome patients with normal salivation. *J. Oral Microbiol.* **2016**, *8*, 31119. [CrossRef]
128. Li, B.; Selmi, C.; Tang, R.; Gershwin, M.E.; Ma, X. The microbiome and autoimmunity: A paradigm from the gut–liver axis. *Cell. Mol. Immunol.* **2018**, *15*, 595–609. [CrossRef] [PubMed]
129. Campanati, A.; Ganzetti, G.; Giuliodori, K.; Marra, M.; Bonfigli, A.; Testa, R.; Offidani, A. Serum levels of adipocytokines in psoriasis patients receiving tumor necrosis factor-α inhibitors: results of a retrospective analysis. *Int. J. Dermatol.* **2015**, *54*, 39–45. [CrossRef] [PubMed]
130. Campanati, A.; Ganzetti, G.; Giuliodori, K.; Postacchini, V.; Liberati, G.; Azzaretto, L.; Vichi, S.; Guanciarossa, F.; Offidani, A. Homocysteine plasma levels in psoriasis patients: our experience and review of the literature. *J. Eur. Acad. Dermatol. Venereol.* **2015**, *29*, 1781–1785.
131. Ganzetti, G.; Campanati, A.; Santarelli, A.; Pozzi, V.; Molinelli, E.; Minnetti, I.; Brisigotti, V.; Procaccini, M.; Emanuelli, M.; Offidani, A.; et al. Periodontal disease: an oral manifestation of psoriasis or an occasional finding? *Drug Dev. Res.* **2014**, *75*, S56–S59.
132. Ganzetti, G.; Campanati, A.; Santarelli, A.; Pozzi, V.; Molinelli, E.; Minnetti, I.; Brisigotti, V.; Procaccini, M.; Emanuelli, M.; Offidani, A. Involvement of the oral cavity in psoriasis: Results of a clinical study. *Br. J. Dermatol.* **2015**, *172*, 282–285. [CrossRef] [PubMed]
133. Ganzetti, G.; Campanati, A.; Santarelli, A.; Sartini, D.; Molinelli, E.; Brisigotti, V.; Di Ruscio, G.; Bobyr, I.; Emanuelli, M.; Offidani, A. Salivary interleukin-1β: Oral inflammatory biomarker in patients with psoriasis. *J. Int. Med. Res.* **2016**, *44*, 10–14. [CrossRef]

13

Enhanced Inflammation and Nitrosative Stress in the Saliva and Plasma of Patients with Plaque Psoriasis

Anna Skutnik-Radziszewska [1], Mateusz Maciejczyk [2], Iwona Flisiak [3], Julita Krahel [3], Urszula Kołodziej [4], Anna Kotowska-Rodziewicz [4], Anna Klimiuk [5] and Anna Zalewska [5,*]

1 Experimental Dentistry Laboratory, Medical University of Bialystok, 1 Jana Kilinskiego Street, 15-089 Bialystok, Poland; anna.skutnik@o2.pl
2 Department of Hygiene, Epidemiology and Ergonomics, Medical University of Bialystok, 2c Mickiewicza Street, 15-022 Bialystok, Poland; mat.maciejczyk@gmail.com
3 Department of Dermatology and Venereology, Medical University of Bialystok, 14 Zurawia Street, 15-540 Bialystok, Poland; iwona.flisiak@umb.edu.pl (I.F.); julita.leonczuk@gmail.com (J.K.)
4 Department of Restorative Dentistry, Medical University of Bialystok, 24A M. Sklodowskiej-Curie Street, 15-276 Bialystok, Poland; ulakol@poczta.onet.pl (U.K.); kotowskanna@wp.pl (A.K-R.)
5 Experimental Dentistry Laboratory, Medical University of Bialystok, 24A M. Sklodowskiej-Curie Street, 15-276 Bialystok, Poland; annak04@poczta.onet.pl
* Correspondence: azalewska426@gmail.com

Abstract: Psoriasis is the most common inflammatory skin disease, characterized by the release of proinflammatory cytokines from lymphocytes, keratinocytes, and dendritic cells. Although psoriasis is considered an immune-mediated inflammatory disease, its effect on secretory activity of salivary glands and quantitative composition of saliva is still unknown. The aim of this study was to evaluate the secretion of saliva as well as several selected inflammation and nitrosative stress biomarkers in unstimulated and stimulated saliva as well as plasma of psoriasis patients. We demonstrated that, with progressing severity and duration of the disease, the secretory function of the parotid and submandibular salivary glands is lost, which is manifested as decreased unstimulated and stimulated saliva secretion and reduced salivary amylase activity and total protein concentration. The levels of tumor necrosis factor-alpha (TNF-α), interleukin-2 (IL-2), and interferon-gamma (INF-γ) were significantly higher, whereas interleukin-10 (IL-10) content was considerably lower in unstimulated and stimulated saliva of patients with psoriasis compared to the controls, and the changes increased with the disease duration. Similarly, we observed that the intensity of nitrosative stress in the salivary glands of psoriasis patients depended on the duration of the disease. By means of receiver operating characteristic (ROC) analysis, we showed that the evaluation of nitric oxide (NO), nitrotyrosine, and IL-2 concentration in non-stimulated saliva with high sensitivity and specificity differentiated psoriasis patients on the basis of the rate of saliva secretion (normal salivation vs. hyposalivation). In summary, the dysfunction of salivary glands in psoriasis patients is caused by inflammation and nitrosative stress.

Keywords: plaque psoriasis; salivary glands; saliva; cytokines; nitrosative stress

---

1. Introduction

Psoriasis vulgaris is a skin inflammatory disease, the third most common among autoimmune diseases [1]. The pathogenesis of psoriasis involves the combination of genetic susceptibility, aberrant immune response, and several environmental factors (injuries, viral infections, medications taken, food intolerances). Typical features of psoriasis vulgaris include an immune-mediated process in which the key role is played by Th1 cells (T-helper 1). The presence of antigen-specific CD4+ (dendritic cell) T cells secreting type 1 cytokines: interferon-gamma (INF-γ), interleukin-2 (IL-2), and tumor necrosis factor-alpha (TNF-α) was observed in psoriatic skin lesions [2,3]. Moreover, the imbalance between Th1 and Th2 cells in psoriasis was confirmed by studies that showed interleukin-10 (IL-10) deficiency in psoriatic skin lesions [4]. Recent findings suggest that redox imbalance in the blood and skin of patients with psoriasis, resulting from the immune system stimulation, plays as important role in the pathogenesis of plaque psoriasis as the inflammatory process itself. It has been shown that, in the course of psoriasis, oxidative stress (OS) is primarily caused by reduced activity/concentration of antioxidants [5–9] and leads to increased oxidative modification of cellular elements of skin and plasma [6,10,11]. Plasma and erythrocyte product of lipid peroxidation (malondialdehyde, MDA) is considered a biomarker of plaque psoriasis exacerbation [12,13].

The detrimental inflammatory milieu and increased production of free radicals (ROS) associated with plaque psoriasis are not limited to the skin, but are also responsible for the growing number of comorbidities, including cardiological diseases, metabolic syndrome, chronic kidney disease, mood disorders, and salivary gland diseases [5,14–17].

Saliva produced by salivary glands performs numerous important functions in the oral cavity: hydrating it, removing harmful waste products and bacteria, participating in the remineralization of dental hard tissues, maintaining redox balance, and being involved in immune responses [18–20]. Disorders of both the composition and amount of saliva secreted into the oral cavity have physiological and psychological consequences. Therefore, it is very important to understand the mechanisms leading to salivary gland dysfunction in the course of systemic diseases. Unfortunately, the pathophysiology of salivary gland disorders in psoriasis is still unknown. In our previous work, we demonstrated that plaque psoriasis is accompanied by salivary redox imbalances with the prevalence of oxidation reactions. We observed that redox equilibrium in the submandibular glands was more vulnerable, and antioxidant capacity of the submandibular glands decreased with the disease duration [15]. There have been very few studies on the modification of saliva inflammatory components in psoriatic patients. Ganzetti et al. [21] demonstrated higher levels of TNF-α, transforming growth factor-beta (TGF-β), and interleukin-1 (IL-1β) in the saliva of psoriatic subjects vs. the controls. Unfortunately, most patients with psoriasis had also been diagnosed with periodontitis or gingivitis. Consequently, the observed cytokine changes in saliva reflected periodontal inflammation and not psoriasis-related salivary changes, and thus they did not explain the pathophysiology of salivary gland dysfunctions in the course of this disease. It has been evidenced that pro-inflammatory cytokines boost the expression of the inducible nitric oxide (NO) synthase (*i*NOS) in the cells, which results in increased NO synthesis in inflamed joints [22]. It was proven that NO and other reactive nitrogen intermediates affect a vast number of physiological functions of salivary glands, including exocytosis, water secretion, salivary blood flow, and non-specific immunological reactions [23–25]. The contribution of nitrosative stress to the pathophysiology of salivary glands in the course of psoriasis is unknown.

An ideal biomarker is characterized by simple determination as well as high sensitivity, specificity, and repeatability. It should also enable the identification of the patient's physiological and pathological status and response to the applied treatment [26]. Numerous biomarkers have been suggested for easier diagnosis of psoriasis and monitoring of its treatment. However, studies on psoriasis biomarkers have been based on blood tests, examining skin fragments, conducting genetic tests, and transcriptomics. The results of these studies were divergent, and therefore neither was considered reliable nor was accepted as a psoriasis marker [27]. Saliva is a mixture of secretions of large salivary glands and gingival fluid. It also contains almost all the elements present in the blood and passing through the spaces between cells as part of an inter- and paracellular transport. It is also relatively easy and safe to collect, providing a new, non-invasive way to diagnose numerous general diseases [28–32].

Thus, the aim of this work was to explore the mechanisms responsible for salivary gland dysfunction in psoriasis. We compared the concentrations of TNF-α, IL-2, INF-γ, IL-10, NO, peroxynitrite, S-nitrosothiols, and nitrotyrosine in the saliva and blood of psoriatic subjects with hyposalivation and normal salivation vs. healthy controls. The goal of our study was also to search for salivary biomarkers to assess the severity of psoriasis and the accompanying salivary complications.

2. Materials and Methods

We obtained the consent of the Local Research Ethics Committee in Bialystok (permission number: R-I-002/563/2018). All patients as well as healthy subjects were informed about the purpose of the study and its risks and benefits, and they all consented to the collection of saliva and blood samples.

This experiment included psoriatic patients applying for treatment to the Department of Dermatology and Venereology of the Medical University of Bialystok. The reason for reporting to the hospital was exacerbation of psoriasis symptoms. Patients had not undergone general treatment of psoriasis within 2 preceding years. The only acceptable forms of treatment included local application of ointment with glucocorticosteroids, but not during 3 preceding months. The severity of skin lesions was assessed using the previously described Psoriasis Area and Severity Index (PASI) [15].

A total of 60 healthy patients participated in the study, who were individuals reporting for check-up visits to the Department of Restorative Dentistry at the Medical University of Bialystok, and were matched to the group of patients in terms of age and sex.

Within 6 preceding months, participants did not take any medicines that could affect the composition and secretion of saliva, as well as vitamins, antioxidants, and antibiotics. The participants from the control group were generally healthy, and patients with psoriasis did not have any accompanying diseases. The inclusion criteria was absence of periodontal pathology (periodontal pocket depth (PPD) < 2 mm, did not bleed during the probing) and no inflammatory or fungal changes on the oral mucosa. Only subjects without acrylic dentures were included in the study. The patients as well as healthy controls were not addicted to alcohol and did not smoke cigarettes.

One of the criteria differentiating the dysfunction of salivary glands is reduced flow of unstimulated saliva (NWS) [18]. Therefore, to delineate the influence of psoriasis vulgaris on the parotid and submandibular glands, psoriatic patients were divided into two groups: with reduced NWS (psoriasis hyposalivation-PH, $n = 30$) and normal NWS (psoriasis normal secretion- PN, $n = 30$). The limit value for NWS was assumed at ≤ 0.2 mL/min, which is considered the minimum value of NWS for healthy population [18]. Moreover, the minimum value of NWS in our control group was 0.21 mL/min.

The number of patients was confirmed by the test as sufficient, and the test power was 0.9. Clinical characteristics of the patients are presented in Table 1.

Table 1. Clinical characteristics of plaque psoriasis patients and control subjects.

Patient Characteristics		**Control** *n* = 60	**PN** *n* = 30	**PH** *n* = 30
Sex	Male *n* (%)	23 (38.33%)	13 (43.33%)	10 (33.33%)
	Female *n* (%)	37 (61.67%)	17 (56.67%)	20 (66.67%)
Age (years)		52 ± 5	49 ± 6	51 ± 3
Height (cm)		172 ± 6	176 ± 3	169 ± 8
Weight (kg)		75 ± 1	72 ± 3	74 ± 1
Duration of psoriasis (years)		ND	9.7 ± 3.4	18.52 ± 7.8
PASI		ND	10.39 ± 2.4	18.29 ± 4.6
Psoriasis in the family	<1 *n* (%)	ND	18 (60%)	6 (20%)
	≥1 *n* (%)	ND	12 (40%)	24 (80%)

Table 1. *Cont.*

Patient Characteristics	Control $n = 60$	PN $n = 30$	PH $n = 30$
	Blood Tests		
RBC ($10^6/\mu L$)	4.54 ± 0.54	4.23 ± 0.65	4.89 ± 0.87
HCT (%)	40.25 ± 6.5	42.45 ± 4.25	45.21 ± 0.89
PLT ($10^3/\mu L$)	275 ± 56	245 ± 87	292 ± 23
WBC ($10^3/\mu L$)	6.5 ± 2.2	7.05 ± 1.8	6.98 ± 1.86
CRP (mg/L)	1.5 ± 0.5	8.56 ± 6.3	6.32 ± 7.56
Glc (mg/dL)	69 ± 9.8	72 ± 9.8	75 ± 6.5
ALT (U/L)	27.56 ± 12.3	24.36 ± 9.68	27.24 ± 6.35
AST (U/L)	28.54 ± 12.25	30.23 ± 6.52	28.98 ± 8.64
	Dental Characteristics		
DMFT	20 ± 3	19 ± 6	21 ± 2
GI	0.2 ± 0.1	0.2 ± 0.2	0.1 ± 0.2
PPD	1.5 ± 0.5	1.0 ± 0.5	1.0 ± 0.5
Dental implants	0	0	0

Abbreviations: ALT—alanine transferase; AST—aspartate transaminase; CRP—C-reactive protein; DMFT—decayed, missing, filled teeth index; GI—gingival index; Glc—D-glucose; HCT—hematocrit; *n*—number of patients; PASI—Psoriasis Area and Severity Index; PBI—papilla bleeding index; PLT—platelets; RBC—red blood cells; WBC—white blood cells. ND-not defined.

2.1. Blood Collection

Blood was collected at fasting, either at the admission of a patient to the hospital or during routine tests in case of control subjects. Blood was collected at 5 mL using an S-Monovette EDTA K3 tube (Sarstedt, Nümbrecht, Germany). The samples were then centrifuged (3000 × *g*, 10 min, 4 °C). No hemolysis was observed in any of the obtained plasma samples. To prevent sample oxidation, 0.5 M Butylated hydroxytoluene BHT (Sigma-Aldrich, Saint Louis, MO, USA; 10 μL/mL blood) was added [28]. Plasma was frozen (−82 °C). The samples were stored deep-frozen for no longer than 6 months.

2.2. Saliva Collection

The examined material was unstimulated and stimulated (SWS) total saliva collected from the patient by the spitting method [28]. Saliva was collected in the morning, on an empty stomach, between 8 a.m. and 10 a.m. in order to minimize the effect of daily changes on saliva secretion. The participants had refrained from taking any drugs for 8 hours prior to the examination. Saliva was collected in a separate room, in a sitting position with the head slightly inclined downwards, with minimized face and lip movements, and after a 5-minute adaptation period. Next, the patient rinsed the mouth three times with water at room temperature. The saliva collected during the first minute was discarded. The subsequent batches of saliva (the patient actively spat out the saliva accumulated in the bottom of the oral cavity) were collected into a plastic centrifuge tube placed in an ice container. NWS was collected for 15 minutes, and SWS was collected after a 5-minute break. Stimulation was performed by dropping 100 μL of 2% citric acid on the tip of the tongue every 20 seconds, for 5 minutes. To prevent sample oxidation, 0.5 M BHT (Sigma-Aldrich, Saint Louis, MO, USA; 10 μL/mL blood) was added to the saliva [33]. The volume of each sample was measured with a pipette calibrated to 0.1 mL. Saliva secretion was calculated by dividing the volume of the obtained saliva by the number of minutes of its collection. The collected saliva was centrifuged (20 minutes, 4 °C, 10,000 × *g*) [33]. The sediments were discarded, and supernatant fluid was divided into portions of 200 μL each, frozen in −80 °C, and stored until assayed, but for no longer than 6 months.

2.3. Stomatological Examination

After saliva collection, stomatological examinations were performed by one dentist (A.S.-R.), in artificial light, using a dental mirror, probe, and periodontal probe (Hossa International, Warsaw, Poland; design and construction in accordance with WHO guidelines) according to WHO criteria [34]. The dental status of each participant was assessed on the basis of the DMFT index (decayed, missing, filled teeth). The condition of periodontal tissues was assessed using GI (gingival index) and probing pocket depth (PPD) were assessed at teeth 16, 21, 24, 36, 41, and 44. The PPD and occurrence of bleeding were assessed after gently introducing the probe into the gingival space parallel to the long axis of the tooth, to the depth of perceived resistance posed by the bottom of the gingival gap. Four surfaces of each examined tooth (mesial, distal, buccal, and lingual) were examined. In the case of GI, we used a scale of 0 to 3. The sum of the values, from four surfaces divided by 4, determined the level of the PPD/ gingival index for a given tooth. Then, the results were added and divided by the number of teeth examined. In 25 participants, the inter-rater agreement between the examiner (A.S.-R.) and other experienced dentists (U.K., A.K.) was performed. The reliability for DMFT was $r = 0.99$, for GI was $r = 0.89$, and for PPD was $r = 0.94$. If bleeding during probing or PPD deeper than 2 mm were found, previously collected saliva was discarded and the patient was excluded from the study. Thus, 53 patients with psoriasis and 37 healthy controls who had bleeding of probing and/or PPD > 2 mm were disqualified from the study.

2.4. Biochemical Assays

All determinations of plasma, NWS, and SWS were performed in duplicate samples. The absorbance/fluorescence was measured using an Infinite M200 PRO Multimode Microplate Reader (Tecan Group Ltd., Männedorf, Switzerland). The results were standardized to 1 mg of protein.

2.5. Pro-Inflammatory Cytokines

The concentrations of TNF-α, IL-2, IL-10, and INF-γ were determined by the ELISA method using commercial kits from EIAab Science Inc. Wuhan (Wuhan, China), according to the manufacturer's instructions.

2.6. Nitrosative Stress

The concentration of NO was determined spectrophotometrically using the Griess reagent—a solution of sulfanilic acid and α-naphthylamine in acetic acid [35]. The reaction of nitrates with sulfanilamide produces *N*-(1-naphthyl)-ethylenediamine dihydrochloride, the absorbance of which was measured at 490 nm wavelength.

The concentration of S-nitrosothiols was determined spectrophotometrically on the basis of the reaction of the Griess reagent with Cu^{2+} copper ions [36]. The solution was shaken and set aside for 20 minutes, and then the absorbance was measured at 490 nm [37].

Peroxynitrite concentration was determined spectrophotometrically via a test using peroxynitrite decomposition followed by nitration of 4-hydroxyphenylacetic acid (4-HPA) and glycyltyrosine [38]. The reaction resulted in the production of nitrophenol, the absorbance of which was measured at 320 nm wavelength.

The concentration of nitrotyrosine was determined by ELISA using the Nitrotyrosine ELISA kit from Immunodiagnostik AG (Bensheim, Germany), following the manufacturer's instructions provided in the package.

2.7. *Salivary Protein*

Salivary protein content was determined using the bicinchoninic acid (BCA) method (Pierce BCA Protein Assay; Thermo Scientific (Rockford, IL, USA)). Bovine serum albumin was used as a standard.

2.8. *Salivary Amylase*

The activity of salivary amylase (EC 3.2.1.1.) was determined colorimetrically using 3,5-dinitrosalicylic acid (DNS) as a substrate [39]. By this method, starch was transformed by amylase to maltose, and was measured at 540 nm by the complex with DNS.

2.9. *Statistical Analysis*

The obtained results were assessed statistically by means of one-way analysis of variance (ANOVA). The significance of differences between individual groups was determined with the post-hoc Tukey's HSD test, and normal distribution was confirmed via the Shapiro–Wilk test. The correlations between the examined parameters were described using the Pearson correlation coefficient. The value of $p < 0.05$ was considered statistically significant. In order to assess the diagnostic usefulness between plaque psoriasis patients with normal salivary secretion and hyposalivation, receiver operating characteristic (ROC) curves were generated and then the area under the curve (AUC) was calculated. Every parameter had its optimal limit values determined, which simultaneously provided high sensitivity and specificity. The analysis of the data was performed in the statistical program GraphPad Prism 8.3.0 for MacOS.

3. Results

3.1. *Inflammatory Cytokines*

3.1.1. NWS

The concentration of IL-2 (↑10.91%, $p = 0.007$; ↑33.64%, $p < 0.0001$, respectively) and INF- γ (↑33.11%, $p \leq 0.0001$; ↑57.34%, $p \leq 0.0001$, respectively) in NWS of psoriasis patients with normal and decreased saliva secretion was significantly higher than in the control group. Moreover, concentrations of IL-2 (↑20.50%, $p \leq 0.0001$) and INF-γ (↑18.21%, $p = 0.005$) in NWS of patients with hyposalivation were considerably higher than in psoriasis patients with normal saliva secretion. TNF-α concentration in the NWS of psoriasis patients with hyposalivation was significantly higher than in the control group (↑61.38%, $p \leq 0.0001$) and in the group of psoriasis patients with normal salivation (↑30.47%, $p = 0.009$). The concentration of IL-10 (↓25.68%, $p = 0.002$; ↓47.30%, $p \leq 0.0001$, respectively) in the NWS of psoriasis patients with normal and decreased saliva secretion was considerably lower than in the control group. Moreover, the concentration of IL-10 (↓29.09%, $p = 0.03$) in NWS of patients with hyposalivation was significantly lower than in the group of psoriasis patients with normal saliva secretion (Figure 1).

3.1.2. SWS

TNF-α concentration (↑69.77%, $p \leq 0.0001$; ↑103.32%, $p \leq 0.0001$, respectively) and IL-2 (↑45.10%, $p \leq 0.0001$; ↑67.65%, $p \leq 0.0001$, respectively) in SWS of patients with psoriasis with normal and decreased saliva secretion was significantly higher than in the control group. The concentration of TNF-α (↑19.77%, $p = 0.0002$) and IL-2 (↑15.54%, $p = 0.03$) in SWS of patients with hyposalivation was considerably higher than in psoriasis patients with normal saliva secretion. INF-γ content in SWS of psoriasis patients with hyposalivation was significantly higher than in the control group (↑66.28%, $p \leq 0.0001$) and in the group of psoriasis patients with normal saliva secretion (↑31.19%, $p = 0.03$). The level of IL-10 (↓44.23%, $p \leq 0.0001$; ↓61.54%, $p \leq 0.0001$, respectively) in SWS in psoriasis patients with normal and decreased saliva secretion was significantly lower than in the control group, with IL-10 content (↓31.23%, $p \leq 0.0001$; ↓61.54%, $p \leq 0.0001$, respectively) in SWS in hyposalivation patients significantly lower than in psoriasis patients with normal saliva secretion (Figure 1).

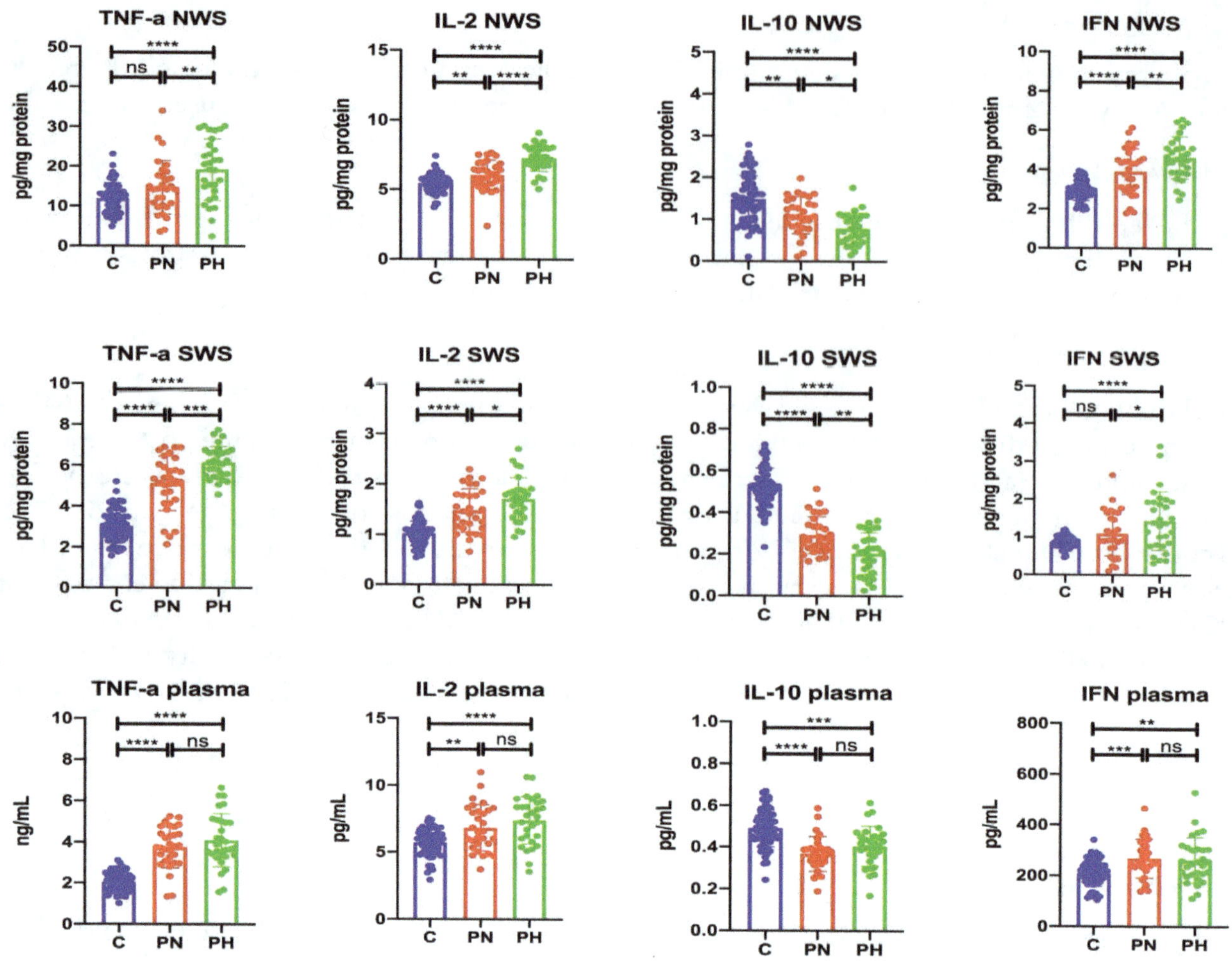

Figure 1. Cytokine levels in unstimulated and stimulated saliva as well as plasma of plaque psoriasis patients with normal salivation and hyposalivation. Abbreviations: C—the control; IL-2—interleukin 2; IL-10—interleukin-10; INF-γ—interferon-gamma; ns—not significant; NWS—non-stimulated whole saliva; PN—psoriasis patients with normal salivation; PH—psoriasis patients with hyposalivation; SWS—stimulated whole saliva; TNF-α—tumor necrosis factor-alpha. * $p < 0.05$, ** $p < 0.01$, *** $p < 0.001$, and **** $p < 0.0001$.

3.1.3. Plasma

TNF-α concentration in plasma of psoriasis patients with normal secretion (↑83.25%, $p \leq 0.0001$) and in plasma of psoriasis patients with hyposalivation (↑100.49%, $p \leq 0.0001$) was significantly higher than in the control group. Similarly, plasma concentration of IL-2 and INF-γ in psoriasis patients with normal secretion (↑19.68%, $p = 0.002$; ↑28.51%, $p = 0.0006$, respectively) and hyposalivation (↑29.70%, mboxemphp ≤ 0.0001; ↑25.29%, $p = 0.003$, respectively) were significantly higher vs. control. Plasma concentration of IL-10 in psoriasis patients with normal secretion (↓24.49%, $p \leq 0.0001$) and hyposalivation (↓18.37%, $p = 0.0001$) was significantly lower than in the control group (Figure 1).

3.2. Nitrosative Stress

3.2.1. NWS

The concentration of NO (↑14.31%, $p = 0.009$; ↑35.14%, $p \leq 0.0001$, respectively) and nitrotyrosine (↑12.41%, $p = 0.04$; ↑39.60%, $p \leq 0.0001$, respectively) in NWS of psoriasis patients with normal secretion and with hyposalivation was significantly higher than in the control group. Moreover, the levels of NO (↑18.23%, $p = 0.0006$) and nitrotyrosine (↑24.19%, $p \leq 0.0001$) in NWS of patients with hyposalivation was considerably higher than in psoriasis patients with normal salivary secretion.

The concentration of S-nitrosothiols and peroxynitrite in NWS of psoriasis patients with hyposalivation was significantly higher than in the control group (↑11.59%, $p = 0.04$; ↑30.70%, $p \leq 0.0001$, respectively) and the group of psoriasis patients with normal salivation (↑16.64%, $p = 0.01$; ↑17.63%, $p = 0.003$, respectively) (Figure 2).

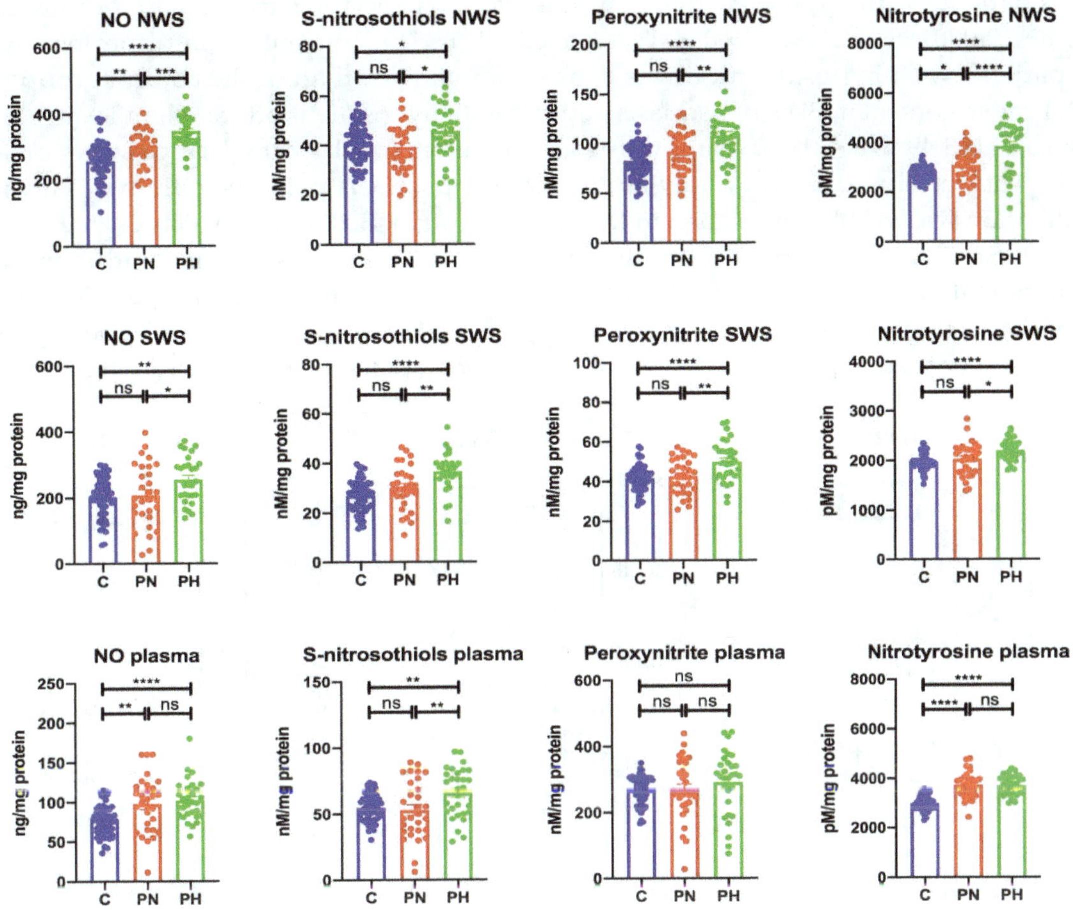

Figure 2. Nitrosative stress in non-stimulated and stimulated saliva as well as plasma of plaque psoriasis patients with normal salivation and hyposalivation. Abbreviations: C—the control; NO—nitric oxide; ns—not significant; NWS—non-stimulated whole saliva; PN—psoriasis patients with normal salivation; PH—psoriasis patients with hyposalivation; SWS—stimulated whole saliva. * $p < 0.05$, ** $p < 0.01$, *** $p < 0.001$, and **** $p < 0.0001$.

3.2.2. SWS

The concentration of NO, S-nitrosothiols, peroxynitrite, and nitrotyrosine in SWS of psoriasis patients with hyposalivation was significantly higher than in the control group (↑25.56%, $p = 0.006$; ↑35.93%, $p \leq 0.0001$; ↑11.47%, $p \leq 0.0001$; ↑11.80%, $p \leq 0.0001$, respectively), as well as compared to the group of psoriasis patients with normal salivation (↑22.71%, $p = 0.04$; ↑21.53%, $p = 0.002$; ↑17.26%, $p = 0.002$; ↑8.26%, $p = 0.02$, respectively) (Figure 2).

3.2.3. Plasma

The concentration of NO (↑27.19%, $p = 0.001$; ↑33.05%, $p \leq 0.0001$, respectively) and nitrotyrosine (↑25.04%, $p \leq 0.0001$; ↑24.34%, $p \leq 0.0001$, respectively) in plasma of psoriasis patients with normal and decreased saliva secretion was considerably higher than in the control group. Plasma concentration of S-nitrosothiols in psoriasis patients with hyposalivation was significantly higher than in the control group (↑20.41%, $p = 0.008$) and in psoriasis patients with normal saliva secretion (↑24.18%, $p = 0.008$). Plasma concentration of peroxynitrite did not differ between the study and control groups (Figure 2).

3.3. Salivary Gland Function

Unstimulated as well as stimulated saliva secretion was significantly lower in psoriasis patients with hyposalivation compared to the control group (↓57.58%, $p \leq 0.0001$; ↓41.03%, $p \leq 0.0001$, respectively). Similarly, unstimulated as well as stimulated saliva secretion was significantly lower in psoriasis patients with hyposalivation compared to the psoriatic patients with normal salivation (↓56.25%, $p \leq 0.0001$; ↓34.29%, $p = 0.0003$, respectively). The concentration of protein in NWS of psoriasis patients with hyposalivation was considerably lower than in the control group (↓24.90%, $p = 0.008$). Protein content in SWS of psoriasis patients with hyposalivation was significantly lower than in the controls (↓43.49%, $p \leq 0.0001$) and the group of patients with normal saliva secretion (↓13.60%, $p = 0.0008$). The activity of salivary amylase in NWS of psoriasis patients with hyposalivation and normal salivation was visibly lower than in the control group (↓30.00%, $p = 0.0003$; ↓25.00%, $p = 0.002$, respectively). Similarly, salivary amylase activity in SWS of psoriasis patients with hyposalivation and normal salivation was significantly lower than in the control group (↓42.86%, $p \leq 0.0001$; ↓25.00%, $p = 0.0006$, respectively). Moreover, amylase activity in SWS of patients with hyposalivation was considerably lower than in patients with normal salivation (↓23.81%, $p = 0.02$) (Figure 3).

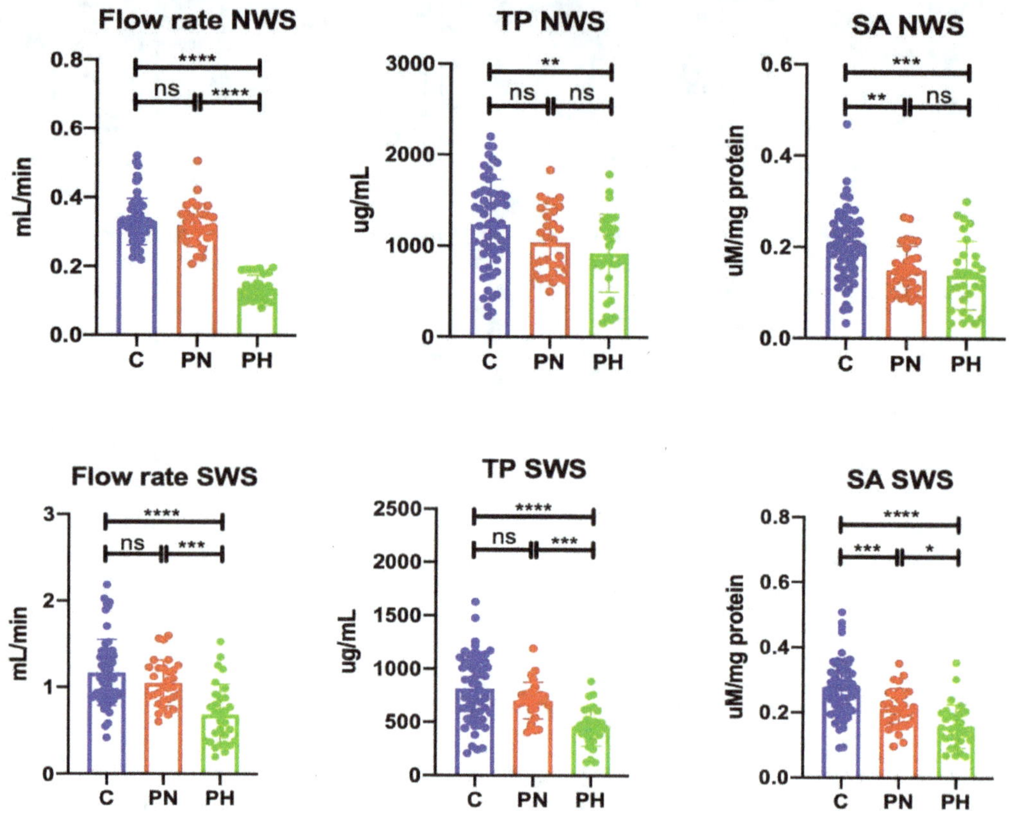

Figure 3. Salivary gland function in plaque psoriasis patients and control subjects. Abbreviations: C—the control; NWS—non-stimulated whole saliva; ns—not significant; PN—psoriasis patients with normal salivation; PH—psoriasis patients with hyposalivation; SA—salivary amylase; SWS—stimulated whole saliva; TP—total protein. * $p < 0.05$, ** $p < 0.01$, *** $p < 0.001$, and **** $p < 0.0001$.

3.4. ROC Analysis

The assessment of diagnostic usefulness of the analyzed biomarkers of inflammation and nitrosative stress is presented in Tables 2 and 3. Many of the assessed parameters clearly differentiated psoriatic patients with hyposalivation from patients with normal salivary flow. Particularly noteworthy is the assessment of NO, nitrotyrosine, and IL-2 levels in NWS, differentiating psoriatic patients with high sensitivity and specificity on the basis of the rate of saliva secretion (Figure 4).

Table 2. ROC analysis of the assessed cytokines and nitrosative stress biomarkers in the saliva of plaque psoriasis patients with normal salivation and hyposalivation.

	NWS						SWS						
Parameter	**AUC**	**95% Confidence Interval**	***p*-Value**	**Cut-Off**	**Sensitivity (%)**	**Specificity (%)**	**AUC**	**95% Confidence Interval**	***p*-Value**	**Cut-Off**	**Sensitivity (%)**	**Specificity (%)**	**AUC**
							Cytokines						
TNF-α (pg/mg protein)	0.68	0.5417–0.8183	**0.0166**	>15.83	63.33	63.33	0.7311	0.6025–0.8597	**0.0021**	>5.717	66.67	66.67	0.5611
IL-2 (pg/mg protein)	0.8111	0.7024–0.9198	**<0.0001**	>6.789	73.33	73.33	0.6478	0.5071–0.7884	**0.0493**	>1.595	63.33	63.33	0.6122
IL-10 (pg/mg protein)	0.7089	0.5760–0.8418	**0.0054**	<0.9704	63.33	63.33	0.7267	0.5997–0.8536	**0.0026**	<0.2410	66.67	66.67	0.6556
INF-γ (pg/mg protein)	0.6622	0.5246–0.7999	**0.0309**	>4.358	60.00	60.00	0.6278	0.4848–0.7708	0.0891	>1.142	60.00	60.00	0.5378
							Nitrosative Stress						
NO (ng/mg protein)	0.77	0.6507–0.8893	**0.0003**	>318.90	66.67	66.67	0.6464	0.5443–0.7885	0.0556	>224.00	60.71	60.00	0.5244
S-nitrosothiols (nM/mg protein)	0.6844	0.5479–0.8209	**0.0141**	>42.73	60.00	60.00	0.7211	0.5857–0.8565	**0.0033**	>34.60	70.00	70.00	0.6644
Peroxynitrite (nM/mg protein)	0.7056	0.5744–0.8367	**0.0062**	>101.50	63.33	63.33	0.69	0.5569–0.8231	**0.0115**	>45.31	60.00	60.00	0.5744
Nitrotyrosine (pM/mg protein)	0.7444	0.6120–0.8769	**0.0011**	>3398.00	70.00	70.00	0.6611	0.5223–0.8000	**0.0321**	>2139.00	60.00	60.00	0.5011

Abbreviations: AUC—area under the curve; C—the control; IL-2—interleukin 2; IL-10—interleukin 10; INF-γ—interferon-gamma; NO—nitric oxide; NWS—non-stimulated whole saliva; SWS—stimulated whole saliva; TNF-α—tumor necrosis factor-alpha.

Table 3. ROC analysis of the assessed cytokines and nitrosative stress biomarkers in the plasma of plaque psoriasis patients with normal salivation and hyposalivation.

			Plasma			
Parameter	**AUC**	**95% Confidence Interval**	***p*-Value**	**Cut-Off**	**Sensitivity (%)**	**Specificity (%)**
			Cytokines			
TNF-α (pg/mL)	0.5611	0.4135–0.7087	0.4161	>3.748	50.00	50.00
IL-2 (pg/mL)	0.6122	0.4685–0.7559	0.1354	>7.201	60.00	60.00
IL-10 (pg/mL)	0.6556	0.5127–0.7984	**0.0385**	>0.3863	63.33	63.33
INF-γ (pg/mL)	0.5378	0.3897–0.6858	0.6152	<251.20	50.00	50.00
			Nitrosative Stress			
NO (ng/mg protein)	0.5244	0.3743–0.6746	0.745	>99.49	46.67	46.67
S-nitrosothiols (nM/mg protein)	0.6644	0.5261–0.8028	**0.0287**	>57.03	60.00	60.00
Peroxynitrite (nM/mg protein)	0.5744	0.4261–0.7228	0.3219	>302.90	60.00	60.00
Nitrotyrosine (pM/mg protein)	0.5011	0.3528–0.6494	0.9882	<3747.00	50.00	50.00

Abbreviations: AUC—area under the curve; C—the control; IL-2—interleukin 2; IL-10—interleukin 10; INF-γ—interferon-gamma; NO—nitric oxide; NWS—non-stimulated whole saliva; SWS—stimulated whole saliva; TNF-α—tumor necrosis factor-alpha.

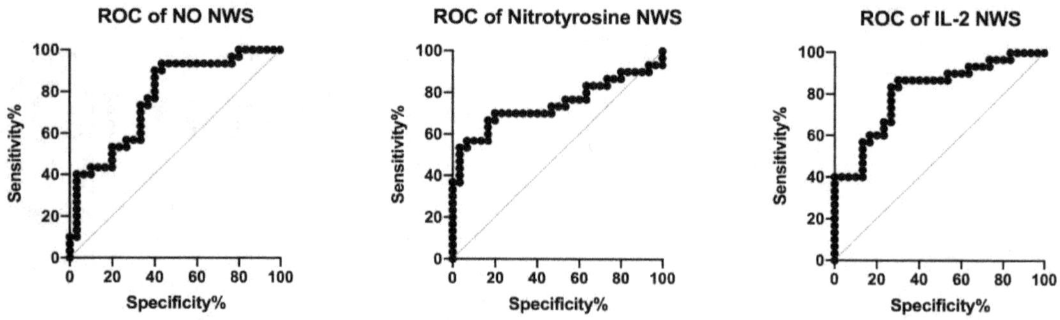

Figure 4. Receiver operating characteristic (ROC) analysis of nitric oxide, nitrotyrosine, and IL-2 in unstimulated saliva of plaque psoriasis patients with normal salivation and hyposalivation. IL-2—interleukin 2; NO—nitric oxide; NWS—non-stimulated whole saliva.

3.5. Correlations

The results of statistically significant correlations are presented in Table 4. We demonstrated a negative correlation between NO concentration and minute secretion of unstimulated saliva as well as between peroxynitrite and protein concentrations in stimulated saliva of patients with hyposalivation. Moreover, we observed a negative correlation between TNF-α level and non-stimulated salivation, as well as in IL-2 content and stimulated salivary flow in patients with hyposalivation. On the other hand, peroxynitrite concentration correlated negatively with α-amylase activity in both unstimulated and stimulated saliva of patients with normal salivation.

We noted a positive correlation between TNF-α and NO concentrations in unstimulated saliva of patients with hyposalivation, as well as between IL-2 and NO contents in unstimulated saliva of psoriasis patients with normal saliva secretion.

We showed a positive correlation between PASI and TNF-α, as well as PASI and IL-2 in unstimulated saliva of patients with hyposalivation. Moreover, we observed a positive correlation between nitrotyrosine concentration and duration of psoriasis in patients with normal as well as reduced salivary flow (both in unstimulated and stimulated saliva).

Table 4. Statistically significant correlations in patients with plaque psoriasis.

Pair of Variables	Group	*r*	*p*
NO NWS and NWS flow rate	PH	−0.68	0.001
Peroxynitrite SWS and total protein SWS	PH	−0.56	0.0015
TNF-α NWS and NWS flow rate	PH	−0.60	0.004
IL-2 SWS and SWS flow rate	PH	−0.54	0.002
Peroxynitrite NWS and amylase NWS	PN	−0.58	0.0008
Peroxynitrite SWS and amylase SWS	PN	−0.68	<0.0001
TNF-α NWS and NO NWS	PH	0.60	0.004
IL-2 NWS and NO NWS	PN	0.64	0.002
TNF-α NWS and PASI	PH	0.59	0.0006
IL-2 NWS and PASI	PH	0.63	0.0029
Nitrotyrosine NWS and disease duration	PN	0.53	0.003
Nitrotyrosine SWS and disease duration	PN	0.58	0.001
Nitrotyrosine NWS and disease duration	PH	0.61	0.004
Nitrotyrosine SWS and disease duration	PH	0.60	<0.0001

Abbreviations: IL-2—interleukin 2; NO—nitric oxide; NWS—non-stimulated whole saliva; PN—psoriasis patients with normal salivation; PH—psoriasis patients with hyposalivation; SWS—stimulated whole saliva; TNF-α—tumor necrosis factor-alpha.

4. Discussion

In the presented study, we evaluated the concentrations of TNF-α, IL-2, INF-γ, IL-10, and selected nitrosative stress parameters (NO, peroxynitrite, S-nitrosothiols, and nitrotyrosine) in NWS and SWS, as well as the plasma of psoriasis patients. The obtained results demonstrated the pathophysiology of salivary gland dysfunction in the course of plaque psoriasis. We were also seeking salivary psoriasis biomarkers that could be helpful in diagnosing the severity of psoriasis and its salivary complications.

The accepted values of normal unstimulated salivary flow are above 0.2 mL/min. Any unstimulated flow rate below 0.2 mL/min is considered salivary gland hypofunction and is referred to as hyposalivation [18]. Hyposalivation has a detrimental effect on numerous aspects of oral health, and thus on general well-being. It decreases the quality of life as it hinders speaking, tasting, chewing, and swallowing food [40]. Reduced saliva secretion is the cause of cracks and fissures in the oral mucosa, which is associated with chronic pain in the oral cavity and the resulting discomfort to the patient. Decreased salivation also contributes to boosted incidence of caries, periodontitis, and fungal infections of the oral cavity [40]. All these may lead to patient malnutrition, social isolation, and even depression, as well as generate high treatment costs. Therefore, it is very important to identify patients with salivation disorders and to prevent the development and effects of salivary gland dysfunction in the course of systemic diseases.

Our findings that plasma concentrations of TNF-α, IL-2, and INF- γ were significantly higher and for IL-10 were significantly lower than in the controls are consistent with the assumption that psoriasis is primarily driven by an aberrant immune response and results from an imbalance between Th1 and Th2 cells [2–4]. Significantly higher concentration of NO, especially nitrotyrosine, and a positive correlation between the latter and the disease duration in psoriatic patients' plasma compared to the controls confirm the contribution of nitrosative stress to the development of the disease [41]. Interestingly, apart from S-nitrosothiols, we did not observe significant differences between patients with hyposalivation and those with normal saliva secretion. On the other hand, patients from the hyposalivation group were characterized by longer duration of psoriasis and higher PASI index compared to those with normal flow of unstimulated saliva.

At this point, it is worth reminding that 90% of saliva is produced by three pairs of large salivary glands: submandibular, parotid, and sublingual. The remaining 10% of saliva is secreted by small salivary glands scattered under the oral cavity mucosa, and gingiva fluid. The submandibular glands are the major contributor to unstimulated salivary flow, and the parotid glands secrete stimulated saliva, that is, saliva secreted mainly in response to stimuli. The contribution of the sublingual glands to unstimulated and stimulated salivation is low [42]. Therefore, any deviation in the composition of unstimulated saliva reflects dysfunction of the submandibular glands, as well as of stimulated saliva, of the parotid glands. The exception here are patients with inflammatory changes in periodontal tissues, in whom changes in saliva composition reflect periodontal diseases. In our work, we excluded patients with periodontitis/gingivitis, and therefore any changes observed in saliva originated from the dysfunction of salivary glands.

Our results revealed significantly increased levels of the tested proinflammatory cytokines and a decrease in IL-10 concentration in unstimulated and stimulated saliva of psoriasis patients with normal salivation (except for TNF-α in NWS and INF-γ in SWS) and hyposalivation compared to the controls. An earlier report suggested that mRNA expression of Th1 and derived inflammatory cytokines IL-2, TNF-α, and INF-γ were also increased in the saliva of the patients with Sjögren's syndrome [43]. The salivary changes were accompanied by clusters of infiltrating cells present in salivary gland biopsy, where 80% were Th1 cells, and the remaining 20% consisted of stimulated B lymphocytes and plasma cells [43]. On the basis of the performed analyses, it was difficult to assess the nature of the developing inflammation in salivary glands of our patients. There were also no histological examinations of the salivary glands of psoriasis patients. By analogy to Sjögren's syndrome, the observed increases in TNF-α, IL-2, and INF-γ concentrations allow us to assume that salivary glands of patients with psoriasis are infested with autoreactive Th1 lymphocytes. Despite the deficiency of Th2 response (↓IL-10) supporting the humoral type response, we do not rule out the presence of stimulated B lymphocytes, as there has been no research to confirm or exclude the existence of the culprit autoantigens. However, increased concentration of the examined proinflammatory cytokines and decreased level of IL-10 in NWS and SWS of patients with hyposalivation compared to psoriasis patients with normal salivation indicates an increase in imbalance between Th1 and Th2 cells, and thus inflammation in salivary glands of patients with hyposalivation vs. those with normal salivary flow.

Human salivary glands contain different kinds of nitric oxide synthase (NOS) isoforms. Neuronal NOS (*n*NOS) was found in the salivary gland parenchyma, ducts, blood vessels, and nerve fibers around acini, mainly in the submandibular glands [44], and—in negligible amounts—in the parotid and sublingual glands [45]. Endothelial NOS (*e*NOS) was identified as localizing to the glandular vascular endothelium of the salivary ducts [45]. *i*NOS has been detected in the salivary ducts of normal tissue [45]. In physiological concentrations, NO does not damage the structures of salivary glands; it regulates oral blood flow and saliva secretion, and participates in non-specific protective mechanisms [23–25], which seems to take place in parotid glands of psoriasis patients without salivation disorders (no changes in the studied nitrosative stress parameters in SWS). We observed excessive amount of NO and peroxynitrite in unstimulated and stimulated saliva of patients with hyposalivation. A positive correlation between TNF-α and NO concentrations in NWS of patients with hyposalivation and between IL-2 and NO content in NWS of patients with normal salivation confirm the previous observations that proinflammatory cytokines lead to the expression of *i*NOS in salivary gland cells, resulting in increased production of NO and its derivatives [46]. We also noted a boost in nitrosative stress (NO, S-nitrosothiols, peroxynitrite) and, primarily, nitrosative damage to protein elements of the salivary glands (S-nitrosothiols and nitrotyrosine) in unstimulated and stimulated saliva of psoriasis patients with hyposalivation vs. those with normal saliva secretion.

Evidence has shown that much larger amounts of NO generated in response to inflammation are connected with the cytotoxic effect of NO due to its interaction with superoxide anions to form peroxynitrite and other free radicals. Research results have revealed that intense production of NO and peroxynitrite in salivary glands acts as a strong proapoptotic agent [46,47]. Moreover, it has been observed that NO, by auto-ADP (adenosyno-diphospate) ribosylation of glyceraldehyde 3-phosphate dehydrogenase, inhibits the production of ATP that is necessary to maintain anabolic processes in the cell [23]. It has been demonstrated that apoptosis of salivary gland structures disturbs their function, and ATP deficiency impairs mechanisms responsible for replacing damaged or lost cellular elements [46,48]. We noted a negative correlation between NO and NWS secretion, and between peroxynitrite and protein concentrations in SWS of hyposalivation patients. These results suggest that decreased salivary secretion and protein synthesis/selection could be caused by the proapoptotic effect of NO on the salivary gland cells. This hypothesis requires further confirmation in histological studies. On the other hand, it is known that TNF-α and IL-2 stimulate the production of metalloproteinases, which results in structural changes in the basement membrane of the salivary glands [49]. A negative correlation between TNF-α and NWS secretion, and IL-2 and SWS secretion in patients with hyposalivation may result from damage to acinar cell-basement membrane interaction resulting from overproduction of MMPs (metalloproteinases) followed by decreased number of secretory units (acini and ducts) [50,51]. This phenomenon has been recently demonstrated in the saliva of Sjögren's syndrome patients [52]. Remodeling of the extracellular matrix, alongside apoptosis, could be the reason for the observed drop in the synthesis/secretion of proteins and reduced salivary secretion in psoriasis patients with hyposalivation. It is noteworthy that salivary gland dysfunction occurs in patients with a longer duration and higher intensity of the disease.

The lack of significant differences in the secretion of NWS and SWS as well as proteins between patients with normal salivation (shorter disease duration, lower PASI) and the controls suggests that, at an early stage of the disease, the mechanisms of controlling saliva secretion and protein production/secretion counteract the damaging effects of psoriasis. Interestingly, already at this early stage we observed decreased amylase activity in SWS and UWS of patients with normal salivation, as well as intensification of this phenomenon in the saliva of patients with hyposalivation. These results may explain the negative correlation between peroxynitrite concentration and salivary amylase activity in NWS and SWS of patients with normal salivation. It has been demonstrated that peroxynitrite reacts readily with iron-sulfur cluster of several enzymes and is able to oxidize the sulfhydryl groups of proteins, leading to the formation of disulfides and resulting in their inactivation [53]. Naturally, it should be remembered that exposure to peroxynitrite entails tyrosine nitration of proteins [54]. This mechanism of amylase inactivation should be eliminated, as increased nitrotyrosine concentration was only observed in NWS and SWS of patients with hyposalivation, both compared to the controls and patients with normal saliva secretion.

Salivary glands are surrounded by a dense network of blood vessels that enable the exchange of components between the acinar cells and ducts, as well as blood. Thus, biomarkers present in the blood can permeate into the structures of salivary glands and hence into saliva. Therefore, saliva is more and more frequently considered a potential source of biological markers for systemic diseases. Many of the examined parameters clearly differentiated psoriatic patients with hyposalivation from psoriatic patients with normal saliva flow, and thus the levels of NO, nitrotyrosine, and IL-2 in NWS deserve special attention and should be further evaluated. Additionally, the observed positive correlation of PASI and TNF-α and IL-1β in UWS of patients with hyposalivation could provide a new non-invasive and simple method in the diagnosis of the intensity of the disease.

5. Conclusions

Increased levels of TNF-α, IL-2, and INF-γ, as well as decreased content of IL-10 in NWS and SWS of psoriasis patients compared to the controls indicated an imbalance between Th1 and Th2 cells in the salivary glands.

The severity of inflammation and nitrosative stress in the salivary glands of psoriatic patients depends on the disease duration.

At an early stage of the disease, the mechanisms controlling saliva secretion and protein production/secretion counteract the damaging effects of psoriasis. With the severity and duration of psoriasis, the secretory function of all salivary glands is lost, which is manifested as significant reduction of unstimulated and stimulated saliva secretion as well as protein concentration.

Dysfunction of salivary glands in the course of psoriasis may be attributed to inflammation and nitrosative stress.

Author Contributions: Conceptualization, A.Z., M.M.; data curation, A.S.-R., U.K., A.K., A.K.-R., J.K.; formal analysis, A.Z., M.M., A.S.-R.; funding acquisition, A.S.-R., A.Z.; investigation, A.S.-R., A.Z., M.M.; methodology, A.Z., M.M.; material collection: A.S.-R., U.K., A.K., A.K.-R.; supervision, A.Z., I.F., J.K.; validation, A.S.-R., A.Z., M.M.; visualization, M.M.; writing—original draft, A.S.-R., A.Z., M.M.; writing—review and editing, A.Z., M.M. All authors have read and agreed to the published version of the manuscript.

References

1. WHO. *Global Report on Psoriasis*; WHO Library Cataloguing-in-Publication Data; World Health Organization: Geneva, Switzerland, 2016; pp. 10–11.
2. Kupper, T.S. Immunologic Targets in Psoriasis. *N. Engl. J. Med.* **2003**, *349*, 1987–1990. [CrossRef] [PubMed]
3. Nickoloff, B.J. The immunologic and genetic basis of psoriasis. *Arch. Dermatol.* **1999**, *135*, 1104–1110. [CrossRef] [PubMed]
4. Liu, R.; Yang, Y.; Yan, X.; Zhang, K. Abnormalities in cytokine secretion from mesenchymal stem cells in psoriatic skin lesions. *Eur. J. Dermatol.* **2013**, *23*, 600–607. [CrossRef]
5. Asha, K.; Singal, A.; Sharma, S.B.; Arora, V.K.; Aggarwal, A. Dyslipidaemia & oxidative stress in patients of psoriasis: Emerging cardiovascular risk factors. *Indian J. Med. Res.* **2017**, *146*, 708–713. [PubMed]
6. Kadam, D.P.; Suryakar, A.N.; Ankush, R.D.; Kadam, C.Y.; Deshpande, K.H. Role of oxidative stress in various stages of psoriasis. *Indian J. Clin. Biochem.* **2010**, *25*, 388–392. [CrossRef]
7. Houshang, N.; Reza, K.; Sadeghi, M.; Ali, E.; Mansour, R.; Vaisi-Raygani, A. Antioxidant status in patients with psoriasis. *Cell Biochem. Funct.* **2014**, *32*, 268–273. [CrossRef]

8. Pujari, V.K.M. The Serum Levels of Malondialdehyde, Vitamin E and Erythrocyte Catalase Activity in Psoriasis Patients. *J. Clin. Diagn. Res.* **2014**, *8*, CC14–CC16. [CrossRef]
9. Yildirim, M.; Inaloz, H.S.; Baysal, V.; Delibas, N. The role of oxidants and antioxidants in psoriasis. *J. Eur. Acad. Dermatol. Venereol.* **2003**, *17*, 34–36. [CrossRef]
10. Barygina, V.V.; Becatti, M.; Soldi, G.; Prignano, F.; Lotti, T.; Nassi, P.; Wright, D.; Taddei, N.; Fiorillo, C. Altered redox status in the blood of psoriatic patients: Involvement of NADPH oxidase and role of anti-TNF-α therapy. *Redox Rep.* **2013**, *18*, 100–106. [CrossRef]
11. Ferretti, G.; Bacchetti, T.; Campanati, A.; Simonetti, O.; Liberati, G.; Offidani, A. Correlation between lipoprotein (a) and lipid peroxidation in psoriasis: Role of the enzyme paraoxonase-1. *Br. J. Dermatol.* **2012**, *166*, 204–207. [CrossRef]
12. Drewa, G.; Krzyzynska-Malinowska, E.; Wozniak, A.; Protas-Drozd, F.; Mila-Kierzenkowska, C.; Rozwodowska, M.; Kowaliszyn, B.; Czajkowski, R. Activity of superoxide dismutase and catalase and the level of lipid peroxidation products reactive with TBA in patients with psoriasis. *Med. Sci. Monit.* **2002**, *8*, BR338–BR343. [PubMed]
13. Lin, X.; Huang, T. Oxidative stress in psoriasis and potential therapeutic use of antioxidants. *Free Radic. Res.* **2016**, *50*, 585–595. [CrossRef] [PubMed]
14. Aparicio, V.A.; Nebot, E.; Porres, J.M.; Sánchez, C.; Aranda, P.; García-del Moral, R.; Machado-Vílchez, M. High-protein diets and renal status in rats. *Nutr. Hosp.* **2013**, *28*, 232–237. [PubMed]
15. Skutnik-Radziszewska, A.; Maciejczyk, M.; Fejfer, K.; Krahel, J.; Flisiak, I.; Kołodziej, U.; Zalewska, A. Salivary Antioxidants and Oxidative Stress in Psoriatic Patients: Can Salivary Total Oxidant Status and Oxidative Status Index Be a Plaque Psoriasis Biomarker? *Oxidative Med. Cell. Longev.* **2020**. [CrossRef] [PubMed]
16. Sondermann, W.; Djeudeu Deudjui, D.A.; Körber, A.; Slomiany, U.; Brinker, T.J.; Erbel, R.; Moebus, S. Psoriasis, cardiovascular risk factors and metabolic disorders: Sex-specific findings of a population-based study. *J. Eur. Acad. Dermatol. Venereol.* **2019**. [CrossRef] [PubMed]
17. Ungprasert, P.; Raksasuk, S. Psoriasis and risk of incident chronic kidney disease and end-stage renal disease: A systematic review and meta-analysis. *Int. Urol. Nephrol.* **2018**, *50*, 1277–1283. [CrossRef]
18. Zalewska, A.; Knaś, M.; Gińdzieńska-Sieśkiewicz, E.; Waszkiewicz, N.; Klimiuk, A.; Litwin, K.; Sierakowski, S.; Waszkiel, D. Salivary antioxidants in patients with systemic sclerosis. *J. Oral Pathol. Med.* **2014**, *43*, 61–68. [CrossRef]
19. Desoutter, A.; Soudain-Pineau, M.; Munsch, F.; Mauprivez, C.; Dufour, T.; Coeuriot, J.L. Xerostomia and medication: A cross-sectional study in long-term geriatric wards. *J. Nutr. Health Aging* **2012**, *16*, 575–579. [CrossRef]
20. Zalewska, A.; Knaś, M.; Waszkiewicz, N.; Waszkiel, D.; Sierakowski, S.; Zwierz, K. Rheumatoid arthritis patients with xerostomia have reduced production of key salivary constituents. *Oral Surg. Oral Med. Oral Pathol. Oral Radiol.* **2013**, *115*, 483–490. [CrossRef]
21. Ganzetti, G.; Campanati, A.; Santarelli, A.; Pozzi, V.; Molinelli, E.; Minnetti, I.; Brisigotti, V.; Procaccini, M.; Emanuelli, M.; Offidani, A. Involvement of the oral cavity in psoriasis: Results of a clinical study. *Br. J. Dermatol.* **2015**, *172*, 282–285. [CrossRef]
22. Stichtenoth, D.O.; Frölich, J.C. Nitric oxide and inflammatory joint diseases. *Br. J. Rheumatol.* **1998**, *37*, 246–257. [CrossRef] [PubMed]
23. Brune, B.; Lapetina, E.G. Activation of a cytosolic ADP-ribosyltransferase by nitric oxide-generating agents. *J. Biol. Chem.* **1989**, *264*, 8455–8458. [PubMed]
24. Modin, A.; Weitzberg, E.; Hökfelt, T.; Lundberg, J.M. Nitric oxide synthase in the pig autonomic nervous system in relation to the influence of NG-nitro-L-arginine on sympathetic and parasympathetic vascular control In Vivo. *Neuroscience* **1994**, *62*, 189–203. [CrossRef]
25. Toda, N.; Ayajiki, K.; Okamura, T. Neurogenic and endothelial nitric oxide regulates blood circulation in lingual and other oral tissues. *J. Cardiovasc. Pharmacol.* **2012**, *60*, 100–108. [CrossRef] [PubMed]
26. Asa'ad, F.; Fiore, M.; Alfieri, A.; Pigatto, P.D.M.; Franchi, C.; Berti, E.; Maiorana, C.; Damiani, G. Saliva as a Future Field in Psoriasis Research. *Biomed Res. Int.* **2018**. [CrossRef]
27. Villanova, F.; Di Meglio, P.; Nestle, F.O. Biomarkers in psoriasis and psoriatic arthritis. *Ann. Rheum. Dis.* **2013**, *72*, 104–110. [CrossRef]

28. Klimiuk, A.; Maciejczyk, M.; Choromańska, M.; Fejfer, K.; Waszkiewicz, N.; Zalewska, A. Salivary Redox Biomarkers in Different Stages of Dementia Severity. *J. Clin. Med.* **2019**, *8*, 840. [CrossRef]
29. Brandtzaeg, P. Do salivary antibodies reliably reflect both mucosal and systemic immunity? *Proc. Ann. N. Y. Acad. Sci.* **2007**, *1098*, 288–311. [CrossRef]
30. Choromańska, M.; Klimiuk, A.; Kostecka-Sochoń, P.; Wilczyńska, K.; Kwiatkowski, M.; Okuniewska, N.; Waszkiewicz, N.; Zalewska, A.; Maciejczyk, M. Antioxidant defence, oxidative stress and oxidative damage in saliva, plasma and erythrocytes of dementia patients. Can salivary AGE be a marker of dementia? *Int. J. Mol. Sci.* **2017**, *18*, 2205. [CrossRef]
31. Maciejczyk, M.; Szulimowska, J.; Skutnik, A.; Taranta-Janusz, K.; Wasilewska, A.; Wiśniewska, N.; Zalewska, A. Salivary Biomarkers of Oxidative Stress in Children with Chronic Kidney Disease. *J. Clin. Med.* **2018**, *7*, 209. [CrossRef]
32. Maciejczyk, M.; Szulimowska, J.; Taranta-Janusz, K.; Werbel, K.; Wasilewska, A.; Zalewska, A. Salivary FRAP as a marker of chronic kidney disease progression in children. *Antioxidants* **2019**, *8*, 409. [CrossRef]
33. Maciejczyk, M.; Zalewska, A.; Ładny, J.R. Salivary Antioxidant Barrier, Redox Status, and Oxidative Damage to Proteins and Lipids in Healthy Children, Adults, and the Elderly. *Oxid. Med. Cell. Longev.* **2019**. [CrossRef]
34. Hefti, A.F. Periodontal probing. *Crit. Rev. Oral Biol. Med.* **1997**, *8*, 336–356. [CrossRef]
35. Grisham, M.B.; Johnson, G.G.; Lancaster, J.R. Quantitation of nitrate and nitrite in extracellular fluids. *Methods Enzymol.* **1996**, *268*, 237–246.
36. Wink, D.A.; Kim, S.; Coffin, D.; Cook, J.C.; Vodovotz, Y.; Chistodoulou, D.; Jourd'heuil, D.; Grisham, M.B. Detection of S-nitrosothiols by fluorometric and colorimetric methods. *Methods Enzymol.* **1999**, *301*, 201–211.
37. Borys, J.; Maciejczyk, M.; Antonowicz, B.; Sidun, J.; Świderska, M.; Zalewska, A. Free radical production, inflammation and apoptosis in patients treated with titanium mandibular fixations—An observational study. *Front. Immunol.* **2019**. [CrossRef] [PubMed]
38. Beckman, J.S.; Ischiropoulos, H.; Zhu, L.; van der Woerd, M.; Smith, C.; Chen, J.; Harrison, J.; Martin, J.C.; Tsai, M. Kinetics of superoxide dismutase- and iron-catalyzed nitration of phenolics by peroxynitrite. *Arch. Biochem. Biophys.* **1992**, *298*, 438–445. [CrossRef]
39. Maciejczyk, M.; Kossakowska, A.; Szulimowska, J.; Klimiuk, A.; Knaś, M.; Car, H.; Niklińska, W.; Ładny, J.R.; Chabowski, A.; Zalewska, A. Lysosomal Exoglycosidase Profile and Secretory Function in the Salivary Glands of Rats with Streptozotocin-Induced Diabetes. *J. Diabetes Res.* **2017**. [CrossRef]
40. Jankowska, A.K.; Waszkiel, D.; Kobus, A.; Zwierz, K. Saliva as a main component of oral cavity ecosystem. Part II. Defense mechanisms. *Wiad. Lek.* **2007**, *60*, 253–257.
41. Dilek, N.; Dilek, A.R.; Taskin, Y.; Erkinüresin, T.; Yalçin, Ö.; Saral, Y. Contribution of myeloperoxidase and inducible nitric oxide synthase to pathogenesis of psoriasis. *Postepy Dermatol. Alergol.* **2016**, *33*, 435–439. [CrossRef] [PubMed]
42. Dawes, C.; Pedersen, A.M.L.; Villa, A.; Ekström, J.; Proctor, G.B.; Vissink, A.; Aframian, D.; McGowan, R.; Aliko, A.; Narayana, N.; et al. The functions of human saliva: A review sponsored by the World Workshop on Oral Medicine VI. *Arch. Oral Biol.* **2015**, *60*, 863–874. [CrossRef] [PubMed]
43. Fox, R.I.; Kang, H.I.; Ando, D.; Abrams, J.; Pisa, E. Cytokine mRNA expression in salivary gland biopsies of Sjögren's syndrome. *J. Immunol.* **1994**, *152*, 5532–5539. [PubMed]
44. Looms, D.; Tritsaris, K.; Pedersen, A.M.; Nauntofte, B.; Dissing, S. Nitric oxide signalling in salivary glands. *J. Oral Pathol. Med.* **2002**, *31*, 569–584. [CrossRef] [PubMed]
45. Soinila, J.; Nuorva, K.; Soinila, S. Nitric oxide synthase in human salivary glands. *Histochem. Cell Biol.* **2006**. [CrossRef]
46. De La Cal, C.; Lomniczi, A.; Mohn, C.E.; De Laurentiis, A.; Casal, M.; Chiarenza, A.; Paz, D.; McCann, S.M.; Rettori, V.; Elverdín, J.C. Decrease in salivary secretion by radiation mediated by nitric oxide and prostaglandins. *Neuroimmunomodulation* **2006**, *13*, 19–27. [CrossRef]
47. Slomiany, B.L.; Slomiany, A. Nitric oxide interferes with salivary mucin synthesis: Involvement of ERK and p38 mitogen-activated protein kinase. *J. Physiol. Pharmacol.* **2002**, *53*, 325–336.
48. Zalewska, A.; Ziembicka, D.; Zendzian-Piotrowska, M.; Maciejczyk, M. The impact of high-fat diet on mitochondrial function, free radical production, and nitrosative stress in the salivary glands of wistar rats. *Oxid. Med. Cell. Longev.* **2019**. [CrossRef]

49. Azuma, M.; Aota, K.; Tamatani, T.; Motegi, K.; Yamashita, T.; Ashida, Y.; Hayashi, Y.; Sato, M. Suppression of tumor necrosis factor alpha-induced matrix metalloproteinase 9 production in human salivary gland acinar cells by cepharanthine occurs via down-regulation of nuclear factor kappaB: A possible therapeutic agent for preventing the destruction of the acinar structure in the salivary glands of Sjögren's syndrome patients. *Arthritis Rheum.* **2002**, *46*, 1585–1594.
50. Bozzato, A.; Burger, P.; Zenk, J.; Uter, W.; Iro, H. Salivary gland biometry in female patients with eating disorders. *Eur. Arch. Oto Rhino Laryngol.* **2008**, *265*, 1095–1102. [CrossRef]
51. Heo, M.S.; Lee, S.C.; Lee, S.S.; Choi, H.M.; Choi, S.C.; Park, T.W. Quantitative analysis of normal major salivary glands using computed tomography. *Oral Surg. Oral Med. Oral Pathol. Oral Radiol. Endod.* **2001**, *92*, 240–244. [CrossRef]
52. Hanemaaijer, R.; Visser, H.; Konttinen, Y.T.; Koolwijk, P.; Verheijen, J.H. A novel and simple immunocapture assay for determination of gelatinase-B (MMP-9) activities in biological fluids: Saliva from patients with Sjögren's syndrome contain increased latent and active gelatinase-B levels. *Matrix Biol.* **1998**, *17*, 657–665. [CrossRef]
53. Weiner, D.; Khankin, E.V.; Levy, Y.; Reznick, A.Z. Effects of cigarette smoke borne reactive nitrogen species on salivary alpha-amylase activity and protein modifications. *J. Physiol. Pharmacol.* **2009**, *60*, 127–132. [PubMed]
54. Gryka, D.; Pilch, W.B.; Czerwińska-Ledwig, O.M.; Piotrowska, A.M.; Klocek, E.; Bukova, A. The influence of Finnish sauna treatments on the concentrations of nitric oxide, 3-nitrotyrosine and selected markers of oxidative status in training and non-training men. *Int. J. Occup. Med. Environ. Health* **2020**. [CrossRef] [PubMed]

14

Influence of Myeloperoxidase Levels on Periodontal Disease: An Applied Clinical Study

Alessandro Polizzi *, Salvatore Torrisi, Simona Santonocito, Mattia Di Stefano, Francesco Indelicato and Antonino Lo Giudice

Department of General Surgery and Surgical-Medical Specialties, School of Dentistry, University of Catania, AOU Policlinico—P.O. Vittorio Emanuele, Via Plebiscito 628, 95124 Catania, Italy; ture_torrisi@hotmail.it (S.T.); simonasantonocito.93@gmail.com (S.S.); mattiadistefano@live.it (M.D.S.); indelicato@policlinico.unict.it (F.I.); nino.logiudice@gmail.com (A.L.G.)

* Correspondence: alexpoli345@gmail.com

Abstract: In this trial, we evaluated the influence on plasma and salivary myeloperoxidase (MPO) levels of periodontal health, coronary heart disease (CHD), periodontitis, or both periodontitis and CHD. Clinical and periodontal parameters were collected from periodontitis patients (n = 31), CHD patients (n = 31), patients with both periodontitis and CHD (n = 31), and from healthy patients (n = 31) together with saliva and plasma samples. The median concentrations of salivary and plasma MPO were statistically higher in the CHD patients [plasma: 26.2 (18.2–34.4) ng/mg; saliva 83.2 (77.4–101.5) ng/mL, $p < 0.01$] and in the periodontitis plus CHD patients [plasma: 27.8 (22.5–35.7) ng/mg; saliva 85.6 (76.5–106.7) ng/mL, $p < 0.001$] with respect to periodontitis and control patients. Through a univariate regression analysis, c-reactive protein (CRP) and CHD (both $p < 0.001$) and periodontitis ($p = 0.024$) were statistically correlated with MPO in plasma. The multivariate regression analysis demonstrated that only CRP was statistically the predictor of MPO in plasma ($p < 0.001$). The multivariate regression analysis in saliva demonstrated that, regarding MPO levels the only predictors were CRP ($p < 0.001$) and total cholesterol ($p = 0.035$). The present study evidenced that subjects with CHD and periodontitis plus CHD had higher plasma and salivary levels of MPO compared to subjects with periodontitis and healthy controls.

Keywords: myeloperoxidase; periodontitis; cardiovascular disease; applied model

1. Introduction

Periodontal disease is a common oral inflammatory multifactorial disease that causes the disruption of the periodontium and the tissues that support the tooth, such as bone and cementum main caused by oral bacteria, that ultimately leads to the loss of the tooth [1]. Almost all adults in the USA present periodontal disease forms and nearly ten percent of the population worldwide express severe type of periodontal disease [2,3].

More recently, observational reports have shown a correlation between periodontal disease and cardiovascular disease, such as stroke, heart disease and endothelial dysfunction [4,5]. Moreover, some studies demonstrated a specific correlation among periodontal disease and an augmented risk of stroke [6] and, coronary heart disease (CHD) [7,8].

The pathogenesis of periodontal disease includes inflammatory and bacteria responses which may determine an increased host response subsequent to the presence of pathogenic oral biofilm in gingival tissues [9]. More specifically, periodontal disease has been correlated with an increase of levels of some systemic inflammatory mediators in serum, such as prostaglandin, interleukin 1 (IL-1), IL-6, and C-reactive protein (CRP) [10].

Myeloperoxidase (MPO) is one of the more mediators expressed within tissues during the progression of inflammation [11]. It was demonstrated that MPO, secreted by endothelial cells after exposure to pathogenic bacteria, represents a potent mediator of vascular inflammation and a vasoconstrictor [12].

In this regard, it has been shown that several proinflammatory cytokines, including IL-1, -6, and -8, have been reported to upregulate the secretion of MPO [13]. The expression of MPO was strongly associated in the gingival tissue and endothelial cells during periodontitis [14]. More specifically, a clinical study found that, in gingival crevicular fluid, MPO increased with the progression of the periodontitis, and also that MPO was involved in the regulation of IL-1b expression in gingival tissues [15,16].

During the last few decades, several studies have analyzed the association between periodontal disease endothelial dysfunction, and increased risk of CHD and cardiovascular disease (CVD) [17,18]. More specifically, it has been supposed that the inflammatory mediators that are present and released during the active phase of periodontal disease such as CRP, interleukins, prostaglandins, and metalloproteases, can negatively influence the release of nitric oxide (NO) [19]. The altered release of NO can affect the endothelium which in turn regulates vascular tone, and, finally, dysfunction of the endothelium and enhanced risk of CVD [20,21]. For these causes, there is growing interest to investigate some other oral mediators that can regulate and impact the subclinical endothelial dysfunctions as an early sign of augmented risk of CHD and CVD. In this regard, a correlation between high proportion of MPO, CRP, and endothelial dysfunction was recently reported [22,23].

The production of NO at local level has been shown to be fundamental in the aetiology and progression of periodontitis. The increment and reduction of NO metabolites in saliva production in periodontal tissue against periodontopathogenic microbiota during periodontitis have been demonstrated to be correlated endothelial dysfunction [24,25]. Furthermore, it has been reported that MPO plays an important role in the reduction of NO synthase especially during periodontitis [26].

Based on these findings, the aims of this trial were to consider a possible association of periodontitis, CVD, or both periodontitis plus CVD on serum and salivary MPO. Futhermore, we analyzed the possible correlation between MPO in serum and saliva and if serum CRP mediated the association between salivary or serum MPO levels.

2. Materials and Methods

2.1. Study Design

For the present study, 311 healthy controls and patients with periodontitis or CHD were chosen at the School of Odontostomatology of the University of Catania, Italy, from October 2018 to December 2019. Patients were chosen in a specific range of age (35–65 years old) and on gender in order to have similar proportion of patients in each category characterized by the selection variable. 50% of the patients and controls were males with 45–54 year of age.

The study was performed following the 2016 revision of the Helsinki declaration on medical research. Ethical approval was obtained by the local International Review Board (IRB) (#18-18). The study was registered at clinicaltrials.gov (NCT04152023). An informed written consent was obtained from each enrolled patient. The trial was performed in accordance to the guidelines for the strengthening of reporting of observational studies (STROBE) [27].

The inclusion criteria for the subjects enrolled in the periodontitis group were: (1) at least 16 teeth, (2) at least of 40% of periodontal sites with clinical attachment level (CAL) ≥2 mm and probing depth (PD) ≥4 mm [28]; (3) at least one periodontal site with ≥2 mm of crestal alveolar bone loss confirmed on digital periapical x-rays; (4) at least ≥40% sites with bleeding on probing (BOP) [29]. Healthy controls had any systemic disorder, at least ≤10% sites with BOP, and no periodontal sites with PD or CAL ≥4 mm, or x-ray signs of bone loss.

For the CVD group, the inclusion criteria were: at least ≥18 years; a diagnosis of CVD with ≥50% of stenosis of at least one coronary artery verified by coronary angiography, or past or current percutaneous coronary intervention [30]. Each type of previous disease, taking drugs, or previous CVD exams (e.g., electrocardiography, etc.) were recorded. In all patients, the diagnosis of CVD was performed by the same operator from medical record information. For the periodontitis plus CVD subjects the inclusion criteria were the same of the single disease (periodontitis and CVD).

The exclusion criteria of all subjects, were (1) consumption of contraceptive drugs; (2) consumption of antibiotics, anti-inflammatory or immunosuppressive drugs during the three months previous the trial; (3) presence of gestation or suction; (4) intake of alcohol; (5) anesthetic allergy; (6) intake of nifedipine, hydantoin or cyclosporin a drugs; (7) any type of periodontal treatment in the three months before baseline.

Then, 187 subjects were left out from the study because they did not meet the inclusion criteria (n = 129), failed to join in the study (n = 37), or were lost at the first assessment (n = 21). For these reasons, for the present study, 31 healthy subjects, 31 periodontitis patients, 31 CHD patients, and 31 patients with both diseases (periodontitis plus CHD) were enrolled in the end (Figure 1).

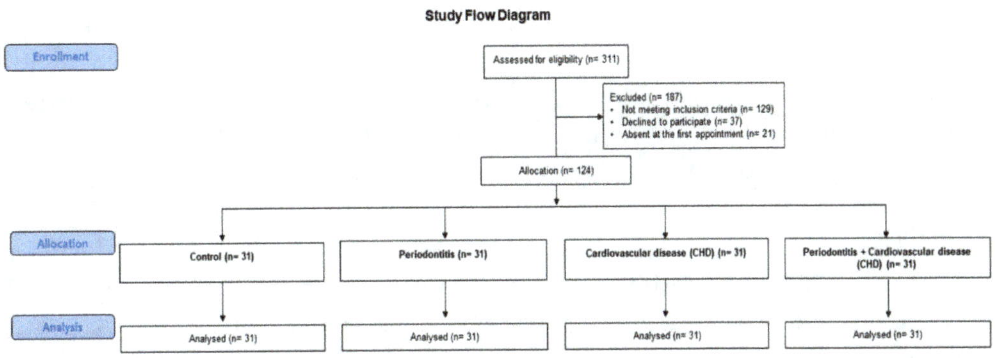

Figure 1. Flowchart of the study.

In each patient, every demographic characteristic (such as educational level) and demographic indices such as age, gender, body mass index (BMI), diabetes and other systemic events were recorded together with the type of drug taken. Diabetes was recorded on the patient's medical story or on fasting blood glucose ≥125 mg/dL. The BMI was recorded by calculating the patient's weight divided by the square of his height in kg/m^2. All enrolled subjects were also classified on their smoking history, such as normal smokers, ex-smokers (subjects who have not smoked for ≥5 years), and non-smokers.

The periodontal evaluation comprised clinical attachment loss (CAL), probing depth (PD), bleeding on probing (BOP), and plaque score (PI) [31]. CAL was verified, such as PD plus gingival recession using the cementoenamel junction as a reference. All periodontal indexes were registered, in all patients, by two independent calibrated examiners (a principal examiner and a control examiner), exonerated in the subsequent study steps, using a periodontal probe (UNC-15, Hu-Friedy, Chicago, IL, USA).

It was assessed the inter- and intra-examiner reliability for PD and CAL through the Intraclass Correlation Coefficient (ICC) analysis. The obtained inter-examiner reliability was in agreement for PD (ICC= 0.819) and CAL (ICC = 0.832) with a good degree of reliability. The intra-examiner reliability of PD and CAL was done only on 24 subjects (six random subjects per group) for both examiners. For the first examiner, the intra-examiner reliability presented an agreement for PD (ICC = 0.819) and CAL (ICC = 0.808); for the second examiner, the intra examiner reliability was good for both PD (ICC = 0.818) and CAL (ICC = 0.801). All periodontal indexes were registered, in each enrolled subject, at six sites in each tooth.

A power analysis was executed in order to evaluate the sample size needed for the study. The sample size was determined considering four groups: an effect size of 0.29 for MPO (primary outcome chosen), a two-sided significance level of 0.05, a standard deviation of 1.5 [23], and a power level of 80%. It was established that would be required around 28 patients per group, with a total number of 114 patients required to obtain a power level of 80%. a total of 124 patients were enrolled, so the study power was 81%. Power and sample size calculation was performed with statistical software (G*Power version 3.1.9.4, Universitat Dusseldorf, Germany).

2.2. Evaluation of Salivary and Serum MPO

All serum and saliva samples were collected on an in all patients between 8:00 and 10:00 a.m., before the periodontal examination, on the same day by the same examiner. All enrolled subjects were requested to refrain from drinking, eating, chewing, brushing their teeth, or other oral hygiene maneuvers in the 12 h preceding the sampling of serum and saliva.

For the collection of serum, a venous blood sample was taken which, after the collection, was immediately cooled with ice and centrifuged at 4 °C (800× g for 10 min). For the collection of saliva samples, the enrolled patients were asked to moisten by chewing a cotton roll for two minutes using the salivette method (Sarsted, Verona, Italy). Subsequently, the saliva sample in each patient was instantaneously centrifuged at 4 °C (1000× g for 2 min). Both saliva and serum samples were stored at −20 °C.

Magnetic bead-based luminex assay (R&D Systems, Minneapolis, MN, and Sigma-Aldrich, Saint Louis, MO, USA) were used to detect serum and salivary concentrations of MPO, following the manufacturers' instructions. Levels of hs-CRP were calculated using a nephelometric assay kit. Levels of hs-CRP >3 mg/L were related to an augmented CVD risk. Routine methods were applied to assess glucose and plasma lipids levels.

2.3. Statistical Analysis

Median, 25%, and 75% percentile were used to express numerical variables while number and % were used to express categorical variables. Nearly all of the variables analyzed (e.g., fasting glucose, triglycerides, all periodontal index) did not have normal distribution, as confirmed by Kolmogorov–Smirnov test. Only age, BMI, and salivary and serum MPO were normally distributed; for this reason, nonparametric tests were used to analyze all data in the present analysis [32]. More specifically, to confront all numerical variables in the 4 groups of patients, was applied the Kruskal Wallis test while the Mann Whitney test was applied to obtain the two-by-two comparisons. Bonferroni's correction was applied for numerous evaluations; the α level of 0.050 was split by the potential comparisons (n = 6), and the adjusted significance level equalled 0.008 (0.050/6).

The p-trend analysis for salivary and serum and MPO levels was obtained using the Jonckheere–Terpstra Test to evaluate whether MPO levels were statistically augmented in the four analyzed groups. To asses any significant interdependence between MPO in saliva and serum and hs-CRP, the Spearman correlation test was used.

Moreover, a univariate and multivariable linear regression analysis were applied in all enrolled patients to evaluate the dependence of MPO levels in serum and saliva (which resulted normally distributed) on possibly explicative outcomes such as sex, education, age, socioeconomic status (SES), triglycerides, total cholesterol, BMI, CRP, and CVD drugs (yes/no). In the multivariate final model, sex, age, and education SES were incorporated such as possible confounders, and tested to analyze if CHD, periodontitis, and hs-CRP influenced MPO in serum. For the evaluation of MPO in saliva, the same analysis was performed using salivary MPO levels as an outcome. All statistical analyses were executed using statistical software (SPSS 22.0 for Windows package, SPS srl, Bologna, Italy). a p-value < 0.05 was set such as significant.

3. Results

The demographic and serological characteristics of the enrolled patients are shown in Table 1. All groups were matched for age and sex, and they did not presented any statistically significant differences regarding education levels, smoking, BMI, and serological features (Table 1).

Table 1. Sample characteristics of enrolled patients. Data are represented as median (25th; 75th percentiles) or number with percentage. * $p < 0.001$ and ** $p < 0.001$ significant differences vs. healthy subjects computed by the Mann Whitney test. §§ $p < 0.001$ significant differences vs. periodontitis patients calculated by the Mann Whitney test. # $p < 0.008$ significant differences vs. coronary heart disease (CHD) patients calculated by the Mann Whitney test.

	Controls (N = 31)	Periodontitis (N = 31)	CVD (N = 31)	Periodontitis + CVD (N = 31)
Age (years)	52 (48; 56)	53 (47; 57)	52 (46; 58)	53 (47; 56)
Gender (male/female)	15/16	16/15	14/17	16/15
Education level				
Primary school, n (%)	11 (35.4)	12 (38.7)	11 (35.4)	12 (38.7)
High school, n (%)	14 (45.1)	13 (41.9)	15 (48.3)	14 (45.1)
College/university, n (%)	6 (19.3)	6 (19.3)	5 (16.1)	5 (16.1)
Body mass index (kg/m^2)	24.4 (21.8; 27.8)	23.9 (22.4; 26.4)	24.8 (21.6; 27.1)	24.5 (22.3; 26.1)
Fasting glucose (mg/dl)	87.9 (82.1; 93.2)	88.7 (82.3; 105.3)	88.1 (80.6; 114.6)	91.1 (85.1; 109.2)
Smokers, n (%)	2 (6.4)	3 (9.6)	2 (6.4)	2 (9.6)
Never smokers, n (%)	27 (88.2)	27 (85.2)	28 (88.2)	26 (85.2)
Past smokers, n (%)	2 (6.4)	1 (3.2)	1 (3.2)	3 (9.6)
Current smokers, n (%)	2 (6.4)	3 (6.4)	2 (6.4)	2 (6.4)
Comorbidities				
Diabetes, n (%)	-	3 (9.6) **	2 (6.4) **	2 (9.6) **
Previous CVD				
Atrial fibrillation, n (%)	-	-	6 (19.3) **,§§	5 (16.1) **,§§
Angina pectoris, n (%)	-	-	12 (38.7) **,§§	13 (41.9) **,§§
Stroke, n (%)	-	-	5 (16.1) **,§§	7 (22.6) **,§§
Heart failure, n (%)	-	-	6 (19.3) **,§§	5 (16.1) **,§§
Antihypertensive, n (%)	-	-	10 (32.2) **,§§	10 (32.2) **,§§
Statins, n (%)	-	-	10 (32.2) **,§§	9 (29) **,§§
Low-dose aspirin, n (%)	-	-	7 (22.6) **,§§	7 (22.6) **,§§
Beta blockers, n (%)	-	-	6 (19.3) **,§§	8 (25.8) **,§§
hs-CRP (mg/L)	2.5 (2.1; 2.9)	3.1 (2.5; 3.9) *	5.6 (4.8; 6.2) **	6.7 (5.8; 7.1) **,§§,#
Total cholesterol (mg/dl)	162 (139; 181)	164 (133; 181)	173 (139; 197)	176 (178; 201)
Triglycerids (mg/dl)	121 (91; 145)	102 (66; 128)	141 (122; 166)	139 (103; 158)

Compared to healthy controls, patients with periodontitis, CDH and a combination of periodontitis and CVD presented a higher value of hs-CRP ($p < 0.001$). Moreover, patients with CHD and periodontitis plus CHD presented no significant differences regarding past CVD events.

In Table 2 are represented dental characteristics of all enrolled patients. Compared with CHD and control patients, subjects with periodontitis and periodontitis plus CVD showed higher periodontal parameters (CAL, PD, BOP, PI) and smaller number of teeth ($p < 0.001$) (Table 2).

Table 2. Periodontal characteristics of enrolled patients. Data are represented as median (25th; 75th percentile). CAL, clinical attachment level; PD, probing pocket depth; BOP, bleeding on probing; PI, plaque index. ** $p < 0.001$ significant differences vs. control subjects. §§ $p < 0.001$ significant differences vs. periodontitis patients. ## $p < 0.001$ significant differences vs. CHD patients.

	Controls (N = 31)	Periodontitis (N = 31)	CVD (N = 31)	Periodontitis + CVD (N = 31)
N° of teeth	26 (21; 27)	20 (15; 21)**	23 (19; 26) **,§§	18 (12; 20) **,##
CAL (mm)	1 (0.9; 1.3)	3.6 (3.1; 4.2) **	2 (1.8; 2.4) **,§§	3.4 (3; 4.1) **,##
CAL 4–5 mm (% sites)	-	38.7 (35.4; 42.9) **	-	40.6 (35.5; 46.1) **,##
CAL ≥6 mm (% sites)	-	18.7 (19.6; 22.3) **	-	17.4 (15.8; 22.7) **,##
PD (mm)	1.5 (1.3; 1.9)	4.4 (3.7; 4.6) **	2.1 (1.8; 2.4) **,§§	3.9 (3.7; 4.4) **,##
PD 4–5 mm (% sites)	-	40.9 (38.6; 45.7) **	-	44.1 (42.7; 55.3) **,##
PD ≥6 mm (% sites)	-	23.1 (19.8; 25.2) **	-	22.7 (20.3; 26.5) **,§§,##
BOP (%)	7.9 (6.5; 8.3)	41.2 (34.3; 46.5) **	8.1 (6.4; 8.9) **,§§	42.3 (41.5; 50.1) **,§§,##
Rx alveolar bone loss (mm)	0.2 (0.1; 0.5)	2.9 (2.5; 3.4) **	0.3 (0.2; 0.9) **,§§	3.3 (2.1; 4.6) **,##
PI (%)	6.5 (4.7; 9.3)	35.4 (31.7; 37.9) **	11.7 (9.1; 12.8) **,§§	32.4 (27.2; 36.1) **,##

Figure 2 represents median (25th; 75th percentile) values of MPO levels in saliva and serum of all enrolled patients. Compared to control subjects, patients with CVD ($p < 0.01$) and with periodontitis plus CVD ($p < 0.001$) had higher median concentrations of MPO in saliva and serum. More specifically, in comparison with periodontitis subjects, patients with periodontitis plus CVD presented increased salivary and serum concentrations of MPO ($p < 0.01$) (Figure 2).

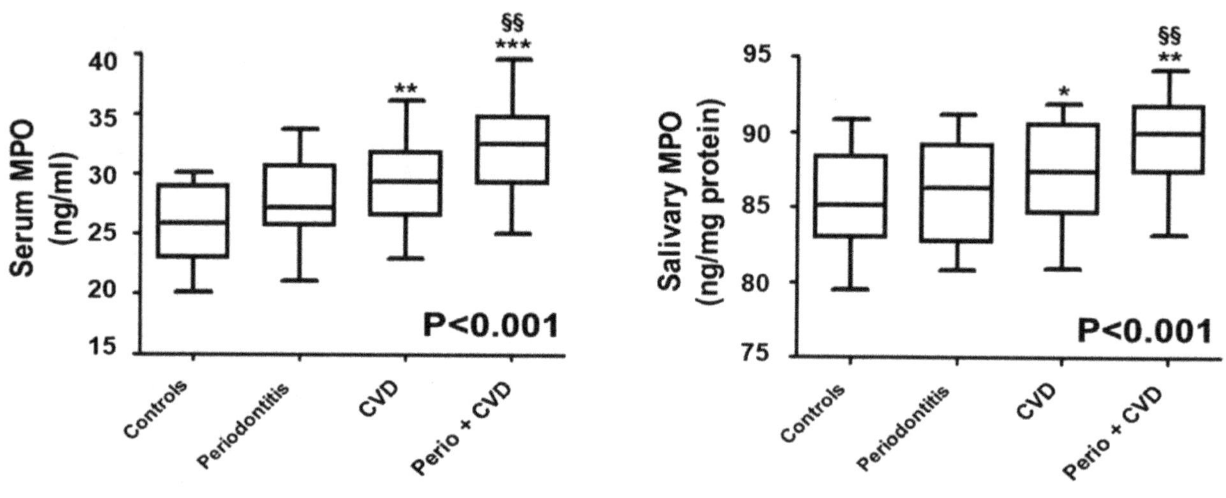

Figure 2. Median values (25%; 75% percentiles) of coronary heart disease (MPO) in saliva and serum. * $p < 0.05$, ** $p < 0.01$ and *** $p < 0.001$ significant differences vs. control subjects (derived by the Kruskal–Wallis test). §§ $p < 0.01$ significant differences vs. periodontitis patients. $p < 0.001$.

Moreover, the p-for trend analysis test evidenced that MPO in serum increased gradually in subjects with periodontitis, CVD, and with periodontitis plus CVD (p-trend <0.001) (Figure 3). No statistically significant associations were found in MPO levels between serum and saliva (rs = 0.213, $p = 0.098$). Moreover, in all enrolled patients presented a positive correlation between serum/salivary MPO and hs-CRP levels (rs = 0.341, $p < 0.001$)/(rs = 0.609, $p < 0.001$) (Figure 3).

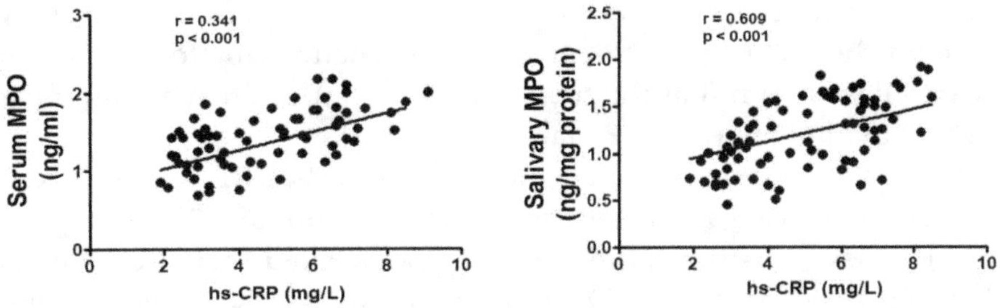

Figure 3. Analysis of correlation of serum and salivary MPO levels with c-reactive protein (CRP) in all patients.

The univariate regression analysis evidenced that there was a significant direct impact of hs-CRP on serum and salivary MPO (both $p < 0.001$). Furthermore, the adjusted multivariate linear regression analysis evidenced that hs-CRP variable was the only significant predictor for serum MPO ($p < 0.001$).

Moreover, hs-CRP ($p < 0.001$) and total cholesterol ($p = 0.035$) were the statistically significant predictor variables for salivary MPO (Table 3).

Table 3. Uni- and multivariate linear regression analysis for MPO levels in serum and saliva in all patients. Age was included as continuous variable. For periodontitis and cardiovascular disease (CVD), controls served as reference. For gender, male served as reference.

Serum MPO Levels		UNIVARIATE			MULTIVARIATE		
	Variable	B	95% CI	*p*	B	95% CI	*p*
	CVD	0.442	0.314; 0.558	**<0.001**	0.122	−0.221; 0.559	0.578
	Periodontitis	0.289	0.18; 0.274	**0.024**	0.231	−0.066; 0.319	0.226
	hs-CRP	0.278	0.028; 0.136	**<0.001**	0.314	0.065; 0.189	**<0.001**
	Age (years)	−0.047	−0.287; 0.056	0.064	−0.039	−0.111; 0.315	0.287
	Female gender	0.212	−0.78; 0.549	0.227	0.219	−0.88; 0.428	0.112
	Education SES	−0.114	−0.178; 0.123	0.287	−0.066	−0.312; 0.398	0.312
Salivary MPO Levels							
	CVD	0.319	0.112; 0.552	**<0.001**	−0.065	−0.412; 0.289	0.451
	Periodontitis	0.078	−0.069; 0.328	0.411	0.007	−0.178; 0.213	0.665
	hs-CRP	0.082	0.027; 0.287	**<0.001**	0.066	0.021; 0.133	**<0.001**
	Age (years)	−0.051	−0.110; 0.036	0.399	0.047	−0.028; 0.087	0.741
	Female gender	0.074	−0.112; 0.211	0.398	0.071	−0.065; 0.412	0.321
	Total Cholesterol	−0.057	−0.151; 0.062	**0.037**	−0.65	−0.041; 0.314	**0.035**
	Serum MPO	0.122	−0.021; 0.557	0.057	−0.036	−0.369; 0.166	0.331

4. Discussion

This trial was aimed at evaluating the impact of conditions such as periodontal disease, CVD, or periodontitis plus CVD on MPO levels in serum and saliva. The present trial evidenced that the occurrence of CVD caused increased levels of MPO and hs-CRP in serum and saliva. Nevertheless, in comparison with periodontitis and healthy controls, only the group of subjects with CVD and periodontitis plus CVD had significantly elevated MPO levels in serum and saliva, endorsing the suggestion that CVD influenced the increment of MPO levels in serum and saliva. Furthermore, results of the present study show that the simultaneous presence of periodontitis in patients with CVD can determine an increased activation of MPO and therefore represent a subclinical stimulus for the purpose of an increase in CVD development.

In accordance with the results of the present study, some reports have shown that high levels of MPO in serum represent real independent risk factors of CVD development and increased mortality index, possibly by inactivating NO signaling [33]. Specifically, it has also been shown that, in patients with atherosclerosis, high systemic levels of MPO are associated with significant carotid epithelial dysfunctions, underlining the fundamental inhibitory role of NO exercised by MPO [34].

Therefore, the simultaneous presence of CVD on the one hand and periodontitis on the other hand can be a real explanation for the deterioration of endothelial function due to high levels of MPO. In this regard, recent research has shown that the treatment of periodontitis has significantly reduced the systemic levels of MPO in patients with coronary disease [35].

Moreover, several reports demonstrated that increased hs-CRP levels in serum can facilitate the increment of MPO levels in serum in several diseases in humans [23,35–38]. In accordance with the results of our study, several studies have been demonstrated that situations which may cause an increase of oxidative stress, such as CVD and periodontal disease, cause the high release of CRP, which in turn, can arouse the production of MPO in saliva and serum in order to defend tissue damage determined by oxidative stress condition [36]. In agreement with the results of the present study, Magan-Fernandez et al. [39] demonstrated that CRP and MPO levels were higher during active phases of periodontal disease.

However, while evidence has previously been demonstrated regarding high serum MPO levels as primary mediators of endothelial dysfunction or in the development of cardiovascular risk, from the authors' knowledge, there is no specific evidence to determine MPO levels in saliva in order to evaluate whether the increased expression of salivary MPO levels determines, by reflection, an increase in MPO in serum and then analyzes the salivary levels of MPO as an index of endothelial dysfunction. In this regard, however, it should be noted that this study did not reveal a significant correlation between serum and saliva MPO levels, as salivary MPO levels are influenced in patients enrolled independently only of hs-CRP and total cholesterol. This explanation can be determined by the way that MPO salivary levels may be due to an exclusive local oral production of MPO.

In this regard, it should be noted that, from the studies currently present in the literature, while the effect of MPO at a systemic level mediated by the reduction of NO on endothelial damage has been previously highlighted, the impact of MPO activation orally (e.g., in saliva) is less clear. However, there are studies that show that periodontal disease is positively correlated with high levels of NO and therefore with related stress-oxidative damage [19,24]. The presence of high levels of NO at salivary level can be explained as NO is produced orally in response by the host as a specific salivary defense in the presence of periodontal pathogenic bacteria that are exacerbated during periodontitis [12,24,40]. Furthermore, some studies suggested that decreasing activities of NO and some other enzymatic antioxidants, such as superoxide dismutase catalase, were associated with periodontitis and high levels of MPO, whereas others claim that antioxidants function as protective agents against free radicals during CP progression [19,24,41].

However, there is no unanimous consensus in the literature on the effects of NO levels on tissue damage during periodontitis. Some reports have shown high levels of NO in periodontal tissue in the active periodontal period [39,42] while, on the other hand, other authors have shown lower levels of NO in saliva of subjects with periodontal disease [25,43]. However, results in the literature may have been determined by the different homogeneity of the patients enrolled in the studies, by the different age ranges of the patients analyzed, or by the excessive presence of patients who smoke; in fact it has been shown that smoking can cause a high increase in salivary NO salivary levels [44–46]. Another explanation for the different results found in the literature can be determined by the different salivary sampling method performed in the different studies. Furthermore, the cause of the different expression of MPO at the salivary and serum level may be due to a different production of NO at the oral level which may be different from the serum one.

As an explanation of the results of the present study, it should be highlighted that the dysfunctional damage at the endothelium level found in patients with periodontitis and with CVD can be determined by a specific inflammatory and immune pathway in which MPO modulates a response towards pathogenic bacteria of the oral biofilm which are exacerbated during the active phases of periodontal damage. It has also been shown that MPO, during periodontal disease, mediates the immune response at the endothelial level through specific heat shock proteins which has been shown to be useful for stimulating the production of cross-reactive T cells [47–52]. In this regard, this process which sees

MPO as a key modulator [53–58], has also been shown to influence the host defense mechanism that determines a subsequent activation of endothelial cell production [55,58–63] which leads to an increased risk of future tissue damage effects due to periodontal pathogens bacteria in several oral diseases [43,64–68]. Moreover, the oral microbiota is a key factor in the protection against the colonization of extrinsic pathogens that could impact systemic health [68]. However, the imbalance of the ecosystem together with high levels of MPO, which can be caused by a weak immune system, lead to a challenge for oral and systemic health [68]. The ecological conditions of these habitats are constantly changing, so ecosystems are subject to frequent variations [68,69].

However, the present trial has some limitations. Among the main limitations there is the type of study, which makes it difficult to analyze the cause and effect on a temporal level of MPO. The small sample size, due to high inclusion and exclusion levels, and to the important excluded confounders, also represents a limitation of the present preliminary study. However, the exclusion of several confounders represents a positive and rigorous aspect for the clear evaluation of these confounders on the concentration of serum and salivary levels of MPO.

Recently, different approaches have been developed with the aim of easily evaluating innovative salivary markers useful for early and subclinically validating the development of different diseases. This study indicates that patients suffering from periodontitis and CVD have higher serum and salivary levels of MPO than subjects with periodontitis and healthy subjects.

The results of this study propose that mostly CVD is a stimulus to the increased serum MPO levels which may be beyond a pathway intermediated by hs-CRP. Therefore, these results are promising but at the same time require further studies with a larger sample of analysis in order to better comprehend the function of MPO during periodontitis.

Author Contributions: Conceptualization, A.P.; methodology, S.T.; validation, S.S., formal analysis, M.D.S.; writing—original draft preparation, F.I.; A.L.G. All authors have read and agreed to the published version of the manuscript.

References

1. Tonetti, M.S.; Greenwell, H.; Kornman, K.S. Staging and grading of periodontitis: Framework and proposal of a new classification and case definition. *J. Periodontol.* **2018**, *89* (Suppl. 1), S159–S172. [CrossRef] [PubMed]
2. Briguglio, F.; Briguglio, E.; Briguglio, R.; Cafiero, C.; Isola, G. Treatment of infrabony periodontal defects using a resorbable biopolymer of hyaluronic acid: a randomized clinical trial. *Quintessence Int.* **2013**, *44*, 231–240. [PubMed]
3. Eke, P.I.; Wei, L.; Thornton-Evans, G.O.; Borrell, L.N.; Borgnakke, W.S.; Dye, B.; Genco, R.J. Risk Indicators for Periodontitis in US Adults: NHANES 2009 to 2012. *J. Periodontol.* **2016**, *87*, 1174–1185. [CrossRef] [PubMed]
4. Isola, G.; Alibrandi, A.; Currò, M.; Matarese, M.; Ricca, S.; Matarese, G.; Ientile, R.; Kocher, T. Evaluation of salivary and serum ADMA levels in patients with periodontal and cardiovascular disease as subclinical marker of cardiovascular risk. *J. Periodontol.* **2020**. [CrossRef]
5. Isola, G.; Giudice, A.L.; Polizzi, A.; Alibrandi, A.; Patini, R.; Ferlito, S. Periodontitis and Tooth Loss Have Negative Systemic Impact on Circulating Progenitor Cell Levels: a Clinical Study. *Genes* **2019**, *10*, 1022. [CrossRef]
6. Holmlund, A.; Holm, G.; Lind, L. Number of Teeth as a Predictor of Cardiovascular Mortality in a Cohort of 7,674 Subjects Followed for 12 Years. *J. Periodontol.* **2010**, *81*, 870–876. [CrossRef]
7. Isola, G.; Polizzi, A.; Alibrandi, A.; Indelicato, F.; Ferlito, S. Analysis of Endothelin-1 concentrations in individuals with periodontitis. *Sci. Rep.* **2020**. [CrossRef]
8. Li, C.; Lv, Z.; Shi, Z.; Zhu, Y.; Wu, Y.; Li, L.; Iheozor-Ejiofor, Z. Periodontal therapy for the management of cardiovascular disease in patients with chronic periodontitis. *Cochrane Database Syst. Rev.* **2017**, *2017*, CD009197. [CrossRef]
9. Isola, G.; Polizzi, A.; Muraglie, S.; Leonardi, R.; Giudice, A.L. Assessment of Vitamin C and Antioxidant Profiles in Saliva and Serum in Patients with Periodontitis and Ischemic Heart Disease. *Nutrients* **2019**, *11*, 2956. [CrossRef]
10. Matarese, G.; Curro, M.; Isola, G.; Caccamo, D.; Vecchio, M.; Giunta, M.L.; Ramaglia, L.; Cordasco, G.; Williams, R.C.; Ientile, R. Transglutaminase 2 up-regulation is associated with RANKL/OPG pathway in

cultured HPDL cells and THP-1-differentiated macrophages. *Amino Acids* **2015**, *47*, 2447–2455. [CrossRef]

11. Aratani, Y. Myeloperoxidase: Its role for host defense, inflammation, and neutrophil function. *Arch. Biochem. Biophys.* **2018**, *640*, 47–52. [CrossRef] [PubMed]
12. Ahmad, S.; Ramadori, G.; Moriconi, F. Modulation of Chemokine- and Adhesion-Molecule Gene Expression and Recruitment of Neutrophil Granulocytes in Rat and Mouse Liver after a Single Gadolinium Chloride or Zymosan Treatment. *Int. J. Mol. Sci.* **2018**, *19*, 3891. [CrossRef] [PubMed]
13. de Souza, R.G.M.; Gomes, A.C.; Navarro, A.M.; Cunha, L.C.D.; Silva, M.A.C.; Junior, F.B.; Mota, J.F. Baru Almonds Increase the Activity of Glutathione Peroxidase in Overweight and Obese Women: a Randomized, Placebo-Controlled Trial. *Nutrients* **2019**, *11*, 1750. [CrossRef] [PubMed]
14. Isola, G.; Matarese, G.; Giudice, G.L.; Briguglio, F.; Alibrandi, A.; Crupi, A.; Cordasco, G.; Ramaglia, L. a New Approach for the Treatment of Lateral Periodontal Cysts with an 810-nm Diode Laser. *Int. J. Periodontics Restor. Dent.* **2017**, *37*, 120–129. [CrossRef] [PubMed]
15. Matarese, G.; Isola, G.; Anastasi, G.P.; Cutroneo, G.; Favaloro, A.; Vita, G.; Cordasco, G.; Milardi, D.; Zizzari, V.L.; Tetè, S.; et al. Transforming Growth Factor Beta 1 and Vascular Endothelial Growth Factor levels in the pathogenesis of periodontal disease. *Eur. J. Inflamm.* **2013**, *11*, 479–488. [CrossRef]
16. Peniche-Palma, D.C.; Carrillo-Avila, B.A.; Sauri-Esquivel, E.A.; Acosta-Viana, K.; Esparza-Villalpando, V.; Pozos-Guillen, A.; Hernandez-Rios, M.; Martinez-Aguilar, V.M. Levels of Myeloperoxidase and Metalloproteinase-9 in Gingival Crevicular Fluid from Diabetic Subjects with and without Stage 2, Grade B Periodontitis. *BioMed Res. Int.* **2019**, *2019*, 5613514. [CrossRef]
17. Currò, M.; Matarese, G.; Isola, G.; Caccamo, D.; Ventura, V.P.; Cornelius, C.; Lentini, M.; Cordasco, G.; Ientile, R. Differential expression of transglutaminase genes in patients with chronic periodontitis. *Oral Dis.* **2014**, *20*, 616–623. [CrossRef]
18. Isola, G.; Williams, R.C.; Lo Gullo, A.; Ramaglia, L.; Matarese, M.; Iorio-Siciliano, V.; Cosio, C.; Matarese, G. Risk association between scleroderma disease characteristics, periodontitis, and tooth loss. *Clin Rheumatol.* **2017**, *36*, 2733–2741. [CrossRef]
19. Andrukhov, O.; Haririan, H.; Bertl, K.; Rausch, W.-D.; Bantleon, H.-P.; Moritz, A.; Rausch-Fan, X. Nitric oxide production, systemic inflammation and lipid metabolism in periodontitis patients: Possible gender aspect. *J. Clin. Periodontol.* **2013**, *40*, 916–923. [CrossRef]
20. Isola, G.; Alibrandi, A.; Rapisarda, E.; Matarese, G.; Williams, R.C.; Leonardi, R. Association of vitamin d in patients with periodontitis: a cross-sectional study. *J. Periodontal Res.* **2020**, in press.
21. Gurav, A.N. The implication of periodontitis in vascular endothelial dysfunction. *Eur. J. Clin. Investig.* **2014**, *44*, 1000–1009. [CrossRef]
22. Tabeta, K.; Hosojima, M.; Nakajima, M.; Miyauchi, S.; Miyazawa, H.; Takahashi, N.; Matsuda, Y.; Sugita, N.; Komatsu, Y.; Sato, K.; et al. Increased serum PCSK9, a potential biomarker to screen for periodontitis, and decreased total bilirubin associated with probing depth in a Japanese community survey. *J. Periodontal Res.* **2018**, *53*, 446–456. [CrossRef]
23. Isola, G.; Ramaglia, L.; Cordasco, G.; Lucchese, A.; Fiorillo, L.; Matarese, G. The effect of a functional appliance in the management of temporomandibular joint disorders in patients with juvenile idiopathic arthritis. *Minerva Stomatol.* **2017**, *66*, 1–8. [PubMed]
24. Kendall, H.K.; Marshall, R.I.; Bartold, P.M. Nitric oxide, and tissue destruction. *Oral Dis.* **2001**, *7*, 2–10. [CrossRef] [PubMed]
25. Aurer, A.; Aleksic, J.; Ivic-Kardum, M.; Aurer, J.; Čulo, F. Nitric oxide synthesis is decreased in periodontitis. *J. Clin. Periodontol.* **2001**, *28*, 565–568. [CrossRef] [PubMed]
26. Ruest, L.B.; Ranjbaran, H.; Tong, E.J.; Svoboda, K.K.H.; Feng, J.Q. Activation of Receptor Activator of Nuclear Factor-κB Ligand and Matrix Metalloproteinase Production in Periodontal Fibroblasts by Endothelin Signaling. *J. Periodontol.* **2016**, *87*, e1–e8. [CrossRef] [PubMed]
27. von Elm, E.; Altman, D.G.; Egger, M.; Pocock, S.J.; Gotzsche, P.C.; Vandenbroucke, J.P. The Strengthening the Reporting of Observational Studies in Epidemiology (STROBE) statement: Guidelines for reporting observational studies. *J. Clin. Periodontol.* **2008**, *61*, 344–349. [CrossRef]
28. Lindhe, J.; Ranney, R.; Lamster, I.; Charles, A.; Chung, C.-P.; Flemmig, T.; Kinane, D.; Listgarten, M.; Löe, H.; Schoor, R.; et al. Consensus Report: Chronic Periodontitis. *Ann. Periodontol.* **1999**, *4*, 38. [CrossRef]
29. Isola, G.; Matarese, M.; Ramaglia, L.; Iorio-Siciliano, V.; Cordasco, G.; Matarese, G. Efficacy of a drug composed of herbal extracts on postoperative discomfort after surgical removal of impacted mandibular

third molar: a randomized, triple-blind, controlled clinical trial. *Clin. Oral Investig.* **2019**, *23*, 2443–2453. [CrossRef]

30. Bassand, J.P.; Hamm, C.W.; Ardissino, D.; Boersma, E.; Budaj, A.; Fernández-Avilés, F.; Fox, K.A.; Hasdai, D.; Ohman, E.M.; Wallentin, L.; et al. Guidelines for the diagnosis and treatment of non-ST-segment elevation acute coronary syndromes: The Task Force for the Diagnosis and Treatment of Non-ST-Segment Elevation Acute Coronary Syndromes of the European Society of Cardiology. *Eur. Heart J.* **2007**, *28*, 1598–1660. [CrossRef]
31. O'Leary, T.J.; Drake, R.B.; Naylor, J.E. The Plaque Control Record. *J. Periodontol.* **1972**, *43*, 38. [CrossRef] [PubMed]
32. Hollander, M.; Wolfe, D.A.; Chicken, E. *Nonparametric Statistical Methods*, 3rd ed.; John Wiley & Sons: Hoboken, NJ, USA, 2013.
33. Lo Giudice, G.; Lo Giudice, R.; Matarese, G.; Isola, G.; Cicciù, M.; Terranova, A.; Palaia, G.; Romeo, U. Evaluation of magnification systems in restorative dentistry. An in-vitro study. *Dental Cadmos* **2015**, *83*, 296–305. [CrossRef]
34. Mazzoli, A.; Crescenzo, R.; Cigliano, L.; Spagnuolo, M.S.; Cancelliere, R.; Gatto, C.; Iossa, S. Early Hepatic Oxidative Stress and Mitochondrial Changes Following Western Diet in Middle Aged Rats. *Nutrients* **2019**, *11*, 2670. [CrossRef]
35. Lahdentausta, L.; Paju, S.; Mäntylä, P.; Buhlin, K.; Pietiäinen, M.; Tervahartiala, T.; Nieminen, M.S.; Sinisalo, J.; Sorsa, T.; Pussinen, P.J. Smoking confounds the periodontal diagnostics using saliva biomarkers. *J. Periodontol.* **2019**, *90*, 475–483. [CrossRef]
36. Isola, G.; Matarese, G.; Ramaglia, L.; Pedullà, E.; Rapisarda, E.; Iorio-Siciliano, V. Association between periodontitis and glycosylated haemoglobin before diabetes onset: a cross-sectional study. *Clin. Oral Investig.* **2019**. [CrossRef]
37. Valenzuela, M.; Draibe, J.; Quero, M.; Fulladosa, X.; Cruzado, J.M.; Bestard, O.; Torras, J.; Valenzuela, L.M. Exploring Frequencies of Circulating Specific Th17 Cells against Myeloperoxidase and Proteinase 3 in ANCA Associated Vasculitis. *Int. J. Mol. Sci.* **2019**, *20*, 5820. [CrossRef]
38. Przepiera-Będzak, H.; Fischer, K.; Brzosko, M. Serum Interleukin-18, Fetuin-A, Soluble Intercellular Adhesion Molecule-1, and Endothelin-1 in Ankylosing Spondylitis, Psoriatic Arthritis, and SAPHO Syndrome. *Int. J. Mol. Sci.* **2016**, *17*, 1255. [CrossRef]
39. Magán-Fernández, A.; O'Valle, F.; Abadía-Molina, F.; Muñoz, R.; Puga-Guil, P.; Mesa, F. Characterization and comparison of neutrophil extracellular traps in gingival samples of periodontitis and gingivitis: a pilot study. *J. Periodontal Res.* **2019**, *54*, 218–224. [CrossRef]
40. Cavuoti, S.; Matarese, G.; Isola, G.; Abdolreza, J.; Femiano, F.; Perillo, L. Combined orthodontic-surgical management of a transmigrated mandibular canine: a case report. *Angle Orthod.* **2016**, *86*, 681–691. [CrossRef]
41. Matejka, M.; Partyka, L.; Ulm, C.; Solar, P.; Sinzinger, H. Nitric oxide synthesis is increased in periodontal disease. *J. Periodontal Res.* **1998**, *33*, 517–518. [CrossRef]
42. Perillo, L.; Isola, G.; Esercizio, D.; Iovane, M.; Triolo, G.; Matarese, G. Differences in craniofacial characteristics in Southern Italian children from Naples: a retrospective study by cephalometric analysis. *Eur. J. Paediatr. Dent.* **2013**, *14*, 195–198. [PubMed]
43. Ozer, L.; Elgün, S.; Özdemir, B.; Pervane, B.; Özmeriç, N. Arginine–Nitric Oxide–Polyamine Metabolism in Periodontal Disease. *J. Periodontol.* **2011**, *82*, 320–328. [CrossRef]
44. Bodis, S.; Haregewoin, A. Significantly reduced salivary nitric oxide levels in smokers. *Ann. Oncol.* **1994**, *5*, 371–372. [CrossRef]
45. Vasconcelos, D.F.P.; Da Silva, F.R.P.; Pinto, M.E.S.C.; Santana, L.D.A.B.; Souza, I.G.; De Souza, L.K.M.; Oliveira, N.C.M.; Ventura, C.A.; Novaes, P.D.; Barbosa, A.L.D.R.; et al. Decrease of Pericytes is Associated with Liver Disease Caused by Ligature-Induced Periodontitis in Rats. *J. Periodontol.* **2017**, *88*, e49–e57. [CrossRef] [PubMed]
46. Isola, G.; Polizzi, A.; Santonocito, S.; Alibrandi, A.; Ferlito, S. Expression of Salivary and Serum Malondialdehyde and Lipid Profile of Patients with Periodontitis and Coronary Heart Disease. *Int. J. Mol. Sci.* **2019**, *20*, 6061. [CrossRef] [PubMed]
47. Isola, G.; Matarese, M.; Ramaglia, L.; Cicciù, M.; Matarese, G. Evaluation of the efficacy of celecoxib and ibuprofen on postoperative pain, swelling, and mouth opening after surgical removal of impacted third molars: a randomized, controlled clinical trial. *Int. J. Oral Maxillofac. Surg.* **2019**, *48*, 1348–1354. [CrossRef] [PubMed]

48. Isola, G.; Perillo, L.; Migliorati, M.; Matarese, M.; Dalessandri, D.; Grassia, V.; Alibrandi, A.; Matarese, G. The impact of temporomandibular joint arthritis on functional disability and global health in patients with juvenile idiopathic arthritis. *Eur. J. Orthod.* **2019**, *41*, 117–124. [CrossRef]
49. Isola, G.; Anastasi, G.P.; Matarese, G.; Williams, R.C.; Cutroneo, G.; Bracco, P.; Piancino, M.G. Functional and molecular outcomes of the human masticatory muscles. *Oral Dis.* **2018**, *24*, 1428–1441. [CrossRef]
50. Isola, G.; Alibrandi, A.; Pedullà, E.; Grassia, V.; Ferlito, S.; Perillo, L.; Rapisarda, E. Analysis of the Effectiveness of Lornoxicam and Flurbiprofen on Management of Pain and Sequelae Following Third Molar Surgery: a Randomized, Controlled, Clinical Trial. *J. Clin. Med.* **2019**, *8*, 325. [CrossRef]
51. Camacho-Alonso, F.; Davia-Peña, R.S.; Vilaplana-Vivo, C.; Tudela-Mulero, M.R.; Merino, J.J.; Martínez-Beneyto, Y. Synergistic effect of photodynamic therapy and alendronate on alveolar bone loss in rats with ligature-induced periodontitis. *J. Periodontal Res.* **2017**, *53*, 306–314. [CrossRef]
52. Isola, G.; Matarese, G.; Alibrandi, A.; Dalessandri, D.; Migliorati, M.; Pedullà, E.; Rapisarda, E. Comparison of Effectiveness of Etoricoxib and Diclofenac on Pain and Perioperative Sequelae After Surgical Avulsion of Mandibular Third Molars: a Randomized, Controlled, Clinical Trial. *Clin. J. Pain* **2019**, *35*, 908–915. [CrossRef]
53. Mohammed, H.; Varoni, E.M.; Cochis, A.; Cordaro, M.; Gallenzi, P.; Patini, R.; Staderini, E.; Lajolo, C.; Rimondini, L.; Rocchetti, V. Oral Dysbiosis in Pancreatic Cancer and Liver Cirrhosis: a Review of the Literature. *Biomedicines* **2018**, *6*, 115. [CrossRef] [PubMed]
54. Patini, R.; Gallenzi, P.; Spagnuolo, G.; Cordaro, M.; Cantiani, M.; Amalfitano, A.; Arcovito, A.; Callà, C.; Mingrone, G.; Nocca, G. Correlation Between Metabolic Syndrome, Periodontitis and Reactive Oxygen Species Production. a Pilot Study. *Open Dent. J.* **2017**, *11*, 621–627. [CrossRef]
55. Caccianiga, G.; Paiusco, A.; Perillo, L.; Nucera, R.; Pinsino, A.; Maddalone, M.; Cordasco, G.; Giudice, A.L. Does Low-Level Laser Therapy Enhance the Efficiency of Orthodontic Dental Alignment? Results from a Randomized Pilot Study. *Photomed. Laser Surg.* **2017**, *35*, 421–426. [CrossRef] [PubMed]
56. Lo Giudice, A.; Nucera, R.; Leonardi, R.; Paiusco, A.; Baldoni, M.; Caccianiga, G. a Comparative Assessment of the Efficiency of Orthodontic Treatment with and Without Photobiomodulation during Mandibular Decrowding in Young Subjects: a Single-Center, Single-Blind Randomized Controlled Trial. *Photobiomodul. Photomed. Laser Surg.* **2020**. [CrossRef]
57. Ferlazzo, N.; Currò, M.; Zinellu, A.; Caccamo, D.; Isola, G.; Ventura, V.; Carru, C.; Matarese, G.; Ientile, R. Influence of MTHFR genetic background on P16 and MGMT methylation in oral squamous cell cancer. *Int. J. Mol. Sci.* **2017**, *18*, 724. [CrossRef]
58. Cutroneo, G.; Piancino, M.G.; Ramieri, G.; Bracco, P.; Vita, G.; Isola, G.; Vermiglio, G.; Favaloro, A.; Anastasi, G.P.; Trimarchi, F. Expression of muscle-specific integrins in masseter muscle fibers during malocclusion disease. *Int. J. Mol. Med.* **2012**, *30*, 235–242. [CrossRef]
59. Isola, G.; Matarese, M.; Briguglio, F.; Grassia, V.; Picciolo, G.; Fiorillo, L.; Matarese, G. Effectiveness of Low-Level Laser Therapy during Tooth Movement: a Randomized Clinical Trial. *Materials* **2019**, *12*, 2187. [CrossRef]
60. Piancino, M.G.; Isola, G.; Cannavale, R.; Cutroneo, G.; Vermiglio, G.; Bracco, P.; Anastasi, G.P.; Grazia, P.M.; Gaetano, I.; Rosangela, C.; et al. From periodontal mechanoreceptors to chewing motor control: a systematic review. *Arch. Oral Boil.* **2017**, *78*, 109–121. [CrossRef]
61. Lo Giudice, A.; Nucera, R.; Perillo, L.; Paiusco, A.; Caccianiga, G. Is low-level laser therapy an effective method to alleviate pain induced by active orthodontic alignment archwire? a randomized clinical trial. *J. Evid. Based Dent. Pract.* **2019**, *19*, 71–78. [CrossRef]
62. Leonardi, R.; Lo Giudice, A.; Rugeri, M.; Muraglie, S.; Cordasco, G.; Barbato, E. Three-dimensional evaluation on digital casts of maxillary palatal size and morphology in patients with functional posterior crossbite. *Eur. J. Orthod.* **2018**, *40*, 556–562. [CrossRef] [PubMed]
63. Giudice, A.L.; Caccianiga, G.; Crimi, S.; Cavallini, C.; Leonardi, R. Frequency and type of ponticulus posticus in a longitudinal sample of nonorthodontically treated patients: Relationship with gender, age, skeletal maturity, and skeletal malocclusion. *Oral Surg. Oral Med. Oral Pathol. Oral Radiol.* **2018**, *126*, 291–297. [CrossRef] [PubMed]
64. Cannavale, R.; Matarese, G.; Isola, G.; Grassia, V.; Perillo, L. Early treatment of an ectopic premolar to prevent molar-premolar transposition. *Am. J. Orthod. Dentofacial Orthop.* **2013**, *143*, 559–569. [CrossRef] [PubMed]

65. Matarese, G.; Isola, G.; Alibrandi, A.; Lo Gullo, A.; Bagnato, G.; Cordasco, G.; Perillo, L. Occlusal and MRI characterizations in systemic sclerosis patients: a prospective study from Southern Italian cohort. *Joint. Bone. Spine.* **2016**, *83*, 57–62. [CrossRef] [PubMed]
66. Isola, G.; Matarese, G.; Cordasco, G.; Rotondo, F.; Crupi, A.; Ramaglia, L. Anticoagulant therapy in patients undergoing dental interventions: a critical review of the literature and current perspectives. *Minerva Stomatol.* **2015**, *64*, 21–46. [PubMed]
67. Matarese, G.; Isola, G.; Ramaglia, L.; Dalessandri, D.; Lucchese, A.; Alibrandi, A.; Fabiano, F.; Cordasco, G. Periodontal biotype: characteristic, prevalence and dimensions related to dental malocclusion. *Minerva Stomatol.* **2016**, *65*, 231–238.
68. Bourgeois, D.; Inquimbert, C.; Ottolenghi, L.; Carrouel, F. Periodontal Pathogens as Risk Factors of Cardiovascular Diseases, Diabetes, Rheumatoid Arthritis, Cancer, and Chronic Obstructive Pulmonary Disease-Is There Cause for Consideration? *Microorganisms* **2019**, *7*, 424. [CrossRef]
69. Khan, A.A.; Alsahli, M.A.; Rahmani, A.H. Myeloperoxidase as an Active Disease Biomarker: Recent Biochemical and Pathological Perspectives. *Med. Sci.* **2018**, *6*, 33. [CrossRef]

15

Comparison of Pain Perception between Clear Aligners and Fixed Appliances

Dinis Pereira [1,2], Vanessa Machado [1,2,*], João Botelho [2], Luís Proença [3], José João Mendes [2] and Ana Sintra Delgado [1,2]

1 Orthodontics Department, CRU, CiiEM, Egas Moniz–Cooperativa de Ensino Superior, 2829-511 Almada, Portugal; adtper@gmail.com (D.P.); anasintradelgado@gmail.com (A.S.D.)
2 Clinical Research Unit (CRU), Centro de Investigação Interdisciplinar Egas Moniz (CiiEM), Instituto Universitário Egas Moniz, 2829-511 Almada, Portugal; jbotelho@egasmoniz.edu.pt (J.B.); jmendes@egasmoniz.edu.pt (J.J.M.)
3 Quantitative Methods for Health Research Unit (MQIS), CiiEM, Egas Moniz—Cooperativa de Ensino Superior, 2829-511 Almada, Portugal; lproenca@egasmoniz.edu.pt
* Correspondence: vmachado@egasmoniz.edu.pt

Featured Application: Clear aligners are associated with significantly less pain than fixed appliances during the first seven days of orthodontic treatment.

Abstract: We aimed to compare the pain discomfort levels between clear aligners and fixed appliances at multiple time points. Four electronic databases (Pubmed, Medline, CENTRAL and Scholar) were searched up to May 2020. There were no year or language restrictions. Randomized clinical trials and case–control studies comparing pain perception through pain visual analog scale (VAS) in patients treated with clear aligners and with fixed appliances were included. Risk of bias within and across studies was assessed using Cochrane tool and Newcastle–Ottawa Scale (NOS) approach. Random-effects meta-analysis were conducted. VAS score and analgesic consumption were collected. Random-effects meta-analyses were used to synthesize available data. Following the review protocol, five articles met the inclusion criteria and were included, with a total of 273 participants (177 females, 96 males). Overall, clear aligners were associated with significantly less pain than fixed appliances during the first seven days of orthodontic treatment. Patients treated with clear aligners experience less pain discomfort than those treated with fixed appliances and consume less analgesics, with SORT A recommendation.

Keywords: clear aligners; fixed appliances; pain perception; VAS (visual analog scale) scale; systematic review; meta-analysis

1. Introduction

With the increase of esthetic requirements, facial's micro and macro-esthetic and smile have become a priority for adolescents and adults [1,2]. Consequently, patients lean to more esthetic and comfortable orthodontic treatments [3].

In 1945, Kesling introduced the concept of clear aligners, that aimed to stress minor tooth movement, usually at the end of orthodontic treatment or to treat minor alignment relapse [4]. Since 1998, clear aligners have become popular and quickly the preferred orthodontic appliances for patients with high esthetic demands [5,6]. In addition, mechanical tooth movement is associated with cognitive, affective and behavioral responses [7] and periodontal mechanoreceptors and chewing muscles (as source of pain receptors) also contribute to pain experience [8,9].

Clear aligners are esthetically more appealing than fixed appliances with brackets and wires [1] and patients benefit by being able to have full access to remove clear aligners to eat and for oral hygiene. Still, patients treated with clear aligners have better periodontal health than those with fixed appliances, and they promote better compliance with oral hygiene in teenagers [10–12].

Moreover, pain experience after initial archwire placement in fixed appliances is well established, comparing multistrand stainless steel and superelastic NiTi archwires [13–20]. However, the difference in the pain perception of clear aligners compared with fixed appliances remains unclear. A recent systematic review concluded that orthodontic patients treated with Invisalign appear to feel lower levels of pain than those treated with fixed appliances during the first few days of treatment, however they were not able to synthetize the magnitude of this difference [21].

Patients choose clear aligners in hope that these appliances will have low impact on their quality of life [22]. Therefore, it becomes relevant to evaluate whether there is a difference in pain perception between fixed appliances and clear aligners. In this sense, we may contribute to a more grounded decision by the patient and the clinician.

Our main objective in this systematic review was to compare the discomfort levels between clear aligners and fixed appliances. Second, we analyzed analgesic consumption difference between the aforementioned orthodontic appliances. The review PICO research question is "Do clear aligners have less pain discomfort impact than fixed appliances treatment in orthodontic patients?", with the following statements: orthodontic patients (patients—P); clear aligners (intervention/exposure—I); fixed appliances (comparison—C); pain discomfort (outcome—O). Our null hypothesis was that clear aligners cause similar pain perception than conventional fixed appliances.

2. Materials and Methods

2.1. Subsection

The present systematic review was conducted and reported according to the preferred reporting items for systematic reviews and meta-analyses (PRISMA) guidelines for reporting studies that evaluate health care interventions [23] (in detail in Supplementary Table S1) and its extension for abstracts [24]. The protocol was previously defined and has been registered in the International Prospective Register of Systematic Reviews (PROSPERO; CRD42019124534).

2.2. Eligibility Criteria

Studies were eligible for inclusion based on the following criteria:

1 Clear aligners treatment comparing with fixed appliances and determined pain discomfort through pain visual analog scale (VAS) at multiple time points;
2 Randomized and non-randomized studies;
3 Studies in humans.

The exclusion criteria were:

1 Studies reporting results emerging from questionnaires;
2 Studies lacking control;
3 Retrospective studies;
4 In vitro and animal studies;
5 Case reports/case series;
6 Editorials, opinions, narrative reviews and technique description articles, without reported sample.

2.3. Search Strategy

A total of four electronic databases (Pubmed, Medline, CENTRAL and Google Scholar) were searched systematically until May 2020. The strategy used for the electronic search was the following:

(VAS OR visual analog scale OR VAS scale OR pain perception OR pain) AND (Invisalign OR Invisalign aligner OR clear aligner) AND (orthodontic brackets OR bracket OR fixed appliance). The reference lists of included articles and relevant reviews were manually searched. Gray literature was searched using the latter strategy in OpenGray (www.opengrey.eu).

2.4. Assessment of Validity

The eligibility of each study was assessed independently by two investigators (VM and DP), who screened the titles and/or abstracts of retrieved studies. Inclusion was dependent on the following eligibility criteria: randomized clinical trials and case–control studies who compare the discomfort level produced by fixed appliances and clear aligners at multiple time points. Final selection of studies was performed by three authors independently (VM, DP, JB) and verified by a fourth and fifth author (JJM, ASD), by reviewing the full text based on inclusion criteria above. Discussion resolved any disagreements. Non-full papers, such as conference abstracts, thesis and letters to editors, were excluded.

2.5. Data Extraction

Characteristics of the included studies and numerical data were extracted in duplicate by two authors (VM and DP) onto a predefined data extraction table: citation, publication status and year of publication, study design, setting, number of cases and characteristics of the participants (mean age, sex), VAS scores at multiple time points, type of fixed appliances and analgesic consumption. Final data were reviewed by a third author (JB).

2.6. Risk of Bias of Included Studies

Risk of bias (RoB) was performed by two independent reviewers (VM and JB). In areas of disagreements, a collective decision was obtained after a discussion between all authors to approach a consensus, with an opinion of a third reviewer (DP). RoB of RCTs was assessed with the Cochrane RoB2 tool [25]. Case–control and cohort studies were appraised with the Newcastle–Ottawa scale. "Stars" (points) were attributed for each methodologic quality criterion and each study could achieve a maximum of 8 points. Studies with 7 to 8 points (80% or more of the domains satisfactorily fulfilled) were arbitrarily considered to be of low RoB, studies with 5 to 6 stars were of medium RoB and studies with less than 5 stars were of high RoB. Disagreements between the review authors over the risk of bias in particular studies were resolved by discussion, with the involvement of a third review author (DP) where necessary.

2.7. Summary Measures & Synthesis of Results

For the conversion of median and interquartile range VAS score values to mean and standard deviations, Hozo et al. [26] procedure was used, under the assumption of normal distribution. All statistical analyses were performed in R version 3.4.1 (R Studio Team 2018, Boston, MA, USA) using a DerSimonian–Laird random-effects model [27]. All random-effects meta-analysis and forest plots were performed using 'meta' package [28].

First, pain discomfort through VAS score of clear aligners versus fixed appliances was appraised through DerSimonian–Laird (DS) random-effect analysis. Of the included studies, the percentage of analgesic consumption was also carried out, through binary random-effects analysis. Quantity I^2 was used to measure to account for homogeneity and calculated through the $\chi 2$ test. Publication bias analysis was planned to be performed if, at least, we had 10 or more studies included [29]. All tests are two-tailed with alpha set at 0.05, except for the homogeneity test whose significance level cutoff will consider to be 0.10 due to the low power of the $\chi 2$ test with a limited amount of studies.

2.8. Strength of Recommendation

The SORT (strength of recommendation taxonomy) was used to judge the strength and quality of the evidence [30]. We discussed the outcomes of the present systematic review, clinical recommendations and future necessary research.

3. Results

3.1. Study Selection

From the databases and other sources, the initial search resulted in a total of 98 record, resulting in 58 after duplicates removal. Following title and abstract screening, 23 studies were selected for full-text evaluation. Nevertheless, after full-text eligibility assessment, 18 studies were excluded (in detail in Supplementary Table S2). Therefore, the meta-analysis was performed on the basis of 5 articles. The flow chart of study selection together with reasons for exclusion is provided in Figure 1.

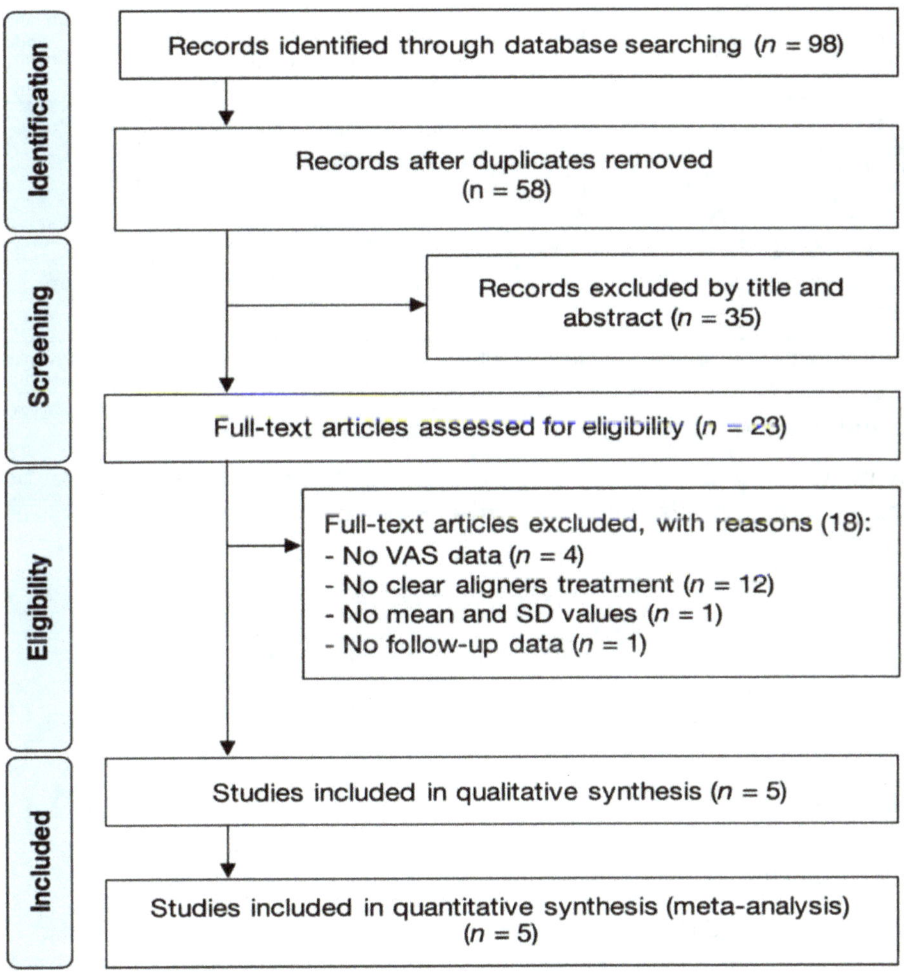

Figure 1. PRISMA (preferred reporting items for systematic reviews and meta-analyses) flowchart.

3.2. Study Characteristics

Three prospective studies evaluated the pain discomfort of clear aligners through the comparison with fixed appliances. A total of 273 participants (177 females, 96 males) were included. The characteristic of the participants is shown in Table 1.

Table 1. Included studies characteristics.

Study	Country	N (F/M)	Participants		Outcome	Funding
			CA	FA		
Miller (2007) [31]	USA	60 (43/17)	33	27	Adults treated with Invisalign aligners experienced less pain and fewer negative impacts on their lives during the first week of orthodontic treatment than did those treated with fixed appliances	NR
Shalish (2012) [32]	USA	68 (45/23)	21	47	The Invisalign patients complained of relatively high levels of pain in the first days after insertion; however this group was characterized by the lowest level of oral symptoms and by a similar level of general activity disturbances and oral dysfunction compared to the Buccal appliance.	NR
White (2017) [6]	USA	41 (24/17)	23	18	Patients treated with traditional fixed appliances reported greater discomfort and consumed more analgesics than patients treated with aligners.	Partially funded by the Robert E. Gaylord Endowed Chair in Orthodontics and by Align Technology
Almasoud (2018) [33]	Saudi Arabia	64 (42/22)	32	32	During the first week of orthodontic treatment, patients treated with Invisalign aligners reported lower pain than did those treated with passive self-ligating fixed appliances.	NR
Piergentili (2019) [34]	Italy	40 (23/17)	20	20	Therapy with traditional fixed orthodontics appliances caused more discomfort to the patients, than clear aligner therapy	NR

CA—clear aligners; FA—fixed appliances; USA—United States of America; NR—not reported.

3.3. *Risk of Bias within Studies*

One RCT was included and was assessed as having some concerns of risk of bias [6] (Figure 2). Table 2 (NOS scale scores) shows the risk of bias assessment for the included studies and all four studies were considered of low risk of bias [31–34].

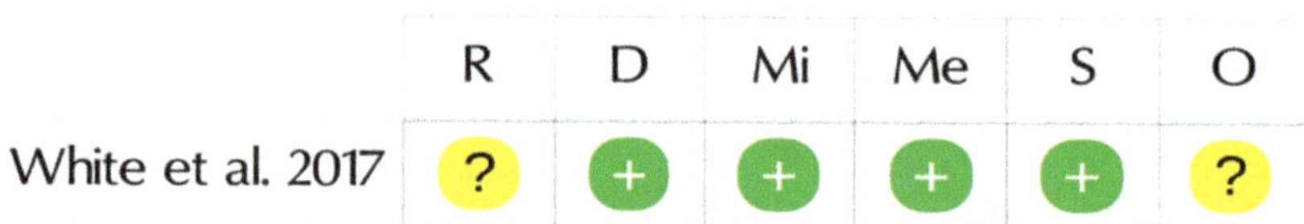

Figure 2. RoB2 assessment. R—bias arising from the randomization process; D—bias due to deviations from intended interventions; Mi—bias due to missing outcome data; Me—bias in measurement of the outcome; S—bias in selection of the reported result; O—overall risk of bias.

Table 2. NOS (Newcastle–Ottawa Scale) score for case–control studies.

	Selection				Comparability	Outcome			TOTAL	
	1	2	3	4	5	6	7	8		Score
Miller (2007) [31]	a	a	a	a	a	a	a	a	8	Low
Shalish (2012) [32]	a	a	a	a	a	a	a	a	8	Low
Almasoud (2018) [33]	c	a	a	a	a	a	a	a	7	Low
Piergentili (2019) [34]	a	a	a	a	a	a	a	a	8	Low

1-case definition adequacy; 2-representativeness of the cases; 3-selection of controls; 4-definition of controls; 5-comparability of cohorts on the basis of the design or analysis; 6-ascertainment of outcome; 7-save method of ascertainment for cases and controls; 8-nonresponse rate.

3.4. Synthesis of Results

Data from three studies including 273 patients reported pain discomfort through VAS score of clear aligners versus fixed appliances [6,31–34]. Four studies provided data on a daily basis [6,31,32,34], while one had data for pain discomfort at day 1, 3 and 7 after [33].

Clear aligners promote lower pain experience than patients using fixed appliances, and the difference is statistically significant for 1, 3, 6 and 7 days of follow-up (Table 3). The overall pain experience also favored clear aligners. Funnel plot analysis revealed no publication bias (Figure 3).

Table 3. Subgroup meta-analysis of VAS score from 1 to 7 days of follow-up.

Subgroup Meta-Analysis	n	MD	95% CI	*p*-Value	I^2 (%)	Tau	*p*-Value
Day 1	**6**	**1.07**	**(0.00; 2.13)**	**<0.001**	**84.9**	**1.16**	**<0.001**
Day 2	5	0.60	(−0.20; 1.41)	>0.05	80.7	0.77	<0.001
Day 3	**6**	**1.25**	**(0.32; 2.17)**	**<0.001**	**83.0**	**0.99**	**<0.001**
Day 4	5	0.79	(−0.07; 1.65)	>0.05	83.8	0.84	<0.001
Day 5	5	0.62	(−0.13; 1.37)	>0.05	83.7	0.71	<0.001
Day 6	**5**	**0.76**	**(0.31; 1.21)**	**<0.001**	**67.6**	**0.38**	**<0.001**
Day 7	**6**	**0.79**	**(0.37; 1.22)**	**<0.001**	**64.2**	**0.36**	**<0.001**
Overall	**6**	**0.33**	**(0.45; 1.57)**	**<0.001**	**80.5**	**0.58**	**<0.001**

Test for subgroup differences (random effects model): Q = 1.62, $p = 0.9514$. MD–Mean Difference.

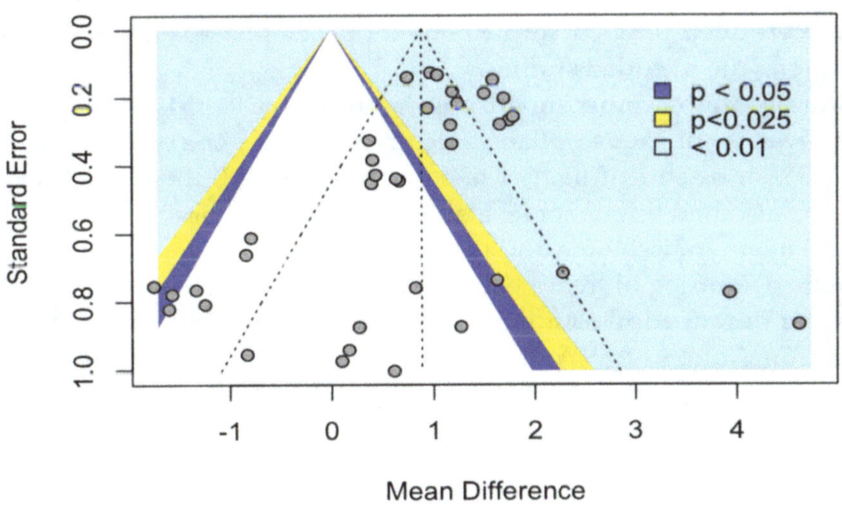

Figure 3. Funnel plot. The outer dashed lines indicate the triangular region within which 95% of studies are expected to lie in the absence of both biases and heterogeneity (fixed effect summary log odds ratio ± 1.96 × standard error of summary log odds ratio). The dashed vertical line corresponds to no intervention effect. The distribution gives a clear visual impression of symmetry, which is confirmed by a $p > 0.05$.

A detailed number of analgesic consumption at day 1, 3 and 7 after, were reported in three studies [6,31,33]. Overall, patients treated with clear aligners have significantly less analgesic consumption compared with fixed appliances group control, one day and seven days after treatment beginning (Table 4). Overall, patients with fixed appliances consume more analgesics at the beginning of treatment.

Table 4. Subgroup meta-analysis of Analgesic consumption at 1, 3 and 7 days of follow-up.

Subgroup Meta-Analysis	n	OR	95% CI	p-Value	I^2 (%)	Tau	p-Value
Day 1	3	0.15	(0.04; 0.50)	<0.001	84.9	49.3	0.14
Day 3	3	0.75	(0.11; 5.10)	<0.001	83.0	81.0	<0.001
Day 7	3	0.23	(0.52; 0.99)	<0.001	64.2	0.0	0.79
Overall	3	0.30	(0.12; 0.72)	<0.001	80.5	58.8	0.01

Test for subgroup differences (random effects model): Q = 1.97, p = 0.3734. OR–Odds Ratio.

3.5. Synthesis of Results

According to the SORT recommendation, the evidence revealed that clear aligners produce less pain experience than fixed appliances, based on consistent findings of at least two good-quality meta-analyses that obtained significant results (SORT A) [30].

4. Discussion

4.1. Summary of Main Findings

This systematic review demonstrate that clear aligners are significantly associated with less pain rather than fixed appliances during the first week of orthodontic treatment, with an overall SORT A recommendation. Clear aligners patients present less risk of analgesics consumption compared to patients with fixed appliances and present significant differences.

4.2. Quality of the Evidence, Limitations and Potential Biases in the Review Process

The strengths of this systematic review include the extensive unrestrictive literature search, with a rigorous and predetermined protocol implemented in each phase. However, there are limitations worth to mention among the included studies.

The included investigations were of small samples, and one of them lack sample size calculation [31]. As well, there are a diversity of fixed appliances description since one did not refer the type of buccal fixed appliances [31], one used self-ligated fixed appliance [33], three used a twin-bracket fixed appliance [6], and one also had lingual brackets [32,34]. Though passive self-ligating systems result in minor periodontal ligament ischemia and therefore less discomfort [35], literature evidences that pain experience in the beginning of treatment is independent of bracket type [36–38]. The type and size of archwires were described in four studies [6], though they differed in type and size among them, which is also a limitation worth mentioning. Nevertheless, previous studies have found no significant differences in the pain perception using different archwires types [36,39,40]. Furthermore, Piergentilli et al. [33] have placed the fixed appliance exclusively in the maxillary arch during the first week of treatment, and this may explain also the observed heterogeneity.

Moreover, only one study [6] performed random selection, while the remaining four [31–34] did not randomly assigned the treatment modalities due to their cohort design nature. However, randomizing adult patients is not simple, since some of whom are unwilling or unable to comply with the random assignment due to esthetic reasons [32]. This difficulty limits the ability to completely randomize the study. The fact that the patient has a choice demonstrates personality traits, which can impair the perception of pain. Notwithstanding, the RCT included in this review [33] lacked allocation concealment contributing to the overall concern on the risk of bias [33]. Allocation concealment is predictably difficult to achieve in this type of studies in which the intervention is a removable appliance and its control a fixed appliance.

Additionally, pain experience is a notoriously subjective response and there is a nonlinear relationship upon multiple factors such as age, gender, individual pain threshold, the magnitude of the force applied, present emotional state and stress, cultural differences and previous pain experiences [14,17,19,41–44]. A hypothetical limitation would be the fact that there is an unbalanced gender ratio. However, gender has no significant effect on orthodontic pain perception [14,17,19,45], except in adolescents, where females have less pain tolerance than males [46,47].

Finally, placing attachments at the beginning of the clear aligner treatment is relevant for pain perception because they cause more pressure during the insertion of the aligner. Among the included studies, Miller et al. [31] did not place attachments, two studies used attachments since they placed the first aligners [6] and Almasoud [33] delayed the attachments placement until the third set of aligners. Despite Shalish et al. [33] did not refer the placement of attachments, patients with clear aligners reported more pain than those using buccal fixed appliances, and alike those using lingual fixed appliances patients. The reason to this pain experience difference could be a greater mechanical force caused by the attachment placement, though they should be investigated deeply in the future. In addition, the importance of the periodontal mechanoreceptors and chewing muscles during clear aligners tooth movement is a matter to be further investigated.

5. Conclusions

Within the limitations of this systematic review, the results show that patients treated with clear aligners experience less pain and discomfort than patients treated with fixed appliances. This information may clarify patients about what to expect during the beginning of orthodontic treatment. In the future, larger randomized clinical trials are needed to demonstrate unequivocally that clear aligners are more comfortable than fixed appliances throughout orthodontics treatment.

Implications for Clinical Practice and Research

These findings may help both patients and clinicians in the treatment modality decision, concerning pain parameters and analgesic consultation, in the first phase of orthodontic treatment.

In the main, randomized clinical trials are needed to perform a robust comparison of clear aligners and buccal fixed appliances. Aspects concerning long-term outcomes appraisal, objective measurements of patient-centered reported outcomes (such as quality of life) and adverse effects (including allergies, periodontal damages and functional impairment) are important factors to consider.

Additionally, the present review encompassed mainly Invisalign® aligners. Future research should be conducted in different clear aligners systems, to find out if exists significant differences between different types of clear aligners systems in pain perception and analgesic drugs intake.

Author Contributions: Conceptualization, D.P., V.M., J.B., L.P., J.J.M., A.S.D.; methodology, V.M. and J.B.; software, V.M. and J.B.; validation D.P., V.M. and J.B.; formal analysis, J.B.; data curation, D.P., V.M. and J.B. All authors have read and agreed to the published version of the manuscript.

References

1. Ziuchkovski, J.P.; Fields, H.W.; Johnston, W.M.; Lindsey, D.T. Assessment of perceived orthodontic appliance attractiveness. *Am. J. Orthod. Dentofac. Orthop.* **2008**, *133*, 68–78. [CrossRef] [PubMed]
2. Sarver, D.M. Interactions of hard tissues, soft tissues, and growth over time, and their impact on orthodontic diagnosis and treatment planning. *Am. J. Orthod. Dentofac. Orthop.* **2015**, *148*, 380–386. [CrossRef]
3. Rosvall, M.D.; Fields, H.W.; Ziuchkovski, J.; Rosenstiel, S.F.; Johnston, W.M. Attractiveness, acceptability, and value of orthodontic appliances. *Am. J. Orthod. Dentofac. Orthop.* **2009**, *135*, e1–e276. [CrossRef]
4. Kesling, H.D. The philosophy of the tooth positioning appliance. *Am. J. Orthod. Oral Surg.* **1945**, *31*, 297–304. [CrossRef]
5. Wong, B.H.; Scholz, R.P.; Turpin, D.L. Invisalign A to Z. *Am. J. Orthod. Dentofac. Orthop.* **2002**, *121*, 540–541. [CrossRef]
6. White, D.W.; Julien, K.C.; Jacob, H.; Campbell, P.M.; Buschang, P.H. Discomfort associated with Invisalign and traditional brackets: A randomized, prospective trial. *Angle Orthod.* **2017**, *87*, 801–808. [CrossRef]
7. Giddon, D.B.; Anderson, N.K.; Will, L.A. Cognitive, Affective, and Behavioral Responses Associated with Mechanical Tooth Movement. *Semin. Orthod.* **2007**, *13*, 212–219. [CrossRef]

8. Piancino, M.G.; Isola, G.; Cannavale, R.; Cutroneo, G.; Vermiglio, G.; Bracco, P.; Anastasi, G.P. From periodontal mechanoreceptors to chewing motor control: A systematic review. *Arch. Oral Biol.* **2017**, *78*, 109–121. [CrossRef]
9. Isola, G.; Anastasi, G.P.; Matarese, G.; Williams, R.C.; Cutroneo, G.; Bracco, P.; Piancino, M.G. Functional and molecular outcomes of the human masticatory muscles. *Oral Dis.* **2018**, *24*, 1428–1441. [CrossRef]
10. Abbate, G.M.; Caria, M.P.; Montanari, P.; Mannu, C.; Orrù, G.; Caprioglio, A.; Levrini, L. Parodontale Gesundheit von Teenagern mit herausnehmbaren Alignern und festsitzenden kieferorthopädischen Apparaturen. *J. Orofac. Orthop.* **2015**, *76*, 240–250. [CrossRef]
11. Azaripour, A.; Weusmann, J.; Mahmoodi, B.; Peppas, D.; Gerhold-Ay, A.; Van Noorden, C.J.F.; Willershausen, B. Braces versus Invisalign®: Gingival parameters and patients' satisfaction during treatment: A cross-sectional study. *BMC Oral Health* **2015**, *15*, 1–5. [CrossRef] [PubMed]
12. Lu, H.; Tang, H.; Zhou, T.; Kang, N. Assessment of the periodontal health status in patients undergoing orthodontic treatment with fixed appliances and Invisalign system. *Medicine* **2018**, *97*, e0248. [CrossRef] [PubMed]
13. Wang, Y.; Liu, C.; Jian, F.; Mcintyre, G.T.; Millett, D.T.; Hickman, J.; Lai, W. Initial arch wires used in orthodontic treatment with fixed appliances. *Cochrane Database Syst. Rev.* **2018**, *7*. [CrossRef] [PubMed]
14. Wilson, S.; Ngan, P.; Kess, B. Time course of the discomfort in young patients undergoing orthodontic treatment. *Pediatr. Dent.* **1989**, *11*, 107–110. [PubMed]
15. Jones, M.; Chan, C. The pain and discomfort experienced during orthodntic treatment: A randomized controlled clinical trial of two intial aligning arch wires. *Am. J. Orthod. Dentofac. Orthop.* **1992**, *102*, 373–381. [CrossRef]
16. Ngan, P.; Kess, B.; Wilson, S. Perception of discomfort by patients undergoing orthodontic treatment. *Am. J. Orthod. Dentofac. Orthop.* **1989**, *96*, 47–53. [CrossRef]
17. Scheurer, P.A.; Firestone, A.R.; Bürgin, W.B. Perception of pain as a result of orthodontic treatment with fixed appliances. *Eur. J. Orthod.* **1996**, *18*, 349–357. [CrossRef]
18. Stewart, F.N.; Kerr, W.J.S.; Taylor, P.J.S. Appliance wear: The patient's point of view. *Eur. J. Orthod.* **1997**, *19*, 377–382. [CrossRef]
19. Krishnan, V.; Davidovitch, Z. Cellular, molecular, and tissue-level reactions to orthodontic force. *Am. J. Orthod. Dentofac. Orthop.* **2006**, *129*, e1–e469. [CrossRef]
20. Grieve, W.G.; Johnson, G.K.; Moore, R.N.; Reinhardt, R.A.; DuBois, L.M. Prostaglandin E (PGE) and interleukin-1β (IL-1β) levels in gingival crevicular fluid during human orthodontic tooth movement. *Am. J. Orthod. Dentofac. Orthop.* **1994**, *105*, 369–374. [CrossRef]
21. Cardoso, P.C.; Espinosa, D.G.; Mecenas, P.; Flores-Mir, C.; Normando, D. Pain level between clear aligners and fixed appliances: A systematic review. *Prog. Orthod.* **2020**, *21*, 3. [CrossRef]
22. Flores-Mir, C.; Brandelli, J.; Pacheco-Pereira, C. Patient satisfaction and quality of life status after 2 treatment modalities: Invisalign and conventional fixed appliances. *Am. J. Orthod. Dentofac. Orthop.* **2018**, *154*, 639–644. [CrossRef] [PubMed]
23. Liberati, A.; Altman, D.G.; Tetzlaff, J.; Mulrow, C.; Gøtzsche, P.C.; Ioannidis, J.P.A.; Clarke, M.; Devereaux, P.J.; Kleijnen, J.; Moher, D. The PRISMA statement for reporting systematic reviews and meta-analyses of studies that evaluate health care interventions: Explanation and elaboration. *PLoS Med.* **2009**, *6*, e1000100. [CrossRef] [PubMed]
24. Beller, E.M.; Glasziou, P.P.; Altman, D.G.; Hopewell, S.; Bastian, H.; Chalmers, I.; Gøtzsche, P.C.; Lasserson, T.; Tovey, D. PRISMA for Abstracts: Reporting Systematic Reviews in Journal and Conference Abstracts. *PLoS Med.* **2013**, *10*, e1001419. [CrossRef]
25. Sterne, J.A.C.; Savović, J.; Page, M.J.; Elbers, R.G.; Blencowe, N.S.; Boutron, I.; Cates, C.J.; Cheng, H.Y.; Corbett, M.S.; Eldridge, S.M.; et al. RoB 2: A revised tool for assessing risk of bias in randomised trials. *BMJ* **2019**, *366*, 1–8. [CrossRef] [PubMed]
26. Hozo, S.P.; Djulbegoviç, B.; Hozo, I. Estimating the mean and variance from the median, range, and the size of a sample. *BMC Med. Res. Methodol.* **2005**, *5*, 1–10. [CrossRef]
27. Schwarzer, G.; Carpenter, J.R.; Rücker, G. *Meta-Analysis with R*; Springer: Berlin/Heidelberg, Germany, 2015, ISBN 9783319214153.
28. Schwarzer, G. Meta: An R Package for Meta-Analysis. *R News* **2007**, *7*, 40–45.

29. Higgins, J.; Green, S. Cochrane Handbook for Systematic Reviews of Interventions; 5.1.0 (updated March 2011); The Cochrane Collaboration: 2011. Available online: https://www.cochrane-handbook.org (accessed on 15 April 2020).
30. Newman, M.G.; Weyant, R.; Hujoel, P. JEBDP Improves Grading System and Adopts Strength of Recommendation Taxonomy Grading (SORT) for Guidelines and Systematic Reviews. *J. Evid. Based. Dent. Pract.* **2007**, *7*, 147–150. [CrossRef]
31. Miller, K.B.; McGorray, S.P.; Womack, R.; Quintero, J.C.; Perelmuter, M.; Gibson, J.; Dolan, T.A.; Wheeler, T.T. A comparison of treatment impacts between Invisalign aligner and fixed appliance therapy during the first week of treatment. *Am. J. Orthod. Dentofac. Orthop.* **2007**, *131*, e1–e302. [CrossRef]
32. Shalish, M.; Cooper-Kazaz, R.; Ivgi, I.; Canetti, L.; Tsur, B.; Bachar, E.; Chaushu, S. Adult patients' adjustability to orthodontic appliances. Part I: A comparison between Labial, Lingual, and Invisalign™. *Eur. J. Orthod.* **2012**, *34*, 724–730. [CrossRef]
33. Almasoud, N.N. Pain perception among patients treated with passive self-ligating fixed appliances and invisalign®aligners during the first week of orthodontic treatment. *Korean J. Orthod.* **2018**, *48*, 326–332. [CrossRef] [PubMed]
34. Piergentili, M.; Bucci, R.; Madariaga, A.C.P.; Martina, S.; Rongo, R.; D'Antò, V. Pain and discomfort associated with labial multibracket appliances vs clear aligners. *J. Aligner Orthod.* **2019**, *3*, 205–212.
35. Wright, N.; Modarai, F.; Cobourne, M.T.; DiBiase, A.T. Do you do Damon ®? What is the current evidence base underlying the philosophy of this appliance system? *J. Orthod.* **2011**, *38*, 222–230. [CrossRef] [PubMed]
36. Fleming, P.S.; DiBiase, A.T.; Sarri, G.; Lee, R.T. Pain experience during initial alignment with a self-ligating and a conventional fixed orthodontic appliance system. *Angle Orthod.* **2009**, *79*, 46–50. [CrossRef]
37. Fleming, P.S.; Johal, A. Self-ligating brackets in orthodontics a systematic review. *Angle Orthod.* **2010**, *80*, 575–584. [CrossRef] [PubMed]
38. Miles, P.G.; Weyant, R.J.; Rustveld, L. A clinical trial of damon 2™ Vs conventional twin brackets during initial alignment. *Angle Orthod.* **2006**, *76*, 480–485.
39. Rahman, S.; Spencer, R.J.; Littlewood, S.J.; O'Dywer, L.; Barber, S.K.; Russell, J.S. A multicenter randomized controlled trial to compare a self-ligating bracket with a conventional bracket in a UK population: Part 2: Pain perception. *Angle Orthod.* **2016**, *86*, 149–156. [CrossRef]
40. Scott, P.; Sherriff, M.; DiBiase, A.T.; Cobourne, M.T. Perception of discomfort during initial orthodontic tooth alignment using a self-ligating or conventional bracket system: A randomized clinical trial. *Eur. J. Orthod.* **2008**, *30*, 227–232. [CrossRef]
41. Bergius, M.; Kiliaridis, S.; Berggren, U. Pain in orthodontics. A review and discussion of the literature. *J. Orofac. Orthop.* **2000**, *61*, 125–137. [CrossRef]
42. Firestone, A.R.; Scheurer, P.A.; Bürgin, W.B. Patients' anticipation of pain and pain-related side effects, and their perception of pain as a result of orthodontic treatment with fixed appliances. *Eur. J. Orthod.* **1999**, *21*, 387–396. [CrossRef]
43. Brown, D.F.; Moerenhout, R.G. The pain experience and psychological adjustment to orthodontic treatment of preadolescents, adolescents, and adults. *Am. J. Orthod. Dentofac. Orthop.* **1991**, *100*, 349–356. [CrossRef]
44. Chow, J.; Cioffi, I. Pain and orthodontic patient compliance: A clinical perspective. *Semin. Orthod.* **2018**, *24*, 242–247. [CrossRef]
45. Erdinç, A.; Dinçer, B. Perception of pain during orthodontic treatment with fixed appliances. *Eur. J. Orthod.* **2004**, *26*, 79–85. [CrossRef] [PubMed]
46. Sandhu, S.S.; Sandhu, J. Orthodontic pain: An interaction between age and sex in early and middle adolescence. *Angle Orthod.* **2013**, *83*, 966–972. [CrossRef] [PubMed]
47. Alhaija, E.S.A.; AlDaikki, A.; Al-Omairi, M.K.; Al-Khateeb, S.N. The relationship between personality traits, pain perception and attitude toward orthodontic treatment. *Angle Orthod.* **2010**, *80*, 1141–1149. [CrossRef]

16

The Oral Microbiome in Children with Black Stained Tooth

Ji Young Hwang [1], Hyo-Seol Lee [2], Jaehyuk Choi [3], Ok Hyung Nam [2], Mi Sun Kim [2,4] and Sung Chul Choi [2,*]

1 Department of Dentistry, Graduate School, Kyung Hee University, Seoul 02447, Korea; berryry@hanmail.com
2 Department of Pediatric Dentistry, School of Dentistry, Kyung Hee University, Seoul 02447, Korea; stberryfield@gmail.com (H.-S.L.); pedokhyung@khu.ac.kr (O.H.N.); pedokms@khu.ac.kr (M.S.K.)
3 Division of Life Sciences, College of Life Sciences and Bioengineering, Incheon National University, Incheon 22012, Korea; jaehyukc@inu.ac.kr
4 Department of Pediatric Dentistry, Kyung Hee University Hospital at Gangdong, Seoul 02447, Korea
* Correspondence: pedochoi@khu.ac.kr

Abstract: Black stain (BS) is a characteristic extrinsic discoloration, which occurs along the third cervical line of the buccal and/or lingual surfaces of teeth, particularly in the primary dentition of humans. BS is produced by oral bacteria and byproducts of saliva, but there is a controversy about related bacteria. The aim of this study was to identify the oral microbiome in tooth BS using pyrosequencing. It was hypothesized that the oral microbiome of BS in children might be related to black-pigment producing bacteria. Supragingival dental plaque was obtained from six children (mean 8.1 years) with BS and four children (mean 8.3 years) without BS. The bacterial metagenome was obtained by pyrosequencing. The BS group contained 348 operative taxonomic units (OTUs), whereas the control group had 293 OTUs. Microbial abundance and diversity were significantly higher in the BS group ($p < 0.05$). In the heatmap, the correlation between samples was the same as the BS scale. At the genus level, six genera—*Abiotrophia, Eikenella, Granulicatella, Neisseria, Porphyromonas* and *Streptococcus*—were significantly different between the two groups ($p < 0.05$). We suggested that compositional changes in the oral microbiome are essential, and several species in the genus *Neisseria, Porphyromonas* and *Streptococcus* may be major contributors for BS formation. Although the number of subjects was relatively limited, our study is the first species-level analysis of pyrosequencing data in BS formation.

Keywords: black stain; oral microbiota; pyrosequencing; *Neisseria*; *Porphyromonas*; *Streptococcus*

1. Introduction

Black stain (BS) is a characteristic, extrinsic dental discoloration that occurs on the cervical third of the tooth and follows the contour of the gingival margin, particularly in primary dentition [1]. BS is thought to be a special form of dental plaque related to calcification because it contains an insoluble ferric salt, which is likely ferric sulfide, and has high calcium and phosphate contents [2]. The ferric sulfide may be formed through a reaction between hydrogen sulfide produced by bacterial action and iron in saliva or gingival exudates.

BS occurs at any age, but there is a higher prevalence in childhood that decreases in adolescence and adulthood [3]. Studies have shown no difference in occurrence between the sexes [1]. Researchers have been interested in BS because of its correlation with the low caries experience [2,4]. However, a recent study of more than 3000 people found no association between dental caries and BS [5].

Many studies have examined BS-related bacteria, but the causative bacteria is still not clear [1,3]. Early ultrastructural examinations of BS demonstrated that the black material is a ferric salt, probably ferric sulfide, formed by the reaction between sulfide produced by bacterial action and iron in the saliva or gingival exudate [2,3]. The most commonly cultivated bacteria from BS teeth were *Actinomycetes* with the detection of rarely pigmented Gram-negative rods [6]. Black-pigmented bacteria were found primarily in extrinsic tooth stains [6,7]. Among black-pigmented bacteria, *Prevotella intermedia* and *Prevotella nigrescens* are the ones most frequently found in the oral cavity and associated with BS [3]. Soukos et al. [6] reported that *Porphyromonas gingivalis*, *P. intermedia* and *P. nigrescens* were related to BS using DNA–DNA hybridization for 40 taxa, whereas Saba et al. [7] suggested that *P. gingivalis* and *Prevotella melaninogenica* were absent and *Actinomycetes* sp. and *Aggregatibacter actinomycetemcomitans* were present in BS by means of polymerase chain reaction (PCR) and electrophoresis gel on the agarose medium for 200 people. This conflict was partly caused by limitations in the analysis methods. As a result, more advanced analysis methods are needed.

Recent advances in sequencing technologies, such as 454 pyrosequencing, have provided a deep understanding of the metagenomic diversity of the human oral microbiome [8]. Pyrosequencing can identify bacterial sequences and their amounts to give both qualitative and quantitative information of the oral microbiome, including uncultivable microorganisms [8]. For example, high-throughput pyrosequencing has revealed that dental plaques pooled from adults contain approximately 10,000 microbial phylotypes, with the ultimate diversity of oral microbiomes being estimated to contain approximately 25,000 phylotypes [9].

The aim of this study was to identify the oral microbiome in BS using pyrosequencing and to test our hypothesis that the oral microbiome of BS in children might be related to black-pigmented bacteria.

2. Material and Methods

2.1. Sampling

This study was approved by the Institutional Review Board of the School of Dentistry, Kyung Hee University (KHD-IRB-1509-5). Ten children were recruited as study subjects. Six of the children had black stained teeth while four children maintained good oral hygiene and had no black stained teeth. Oral examinations were performed on all the children, and decayed-missing-filled teeth (DMFT) indices were estimated. The BS scale was estimated using the Shourie method [10]. The criteria for classifying BS were as follows: 1; no line, 2; incomplete coalescence of pigmented spots and 3; continuous line formed by pigmented spots. After classification, subjects with parental consent were instructed not to brush their teeth for 24 h before sampling. Sampling was performed in the morning from the subjects, who were instructed to skip breakfast. Sterilized dental explorers were used to collect supragingival plaque on the buccal and lingual surfaces of all teeth. The samples were collected in 1 mL of sterile phosphate-buffered saline and stored at −80 °C after liquid nitrogen treatment.

2.2. Genomic DNA Extraction

The following molecular and sequencing procedures were performed in an outside outsourcing research laboratory. Genomic DNA (gDNA) was isolated from the dental plaque samples using a DNA extraction kit for bacteria (iNtRON Biotechnology, Seongnam, Korea) following the manufacturer's protocol. The collected samples were treated with lysozyme at 37 °C for 15 min and lysed with a buffer containing proteinase K and RNase A at 65 °C for 15 min. The lysates were mixed with a binding buffer and then passed through resin columns for purification. The harvested g DNA from the samples was quantified using a NanoDrop ND-1000 spectrophotometer (Thermo Scientific, Waltham, MA, USA).

2.3. PCR Amplification

PCR was performed to amplify the V1 to V3 region of the 16S rRNA gene from the samples' gDNA. 9F (5′-AGAGTTTGATCMTGGCTCAG-3′) and 541R (5′-ATTACCGCGGCTGCTGG-3′) primers were used in the amplification. The amplifications were carried out under the following conditions: initial denaturation at 94 °C for 5 min, followed by 30 cycles of denaturation at 94 °C for 30 s, primer annealing at 55 °C for 30 s and extension at 72 °C for 30 s with a final extension phase at 72 °C for 5 min. The PCR products were visualized under a Gel Doc system (BioRad, Hercules, CA, USA) after electrophoresis on a 2% agarose gel. The amplified products were cleaned with the QIAquick PCR purification kit (Qiagen, Valencia, CA, USA).

2.4. DNA Pyrosequencing

Equal concentrations of the PCR products were pooled together and cleaned with Agencourt Amperes magnetic purification beads (Danvers, MA, USA). The quality and size of the pooled products were assessed on an Agilent Bioanalyzer 2100 (Palo Alto, CA, USA) using a DNA 7500 chip. The pooled products were used for emulsion PCR and then loaded onto Picotiter plates for high-throughput pyrosequencing. The sequencing was performed on the GS FLX Plus system (Roche, Branford, CT, USA) according to the manufacturer's instructions at ChunLab, Inc. (Seoul, Korea).

2.5. Pyrosequencing Data Analysis

Obtained raw data were categorized into samples according to the barcode information. The barcode, linker and primers were trimmed off from the reads and reads showing ambiguous nucleotides (2≤), a low-quality score (<25) or a short length (<300 bp) were removed. Potential chimera sequences detected by the Bellerophon method were filtered. The final reads were compared with sequence and taxonomic information acquired from the EzTaxon-e database. This database has curated 16S rRNA gene sequences of species and phylotypes of either cultured or uncultured entries in the GenBank database with taxonomy information. The read sequences were queried with BLASTN, and a maximum of five best-hit sequences were compared by pairwise alignment to determine species or phylotypes. Operational taxonomic units (OTUs) were obtained at a 97% similarity level by the CL community program (ChunLab, Inc., Seoul, Korea) after comparing with the EZ taxon database. Alpha diversity was determined using the "phyloseq" R package. A heatmap analysis was performed based on microbial abundance in the "heatplus" R package. Principal component analysis (PCA) was performed using "devtools" and "ggbiplot" R packages.

2.6. Statistical Analysis

In clinical findings, dmft indices between the BS and control groups were statistically analyzed by Mann–Whitney test ($p = 0.05$), and the association between BS formation and caries development were statistically analyzed by Chi-squared test ($p = 0.05$). After the pyrosequencing, the diversity of the oral microbiome of the subjects was statistically analyzed by the t-test ($p = 0.05$). In the heatmap, the Bray–Curtis method was used for calculating cluster dissimilarity in the clustering analysis ($p = 0.05$). The abundance of the predominant bacterial groups was analyzed by t-test ($p = 0.05$). Jonckheere's trend test was used for the trend analysis ($p = 0.05$).

3. Results

3.1. Clinical Findings

Children with BS (BS group, n = 6) whose ages ranged from 4 to 11 (mean of 8.1 years) were included in this study. The control (non-BS) group (n = 4) had a mean age of 8.3 (range 6–9) years. The BS group exhibited a mean BS score of 1.5 (BS scale 1 = 3 and BS scale 2 = 3), zero DMFT index and a 3.8 average dmft index. By contrast, four control patients showed zero BS scale, zero DMFT index and a 1.75 average dmft index. The dmft indices between the BS and control groups were not significantly different ($p > 0.05$). No significant association between BS formation and caries development was observed ($p > 0.05$).

3.2. Diversity of the Oral Microbiome

A total of 10 samples were sequenced, and 60,371 reads in total were obtained. Of all the reads, 39,013 reads (64.6%) passed quality filtering (low-quality sequence reads and a minimum length of 300 bp) and remained. Both the BS and control groups contained 28,142 and 10,871 reads with an average length of 472 and 465 bp, respectively (Supplementary Table S1). The microbial abundance based on the read number was significantly higher in the BS group than the control group (Figure 1A, $p < 0.05$). OTUs were identified by pairwise alignment to the EzTaxon database at a 3% distance. Totals of 15 phyla, 28 classes, 45 orders, 80 families, 145 genera and 423 OTUs (species) were identified in these samples. The BS group contained 348 OTUs in total (without duplication), whereas the control group had 293 OTUs. The alpha diversity of the microbiome was estimated by Simpson and Shannon indices, indicating that the diversity in the BS group was significantly higher than in the control group (Figure 1B,C, $p < 0.05$).

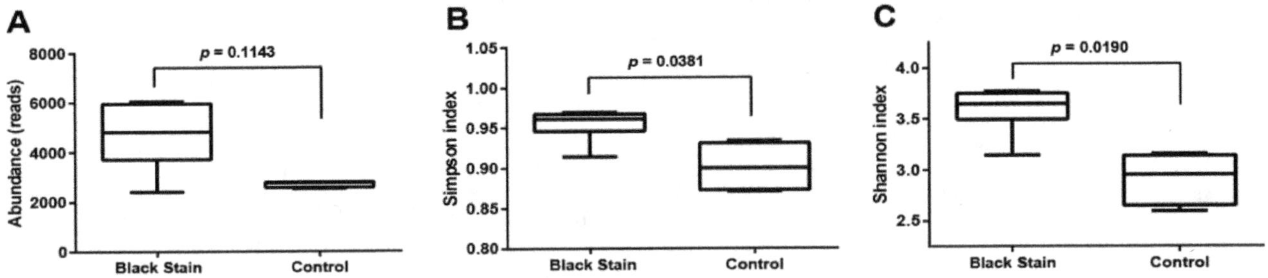

Figure 1. Diversity of the oral microbiome of the subjects. Abundance (**A**), Simpson index (**B**) and Shannon index (**C**) were compared between the black stain and control groups. Significance was determined by *t*-test ($p = 0.05$).

3.3. Different Genera and Species between BS and Control Group

Heatmap analysis was employed to see overall patterns of microbial abundance at different levels of taxonomy. At all levels from species to order, the control group was isolated from the BS group (Figure 2), suggesting that the microbial composition was quite different between the two groups. The only exception was the sample "C12", which formed its own lineage within the BS group. Since the diversity pattern of C12 was much different from the other samples in the control group, we excluded the sample from further statistical analysis. To test the hypothesis that changes in microbial diversity affected BS formation, the abundance (read number) of each OTU was compared between the groups using the Mann–Whitney U test. At the genus level, six genera—*Abiotrophia, Eikenella, Granulicatella, Neisseria, Porphyromonas* and *Streptococcus*—were significantly different between the two groups ($p < 0.05$). *Neisseria, Porphyromonas* and *Streptococcus* contained 11, 14 and 31 species within them, respectively (Figure 3). All six genera were more abundant in the BS group than the control group. In addition, the genus *Selenomonas* exhibited the opposite trend and was more abundant in the control group ($p = 0.053$). At the species level, 19 species were identified as significantly different between the two groups ($p < 0.05$, Table 1). The number of each sample represented the identified OTUs. Except for *Selenomonas noxia, Corynebacterium_uc* and *JQ454562_s* (*Prevotella*), all the species were higher in the BS group than the control group. Twelve out of 19 species were included in the genus showing significance.

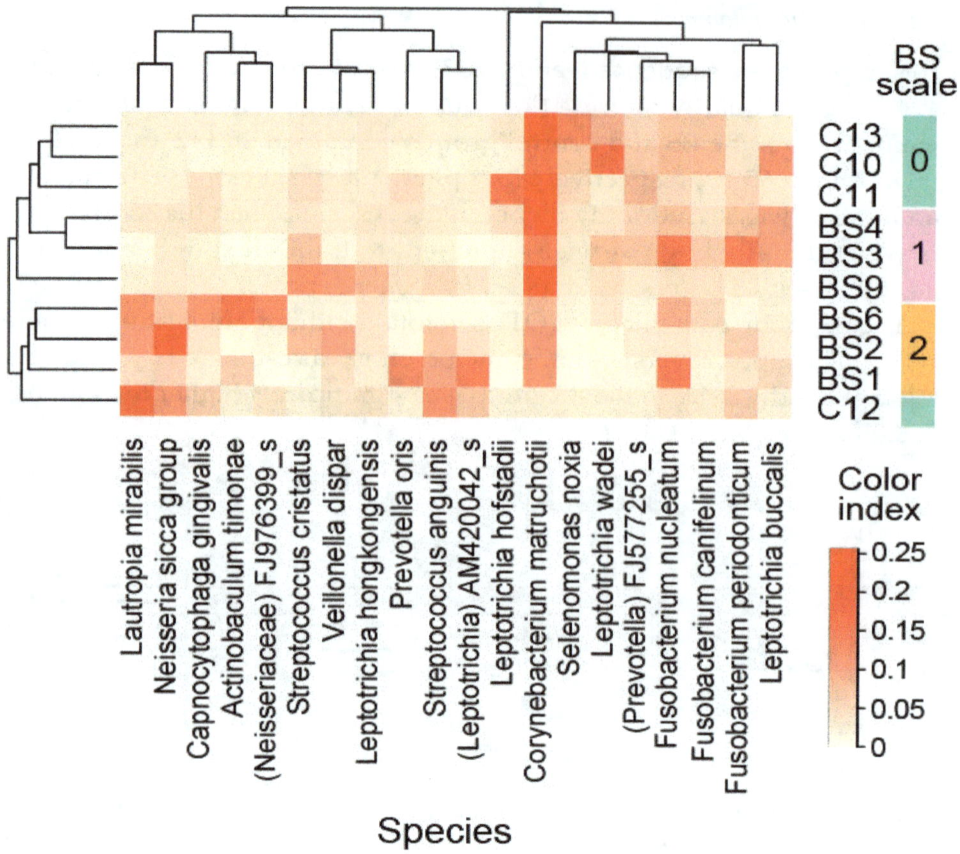

Figure 2. Heatmap of the oral microbiome relative abundance. The species having more than 5% of the total reads are shown. The Bray–Curtis method was used for calculating cluster dissimilarity in the clustering analysis ($p = 0.05$, significantly different). B: black stain group, C: control group.

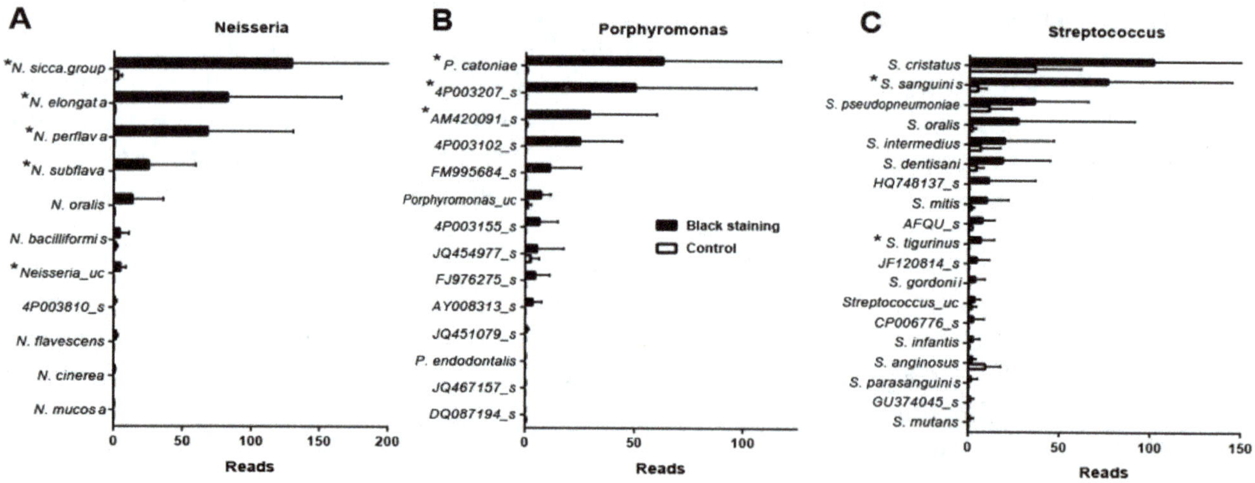

Figure 3. Abundance of the predominant bacterial groups between the black staining and control groups. Genus *Neisseria* (**A**), genus *Porphyromonas* (**B**), *Streptococcus* (**C**). Asterisks indicate species significantly different between the two groups ($p < 0.05$).

Table 1. Species showing a significant difference between the black stain and control groups ($p < 0.05$). The number of each sample representing the identified operative taxonomic units (OTUs).

Taxonomy		Black Stain Group							Control Group				p Value
Genus	**Species**	**B1**	**B2**	**B6**	**B3**	**B4**	**B9**	**Ave.**	**C10**	**C11**	**C13**	**Ave.**	
Abiotrophia	*Ab. defectiva*	25	122	7	7	23	2	31.0	0	0	0	0.0	0.025
Actinomyces	*Ac. naeslundii*	44	14	55	53	5	16	31.2	1	1	2	1.3	0.028
Cardiobacterium	*C. hominis*	20	3	33	53	24	4	22.8	0	1	3	1.3	0.038
Eikenella	*E. corrodens*	8	19	14	21	101	3	27.7	0	1	2	1.0	0.028
Granulicatella	*G. adiacens*	10	67	22	4	33	1	22.8	0	1	1	0.7	0.049
Kingella	*JQ455165_s*	6	4	10	1	19	32	12.0	0	0	0	0.0	0.026
Leptotrichia	*L. hongkongensis*	51	55	68	36	84	143	72.8	21	18	25	21.3	0.028
Neisseria	*N. elongata*	34	97	35	70	242	16	82.3	1	0	1	0.7	0.028
Neisseria	*N. perflava*	5	21	121	121	132	6	67.7	0	0	0	0.0	0.025
Neisseria	*N. sicca group*	107	360	67	32	194	15	129.2	6	2	0	2.7	0.028
Neisseria	*N. subflava*	1	88	6	13	41	1	25.0	0	0	0	0.0	0.025
Porphyromonas	*AM420091_s*	2	33	40	84	3	10	28.7	0	1	0	0.3	0.028
Porphyromonas	*P. catoniae*	19	97	73	38	147	1	62.5	1	0	0	0.3	0.037
Porphyromonas	*4P003207_s*	6	35	99	138	16	5	49.8	0	0	0	0.0	0.026
Selenomonas_g1	*Se. noxia*	0	5	63	37	41	7	25.5	126	85	404	205.0	0.028
Streptococcus	*St. sanguinis*	195	116	43	26	13	63	76.0	3	10	1	4.7	0.028

Species where all the samples had less than 10 reads on average are not included.

3.4. *Trend Analysis among the Three BS Scale Groups*

In the heatmap at the species level, clusters based on microbial abundance were correlated to BS scale severity (Figure 2). For example, the samples "B1", "B2" and "B9", which had been determined as having "BS scale 2" severity according to Shori's method, were clustered together in similarity (Figure 2). A similar correlation was observed at all taxonomical levels, suggesting that BS scale severity may be correlated with the bacterial composition (Figure 2). Therefore, a dose-dependent relationship between the BS scale and abundance was examined using a nonparametric Jonckheere's trend test in the "clinfun" R package. A total of 47 species showed a trend among the BS scale clusters: 39 species exhibited an "increasing" trend when the BS scale increased ($p < 0.05$), whereas eight species were found to exhibit a "decreasing" tendency ($p < 0.05$). Principal component analysis (PCA) for these selected species revealed that species showing an "increasing" trend contributed to an increase in BS scale severity (Figure 4). This microbial community may play an essential role in the formation of BS. The most abundant genera were *Neisseria*, *Porphyromonas*, *Streptococcus* and *Capnocytophaga*. In contrast, the "decreasing" population, which showed abundance in the control group, consisted of *Corynebacterium*, *Prevotella*, *Selenomonas*, *Capnocytophaga* and *Leptotrichia*. Four genera were found in both groups: *Capnocytophaga*, *Corynebacterium*, *Leptotrichia* and *Prevotella*.

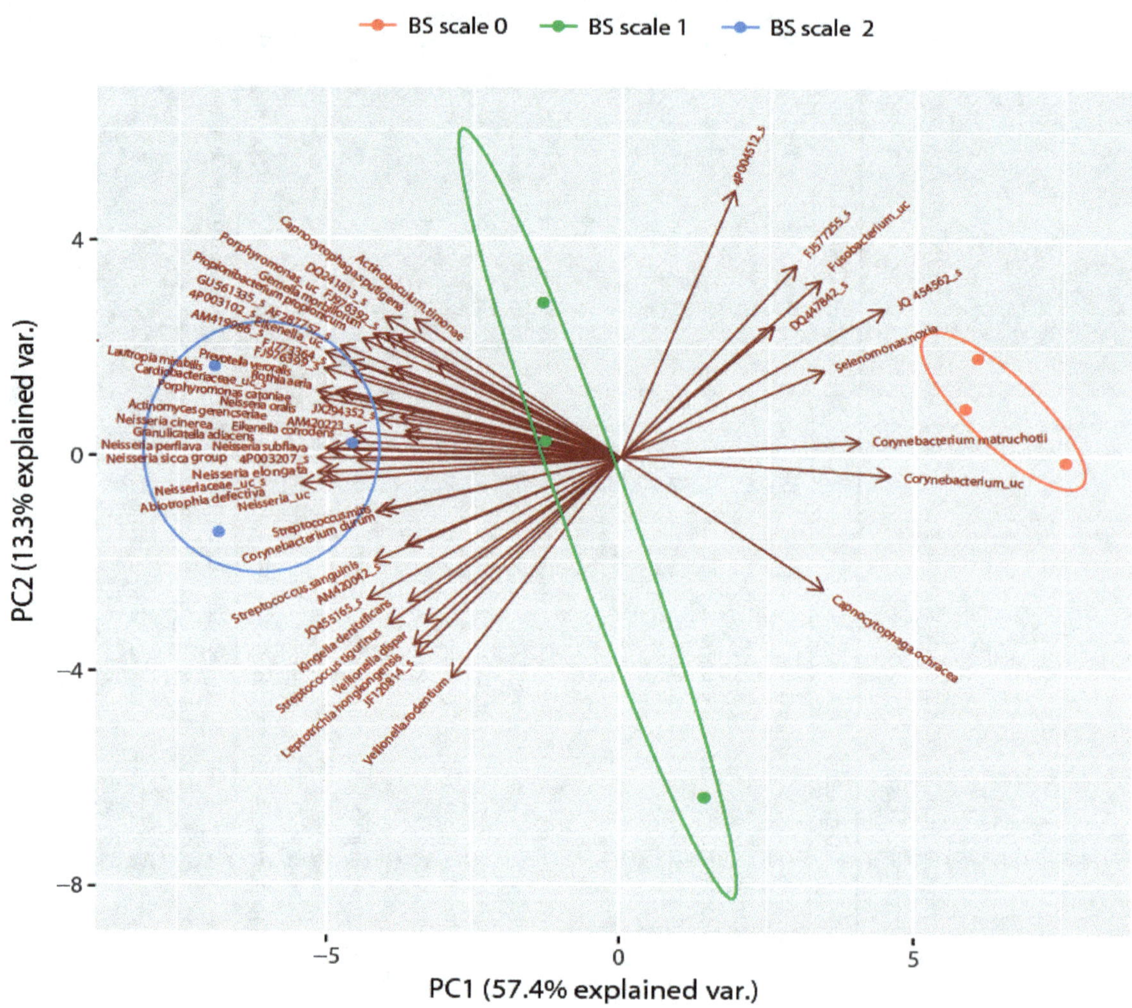

Figure 4. Principle component analysis of the selected species showing an increasing or decreasing trend according to the severity of the black stain (BS) scale. Approximately 71% of the total variance among the individual samples was explained by the first two components.

4. Discussion

Conventional BS therapy has been focused on the mechanical removal of black pigments themselves because the exact mechanism of BS prevalence had yet to be identified [1]. In this study, we used pyrosequencing analysis of supragingival dental plaque of children with and without BS to understand the microbiological aspects of BS, which may lead to better prevention and treatment for BS. The genera *Porphyromonas*, *Streptococcus* and *Neisseria*, were abundant in the microbiome of children with BS, while the genera *Corynebacterium*, *Prevotella* and *Selenomonas_g1* were abundant in children without BS in this study. This study suggests that dynamics in the oral microbiome may cause the formation of BS in children, and the microbial population in the above genera would play important roles in changing microbial dynamics.

The genus *Porphyromonas* was significantly abundant in the BS group (Figure 2). All the species belonging to this genus exhibited a similar pattern in abundance (Figure 3). Four *Porphylromonas* sp. showed a trend to increase as the BS scales increased (Figure 4). *Porphyromonas* is an obligate anaerobic bacterium that produces a black pigment called porphyrin [11]. This pigment can protect the bacterial cell from oxidative stress by reducing oxygen. *P. gingivalis* is one of the most well-known species that produces black pigments [12] and is implicated in the progression of periodontal disease [4]. However, this species was not one of the pathogens observed in this study. *Porphyromonas catoniae* is the most common species in this genus (Figure 3A). It is frequently found in the oral microbiota of healthy children [9] and is known to be a pioneer bacterium that is established in the mouths of babies [13]. In addition, it is a non-pigmented species [14]. However, it is possible that this species may play an opportunistic role in the formation of BS because this species exhibits activities of diverse cellular enzymes like trypsin, which is important in bacterial colonization [13]. The other *Porphyromonas* spp. may contribute to the accumulation of black pigments.

The genus *Streptococcus* was also observed abundantly in the BS group (Figures 2 and 3B). *S. cristatus*, *S. sanguinis*, *S. oralis*, *S. mitis* and *S. gordonii* are known as oral biofilm bacteria that colonize the tooth surface [15,16]. Since these species are normal tooth microbiome and do not produce black pigments, they may contribute to the formation of microbial beds on teeth and interact with other species producing black pigments. Although the genus *Streptococcus* makes up 10% of the total microbiome, *S. mutans* was detected in only one subject (BS2, five reads). This rare detection of *S. mutans* is consistent with a recent report of BS patients where *S. mutans* was not found. This may be due to the antagonistic effect of the predisposed *Streptococcus* spp. *S. sanguinis* and *S. gordonii* that are known to inhibit the growth of *S. mutans* by producing hydrogen peroxide [17]. A recent study using pyrosequencing suggests that the genus *Streptococcus* was most abundant but showed no difference between the groups [18]. Another pyrosequencing study reported that this genus was observed frequently in subjects having both caries and pigments, but not in subjects having only pigments [19]. Interestingly, a recent microbiome study showed that the population of *P. catoniae* was decreased in children with caries and increased in children with healthy oral status [9]. Since the *P. catoniae* population was found to be increased in our BS group, it may have a negative influence on caries development (Figure 3A).

Veillonella dispar and *V. rodentium* were identified as positive candidates for BS formation (Figure 4). *V. dispar* produces hydrogen sulfide (H_2S) from L-cysteine [20]. The genus *Actinomyces* can produce H_2S and has been known to be a strong candidate for BS formation. However, *Actinomyces gerencseriae* was detected in this study, and there is no report about the H_2S production of this species.

Microbial composition is continuously affected by the environment of the oral cavity, and each population interacts with others in the same community. Therefore, a decrease in population density may result in the breakdown of one community, presenting the opportunity for a new population or community to thrive. We hypothesized that different microbial compositions would appear in different BS scales. The BS scale indicates different environmental factors affecting microbial composition. In that hypothesis, our trend analysis exhibited positive or negative candidates in BS formation. In Figure 4, some species decreased as BS scales increased, and the others were increased in proportion to the BS scale. These species may play core roles in BS formation. However, their exact roles must be identified in further studies.

Recently, two pyrosequencing studies were performed to analyze the microbiota of BS [18,19]. One was performed for 25 subjects [18], while the other study consisted of 111 subjects [19]. Li et al. [18] reported that the genera of *Actinomyces*, *Tannerella*, *Treponema*, *Corynebacterium*, *Cardiobacterium* and *Hemophilus* were more abundant in children with BS. In another study, the genera *Leptotrichia* and *Fusobacterium* contributed to BS formation, while the genera *Streptococcus* and *Mogibacterium* were important in the formation of both caries and pigments. Interestingly, three studies, including ours, did not reveal a strong consistency between them. Different ethnic backgrounds and dietary styles may provide confounding effects, suggesting that a more careful sampling design is required for this kind of study.

The limitation of this study is the small sample size. Larger sample size is needed for safe experiments and the potential confounding factor that the pyrosequencing may present. Further research will be designed by reflecting this limitation. In addition, it is meaningful to compare the study with existing healthy subjects in place of the small control group. In the study of healthy children, Proteobacteria was abundant in the group without dental caries, and Firmicutes and Bacteroides were abundant in the group with dental caries [21]. A study of healthy elderly people found that Firmicutes and Veillonella were abundant at the phyla level [22,23]. This was markedly different from the BS group in this study, in which Neisseria, Porphyromonas and Streptococcus were significant.

5. Conclusions

In conclusion, this study investigated the composition of the oral microbiome of supragingival plaque in relation to BS formation. Although the number of subjects was relatively limited, our study is the first species-level analysis of the pyrosequencing data in BS formation. We highlighted that compositional changes in the oral microbiome are essential, and several species in the genus *Neisseria*, *Porphyromonas* and *Streptococcus* may be major contributors to BS formation. The proposed species information will provide a foundation for understanding the complex ecology of BS and for identifying the causal agent for BS formation.

Author Contributions: Conceptualization, J.Y.H. and S.C.C.; methodology, H.-S.L.; software, J.C.; validation, J.C.; formal analysis, O.H.N.; investigation, S.C.C.; resources, M.S.K.; data duration, H.-S.L.; writing—original draft preparation, J.Y.H. and S.C.C.; writing—review and editing, H.-S.L. and S.C.C.; supervision, project administration, funding acquisition, S.C.C. All authors have read and agreed to the published version of the manuscript.

Acknowledgments: We thank the children that participated in this study.

References

1. Zyla, T.; Kawala, B.; Antoszewska-Smith, J.; Kawala, M. Black stain and dental caries: A review of the literature. *Biomed. Res. Int.* **2015**, *2015*, 469392. [CrossRef] [PubMed]
2. Reid, J.S.; Beeley, J.A.; MacDonald, D.G. Investigations into black extrinsic tooth stain. *J. Dent. Res.* **1977**, *56*, 895–899. [CrossRef] [PubMed]
3. Slots, J. The microflora of black stain on human primary teeth. *Scand. J. Dent. Res.* **1974**, *82*, 484–490. [CrossRef] [PubMed]
4. Ximenez-Fyvie, L.A.; Haffajee, A.D.; Socransky, S.S. Microbial composition of supra- and subgingival plaque in subjects with adult periodontitis. *J. Clin. Periodontol.* **2000**, *27*, 722–732. [CrossRef]
5. Garcia Martin, J.M.; Gonzalez Garcia, M.; Seoane Leston, J.; Llorente Pendas, S.; Diaz Martin, J.J.; Garcia-Pola, M.J. Prevalence of black stain and associated risk factors in preschool Spanish children. *Pediatr. Int.* **2013**, *55*, 355–359. [CrossRef]
6. Soukos, N.S.; Som, S.; Abernethy, A.D.; Ruggiero, K.; Dunham, J.; Lee, C.; Doukas, A.G.; Goodson, J.M. Phototargeting oral black-pigmented bacteria. *Antimicrob. Agents Chemother.* **2005**, *49*, 1391–1396. [CrossRef]

7. Saba, C.; Solidani, M.; Berlutti, F.; Vestri, A.; Ottolenghi, L.; Polimeni, A. Black stains in the mixed dentition: A PCR microbiological study of the etiopathogenic bacteria. *J. Clin. Pediatr. Dent.* **2006**, *30*, 219–224. [CrossRef]
8. Keijser, B.J.; Zaura, E.; Huse, S.M.; van der Vossen, J.M.; Schuren, F.H.; Montijn, R.C.; Ten Cate, J.M.; Crielaard, W. Pyrosequencing analysis of the oral microflora of healthy adults. *J. Dent. Res.* **2008**, *87*, 1016–1020. [CrossRef]
9. Crielaard, W.; Zaura, E.; Schuller, A.A.; Huse, S.M.; Montijn, R.C.; Keijser, B.J. Exploring the oral microbiota of children at various developmental stages of their dentition in the relation to their oral health. *BMC Med. Genom.* **2011**, *4*, 22. [CrossRef]
10. Shourie, K.L. Mesenteric line or pigmented plaque; a sign of comparative freedom from caries. *J. Am. Dent. Assoc.* **1947**, *35*, 805–807. [CrossRef]
11. Liu, G.Y.; Nizet, V. Color me bad: Microbial pigments as virulence factors. *Trends Microbiol.* **2009**, *17*, 406–413. [CrossRef] [PubMed]
12. Haffajee, A.D.; Cugini, M.A.; Tanner, A.; Pollack, R.P.; Smith, C.; Kent, R.L., Jr.; Socransky, S.S. Subgingival microbiota in healthy, well-maintained elder and periodontitis subjects. *J. Clin. Periodontol.* **1998**, *25*, 346–353. [CrossRef] [PubMed]
13. Kononen, E.; Kanervo, A.; Takala, A.; Asikainen, S.; Jousimies-Somer, H. Establishment of oral anaerobes during the first year of life. *J. Dent. Res.* **1999**, *78*, 1634–1639. [CrossRef] [PubMed]
14. Willems, A.; Collins, M.D. Reclassification of *Oribaculum catoniae* (Moore and Moore 1994) as *Porphyromonas catoniae* comb. nov. and emendation of the genus *Porphyromonas*. *Int. J. Syst. Bacteriol.* **1995**, *45*, 578–581. [CrossRef]
15. Handley, P.S.; Correia, F.F.; Russell, K.; Rosan, B.; DiRienzo, J.M. Association of a novel high molecular weight, serine-rich protein (SrpA) with fibril-mediated adhesion of the oral biofilm bacterium *Streptococcus cristatus*. *Oral Microbiol. Immunol.* **2005**, *20*, 131–140. [CrossRef]
16. Rickard, A.H.; Gilbert, P.; High, N.J.; Kolenbrander, P.E.; Handley, P.S. Bacterial coaggregation: An integral process in the development of multi-species biofilms. *Trends Microbiol.* **2003**, *11*, 94–100. [CrossRef]
17. Kreth, J.; Zhang, Y.; Herzberg, M.C. Streptococcal antagonism in oral biofilms: *Streptococcus sanguinis* and *Streptococcus gordonii* interference with *Streptococcus mutans*. *J. Bacteriol.* **2008**, *190*, 4632–4640. [CrossRef]
18. Li, Y.; Zhang, Q.; Zhang, F.; Liu, R.; Liu, H.; Chen, F. Analysis of the Microbiota of Black Stain in the Primary Dentition. *PLoS ONE* **2015**, *10*, e0137030. [CrossRef]
19. Li, Y.; Zou, C.G.; Fu, Y.; Li, Y.; Zhou, Q.; Liu, B.; Zhang, Z.; Liu, J. Oral microbial community typing of caries and pigment in primary dentition. *BMC Genom.* **2016**, *17*, 558. [CrossRef]
20. Washio, J.; Shimada, Y.; Yamada, M.; Sakamaki, R.; Takahashi, N. Effects of pH and lactate on hydrogen sulfide production by oral *Veillonella* spp. *Appl. Environ. Microbiol.* **2014**, *80*, 4184–4188. [CrossRef]
21. Yoshiaki, N.; Ryoko, O.; Ryo, H.; Nobuhiro, H. Oral Microbiome of Children Living in an Isolated Area in Myanmar. *Int. J. Environ. Res.* **2020**, *17*, 4033.
22. Yoshiaki, N.; Erika, K.; Ayako, O.; Ryoko, O.; Mieko, S.; Yasuko, T.; Chieko, T.; Kazumune, A.; Hideki, D.; Tamotsu, S.; et al. Oral Microbiome in Four female Centenarians. *Appl. Sci.* **2020**, *10*, 5312.
23. Yoshiaki, N.; Erika, K.; Noboru, K.; Kaname, N.; Akihiro, Y.; Nobuhiro, H. The Oral Microbiome of Healthy Japanese People at the Age of 90. *Appl. Sci.* **2020**, *10*, 6450.

17

Salivary Cytokine Biomarker Concentrations in Relation to Obesity and Periodontitis

Sanna Syrjäläinen [1], Ulvi Kahraman Gursoy [1,*], Mervi Gursoy [1], Pirkko Pussinen [2], Milla Pietiäinen [2], Antti Jula [3], Veikko Salomaa [3], Pekka Jousilahti [3] and Eija Könönen [1,4]

1 Periodontology, Institute of Dentistry, University of Turku, 20520 Turku, Finland; sanna.syrjalainen@utu.fi (S.S.); mervi.gursoy@utu.fi (M.G.); eija.kononen@utu.fi (E.K.)
2 Oral and Maxillofacial Diseases, University of Helsinki, 00014 Helsinki, Finland; pirkko.pussinen@helsinki.fi (P.P.); milla.pietiainen@helsinki.fi (M.P.)
3 Finnish Institute for Health and Welfare, 00271 Helsinki, Finland; antti.jula@thl.fi (A.J.); veikko.salomaa@thl.fi (V.S.); pekka.jousilahti@thl.fi (P.J.)
4 Oral Health Care, Welfare Division, City of Turku, 20101 Turku, Finland
* Correspondence: ulvi.gursoy@utu.fi

Abstract: Systemic low-grade inflammation is associated with obesity. Our aim was to examine the association between obesity and salivary biomarkers of periodontitis. Salivary interleukin (IL)-1-receptor antagonist (IL-1Ra), IL-6, IL-8, IL-10, and tumor necrosis factor (TNF)-α concentrations were measured from 287 non-diabetic obese (body mass index (BMI) of >35 kg/m^2) individuals and 293 normal-weight (BMI of 18.5–25 kg/m^2) controls. Periodontal status was defined according to a diagnostic cumulative risk score (CRS) to calculate the risk of having periodontitis (CRS I, low risk; CRS II, medium risk; CRS III, high risk). In the whole population, and especially in smokers, higher IL-8 and lower IL-10 concentrations were detected in the obese group compared to the control group, while in non-smoking participants, the obese and control groups did not differ. IL-1Ra and IL-8 concentrations were higher in those with medium or high risk (CRS II and CRS III, $p < 0.001$) of periodontitis, whereas IL-10 and TNF-α concentrations were lower when compared to those with low risk (CRS I). In multivariate models adjusted for periodontal status, obesity did not associate with any salivary cytokine concentration. In conclusion, salivary cytokine biomarkers are not independently associated with obesity and concentrations are dependent on periodontal status.

Keywords: obesity; periodontitis; cytokine; inflammation; saliva

---

1. Introduction

Obesity is an increasing health problem in developed countries and is a major risk factor for diabetes, cancer, and cardiovascular diseases [1]. Obesity is linked to both local and systemic inflammation [2–5]. In obese subjects, there is an elevated release of proinflammatory cytokines into serum derived from either adipocytes, stromal vascular fraction cells, or immune cells in adipose tissue [3,5,6]. This elevated cytokine release in obese individuals is a reversible condition, since even mild weight loss can reduce serum cytokine levels [7].

There is substantial evidence showing a positive association between obesity or weight gain and periodontitis [8–11]. The underlying mechanisms explaining this association are not completely elucidated, but one proposed mechanism is that the low-grade systemic inflammation related to obesity could expose obese people to infectious diseases [3,4,12]. Pathogenic bacterial biofilms at the gingival margin trigger the initiation of inflammatory processes in periodontal tissues, including the production of chemokines and proinflammatory cytokines [13,14]. Inflammatory cytokines in the periodontium are low-molecular weight proteins secreted from both periodontal tissue and immune cells [13]. They are the main regulators of inflammation and tissue destruction in periodontitis [15], and their levels in saliva predict periodontal disease progression and remission [16]. To our knowledge, the association between salivary cytokine concentrations and obesity and periodontitis has not been examined in humans so far.

In the present study, we used a novel diagnostic method, the cumulative risk score (CRS), to detect periodontal disease based on three biomarkers in saliva [17]. CRS combines *Porphyromonas gingivalis*, interleukin (IL)-1β, and matrix metalloproteinase (MMP)-8, and categorizes individuals with low, medium, or high risk of having periodontitis. Our hypothesis is that low-grade inflammation related to obesity affects the cytokine biomarker concentrations in saliva. In this context, our cross-sectional study aimed to examine the relation between obesity and periodontitis-associated salivary cytokine concentrations in smoking and non-smoking individuals.

2. Experimental Section

2.1. Study Population

The study consisted of 580 individuals aged 25–74 (mean 55.3) years. They were participants of the Dietary, Lifestyle, and Genetic determinant of Obesity and Metabolic syndrome (DILGOM) study, which was an extension of the population-based National FINRISK2007 health survey to investigate more specifically the effects of diet, lifestyle, and genetic factors on obesity and metabolic syndrome [18,19]. Of the 5024 individuals who participated in the DILGOM study, 287 severely obese (body mass index (BMI) $\geq$35 kg/m^2) and 297 normal-weight (BMI 18.5–25 kg/m^2) controls matched for age and smoking status were included. Exclusion criteria for both cases and controls were diabetes, cardiovascular disease, cancer, or medication for hypercholesterolemia. The protocol of the FINRISK2007 survey included questionnaire data on smoking and other health behaviors, socioeconomic background factors, clinical measurements, and venous blood samples. Participants were categorized by their smoking status as current smokers or non-smokers (smokeless for at least the past 6 months). Height was measured to the nearest 0.1 cm and weight to the nearest 0.1 kg.

2.2. Bacterial and Cytokine Measurements from Salivary Samples

Paraffin-stimulated whole saliva samples were collected by expectoration into plastic tubes from the DILGOM study participants. All samples were stored frozen at −70 °C until laboratory analyses. Before analyses, melted samples were gently mixed, and centrifuged at 10,000 × *g* for 5 min. DNA was isolated from the pellet and used in *P. gingivalis* quantification, while the supernatant was used in cytokine determinations.

Salivary concentrations of IL-1β, IL-1 receptor antagonist (IL-1Ra), IL-6, IL-8, IL-10, tumor necrosis factor alpha (TNF–α), and MMP-8 were analyzed with the flow-cytometric Luminex xMAP technique with commercially available kits by Bio-PlexTM 200 (Bio-Rad Laboratories Incorporation, Santa Rosa, CA, USA).

The amounts of *P. gingivalis* were determined with a quantitative real-time PCR (qPCR) assay as previously described [20] with modifications. Reaction mixtures (total volume 20 μL) contained 2 μL of template DNA, 200 nM primers (Thermo Fisher Scientific, Waltham, MA, USA), and 1 × Universal KAPA SYBR FAST qPCR mastermix (KAPA Biosystems, Wilmington, MA, USA) supplemented with 1 × ROX Low reference dye. qPCR analyses were performed with the Mx3005P Real-Time qPCR System (Stratagene, La Jolla, CA, USA) via the following steps: Initial denaturation at 95 °C for 3 min, followed by 40 cycles of 3 s at 95 °C and 20 s at 60 °C. A dissociation curve was generated from one cycle of 1 min at 95 °C, then lowering the temperature gradually to 60 °C, 30 s at 60 °C, then raising the temperature gradually to 95 °C, and 30 s at 95 °C. The data were analyzed with the Mx3005P Real-Time qPCR System software and the results were presented as genomic equivalents (GE)/mL saliva.

For the standard curve, the whole *P. gingivalis waaA* gene, encoding 3-deoxy-Dmanno-oct-2-ulosonic acid (Kdo) transferase, was cloned to pJet1.2/blunt vector (Thermo Fisher Scientific, Waltham, MA, USA). The cloned fragment was PCR-amplified in the reaction containing 500 nM primers (Fwd-ATGCGATTCCTTTTCAG and Rew-CTATTTCATGATTCGGTG), 200 μM dNTPs, Phusion DNA Polymerase (Thermo Fisher Scientific, Waltham, MA, USA) 0.04 U/μL, 1 × Phusion High-Fidelity Buffer, and 10 ng of chromosomal DNA of *P. gingivalis* strain W50. The cycling conditions followed the manufacturer's instructions. The purified PCR fragment was ligated into pJet1.2/blunt vector with CloneJET PCR Cloning Kit (Thermo Fisher Scientific, Waltham, MA, USA) according to the manufacturer's instructions and ligation mixture was transformed into *Escherichia coli* DH5a competent cells. The correct insert was verified by sequencing. The constructed plasmid, pJet1.2/blunt-Pg, was linearized with FastDigest HindIII restriction enzyme (Thermo Fisher Scientific, Waltham, MA, USA) and used for a tenfold dilution series for the qPCR analysis. The plasmid copy number was determined with "DNA Copy Number and Dilution Calculator" (www.thermofisher.com).

2.3. Periodontal Status Assessment Based on Cumulative Risk Score (CRS)

Periodontal status of the study population ($n = 580$) was defined according to CRS as described in detail by Gursoy et al. [17]. Briefly, for calculating CRS, the salivary concentrations of *P. gingivalis*, IL-1β, and MMP-8 were independently divided into tertiles and each participant was categorized to one of the three tertiles according to the level of the biomarker in the saliva. The person's cumulative score was calculated by multiplication of three biomarkers' tertile values. Based on these calculations, the study participants were categorized into three periodontal status groups, as follows: CRS I: low risk; CRS II: medium risk; CRS III: High risk [17,21,22].

2.4. Statistical Analyses

All statistical analyses were conducted using the IBM SPSS Statistic 23.0 software (IBM, Armonk, North Castle, NY, USA). In descriptive statistics, continuous variables were reported as means and standard deviations and the differences between the groups were analyzed by independent *t*-test. Categorical variables were reported as the number of individuals and as percentages. Differences between the groups in categorical variables were analyzed using the chi-square test. Statistical significance was set at a p-value of < 0.05.

Results of two saliva samples were not included in analyses due to the low sample quality. Due to skewed distribution, salivary cytokine concentrations were reported as medians and interquartile ranges. Differences of salivary cytokine concentrations between the obese and normal-weight participants and a pairwise comparison between the groups among different CRS categories were conducted using the Mann–Whitney *U* test. A p-value significance level of < 0.05 was used. Multinomial logistic regression was used to determine whether salivary cytokines were associated with obesity, before and after adjusting the model for smoking and periodontal status (CRS). For multinomial logistic regression, cytokine concentrations were converted into tertiles, and the lowest tertile was used as the reference group.

2.5. Ethical Issues

The study was conducted in accordance with the Declaration of Helsinki and approved by the Ethical Committee of the Hospital District of Helsinki and Uusimaa. Written informed consent was obtained from each participant.

3. Results

There was no difference in age, gender, or smoking status between the two study groups, whereas mean BMI was significantly higher in the obese (39.0 kg/m^2) than in the normal-weight (22.9 kg/m^2) groups ($p < 0.001$) (Table 1). Obese individuals were lower educated ($p = 0.005$) and were more likely to have periodontal disease than their controls ($p = 0.015$).

Table 1. Characteristics of the study groups according to their weight status. Significant differences ($p < 0.05$) are presented in bold.

Demographic and Clinical Parameters	Obese $n = 287$	Normal Weight $n = 293$	p
Age, mean (SD)	55.0 (11.9)	55.5 (12.0)	0.604
Males, n (%)	98 (34.1)	98 (33.4)	0.859
Smokers, n (%)	51 (17.8)	47 (16.0)	0.578
Education level, n (%)			
Low	105 (37.1)	74 (25.3)	**0.005**
Average	94 (33.2)	104 (31.7)	
High	84 (29.7)	115 (39.2)	
BMI, mean (SD)	39.0 (4.1)	22.9 (1.6)	**<0.001**
Periodontitis, n (%)			
Cumulative Risk Score (CRS) I	58 (20.2)	80 (27.3)	**0.015**
Cumulative Risk Score (CRS) II	82 (28.6)	97 (33.1)	
Cumulative Risk Score (CRS) III	147 (51.2)	116 (39.6)	

p-values: Independent samples T-test (age, body mass index (BMI)) and chi-square test (gender, smoking status, educational level, periodontitis).

In the whole population and in smokers, the salivary concentrations of IL-8 were higher (whole population $p = 0.033$; smokers $p = 0.005$) and those of IL-10 were lower (whole population $p = 0.022$; smokers $p = 0.018$) in the obese group than in their controls (Table 2). Other salivary cytokine concentrations did not differ according to weight status. In non-smokers, there was no difference in salivary cytokine concentrations between the groups.

When the study participants were stratified only according to their periodontal status and not by their weight, IL-1Ra and IL-8 concentrations were higher in those with medium or high risk (CRS II and CRS III, $p < 0.001$) of periodontitis, whereas IL-10 and TNF-α concentrations were lower when compared to those with the low risk (CRS I). After weight was taken into account, obese individuals with CRS I had lower IL-10 ($p = 0.043$) and TNF-α ($p = 0.35$) concentrations than their normal-weight controls, while obese individuals with CRS III had higher IL-6 concentrations ($p = 0.011$). Other cytokine concentrations in saliva did not differ between the obese and control groups according to their periodontal status (Table 3).

Table 2. Salivary cytokine concentrations (pg/mL) in the study population and as divided according to smoking status. Significant differences ($p < 0.05$) are presented in bold.

	Whole Population			Smokers			Non-Smokers		
	Obese n = 285	**Normal Weight n = 293**	p	**Obese n = 50**	**Normal Weight n = 47**	p	**Obese n = 235**	**Normal Weight n = 246**	p
IL-1Ra	7979 (8712)	7782 (8962)	0.097	7018 (7885)	4877 (4915)	0.036	8566 (9141)	8098 (9136)	0.307
IL-6	3.6 (5.2)	3.3 (4.2)	0.095	3.6 (5.7)	3.6 (6.1)	0.948	3.6 (5.2)	3.2 (4.0)	0.071
IL-8	378 (472)	300 (365)	**0.033**	345 (431)	241 (152)	**0.005**	380(472)	375 (400)	0.257
IL-10	1.5 (3.0)	2.0 (3.7)	**0.022**	1.7 (3.2)	2.7 (6.5)	**0.018**	1.5 (2.9)	1.9 (3.7)	0.132
TNF-α	10.4 (17.4)	12.6 (18.8)	0.103	10.7 (18.5)	18.3 (23.4)	0.094	10.1 (17.5)	12.4 (17.7)	0.291

All values are given as medians (interquartile ranges). p-values: Mann–Whitney U test.

Table 3. Salivary cytokine concentrations (pg/mL) in the study population divided according to periodontal status. Significant differences ($p < 0.05$) are presented in bold.

	CRS I			CRS II			CRS III		
	Obese n = 58	**Normal Weight n = 80**	p	**Obese n = 82**	**Normal Weight n = 97**	p	**Obese n = 147**	**Normal Weight n = 116**	p
IL-1Ra	4419 (2829)	3727 (3497)	0.064	6582 (5478)$^{a.}$	7224 (5402)^{a}	0.666	12136 (9387)^{a,b}	13045 (10240)^{a,b}	0.212
IL-6	3.6 (4.3)	4.5 (4.7)	0.341	2.9 (3.3)	3.0 (3.0)^{a}	0.993	4.8 (6.8)^{a,b}	3.0 (5.5)	**0.011**
IL-8	169 (127)	168 (125)	0.440	274 (292)^{a}	284 (242)^{a}	0.682	573 (443)^{a,b}	566 (464)^{a,b}	0.784
IL-10	3.5 (5.8)	5.7 (8.1)	**0.043**	1.5 (2.8)^{a}	2.0 (3.0)^{a}	0.078	1.3 (2.2)^{a}	1.2 (1.9)^{a,b}	0.698
TNF-α	14.4 (23.9)	26.4 (26.4)	**0.035**	9.8 (14.5)^{a}	12.4 (13.9)^{a}	0.460	8.9 (15.8)^{a,b}	10.3 (10.9)^{a}	0.841

All values are given as medians (interquartile ranges). In each CRS group, cytokine concentrations were compared between obese and normal-weight groups (p-values). Superscript letters indicate significant differences between the CRS groups in obese and normal-weight individuals as follows: a) A difference in CRS I and b) a difference in CRS II. P-values and superscripts: Mann–Whitney U test.

The multinomial regression model revealed a significant association between obesity and IL-10 concentrations, but the significance was lost after the model was adjusted for smoking and periodontal status (Table 4).

Table 4. Associations of salivary IL-1Ra, IL-6, IL-8, IL-10, and TNF-α tertiles with obesity, before and after adjusting the model for smoking and periodontal status (CRS). Significant associations ($p < 0.05$) are presented in bold.

	Middle Tertile		Highest Tertile	
	Unadjusted	Adjusted	Unadjusted	Adjusted
IL-1Ra	1.5 (1.0–2.3), **0.033**	1.3 (0.9–2.1), 0.194	1.5 (0.9–2.2), 0.06	1.1 (0.7–1.8), 0.722
IL-6	1.3 (0.9–1.9), 0.222	1.3 (0.8–1.9), 0.247	1.2 (0.8–1.8), 0.334	1.2 (0.8–1.8), 0.359
IL-8	1.1 (0.7–1.6), 0.760	0.9 (0.5–1.3), 0.514	1.4 (0.9–2.1), 0.114	0.9 (0.6–1.6), 0.852
IL-10	0.8 (0.5–1.2), 0.264	0.8 (0.5–1.2), 0.287	0.7 (0.4–0.9), **0.042**	0.8 (0.5–1.2), 0.247
TNF-α	0.8 (0.5–1.2), 0.263	0.8 (0.5–1.2), 0.306	0.7 (0.5–1.1), 0.114	0.8 (0.5–1.2), 0.327

Odds ratios (95% confidence intervals) and p-values: Multinomial logistic regression model.

4. Discussion

The main finding of the present study was that, despite periodontal status being worse in obese individuals (BMI of ≥35kg/m^2) compared to normal-weight controls (BMI of 18.5–25 kg/m^2), the association was not consistently reflected in salivary cytokine concentrations. Instead, the concentrations were merely affected by periodontal status rather than obesity. To our knowledge, this was the first study to investigate potential associations of salivary cytokines with obesity by taking periodontal and smoking states into account.

The relatively large sample size, including 287 severely obese and 293 normal-weight individuals, allowed us to make reliable comparisons of cytokine concentrations in saliva between these groups. However, the cross-sectional study design does not provide any information about the causality between periodontitis, obesity, and cytokines. In addition, the relatively large age range of the study population may have displayed an underestimated effect, since the immune response undergoes remodeling with age. To define the presence of periodontal disease, a novel salivary diagnostic tool, CRS, was used [17]. Its capability has been validated in independent populations twice, showing that the CRS index is more strongly associated with moderate to severe periodontitis than any of the salivary biomarkers alone [21,22]. Finally, as part of the sample collection protocol of this survey study, stimulated saliva samples were collected. The protein concentration was higher in the unstimulated saliva samples than the stimulated saliva samples, however, the unstimulated saliva samples possessed greater inter- and intraindividual variation than the stimulated saliva samples [23].

According to the present study, obese individuals expressed enhanced IL-8 and IL-1Ra but reduced IL-10 concentrations in saliva when compared to normal-weight individuals. This finding was observed especially in smokers. Studies dealing with salivary cytokines in relation to weight are sparse. In a recent small-scale study ($n = 44$), TNF-α concentrations in saliva were shown to be significantly higher in obese than non-obese adults [24]. In obese and non-obese children, on the other hand, salivary TNF-α concentrations did not differ [25]. As both obesity and periodontitis are inflammatory states, it was proposed that obesity-related inflammation could predispose obese subjects to periodontal tissue destruction [12,26]. In the present study, obese individuals displayed mainly CRS II and III, indicating worsened periodontal conditions, more frequently than their normal-weight controls. Nevertheless, there were no consistent differences in the salivary cytokine concentrations between the groups.

In periodontitis, cytokines are mainly released from periodontal tissues after pathogenic bacterial recognition [13,14]. There is also some evidence that adipose tissue-derived cytokines act in a paracrine more than an endocrine manner, and hence do not contribute to cytokine concentrations in the oral cavity [27,28]. It is therefore possible that the local infection of the periodontium has such a strong effect on salivary cytokine concentrations that it overpowers the systemic influence of obesity in statistical analyses. Still, obesity may reinforce the inflammatory response to periodontal pathogens in the periodontium, resulting in an increased susceptibility to periodontitis. It is also possible that the link between obesity and periodontitis is not explained by inflammatory factors.

Obesity and periodontitis share other risk factors, including low socioeconomic status [29]. In the present study, obese individuals were less educated than their controls. This is in line with studies linking educational status to health behaviors as well as eating habits to the prevalence of periodontal disease [29–31]. Obesity-related comorbidities, for example, diabetes mellitus, which is a well-known risk factor for periodontitis [26], could also explain the association between obesity and periodontitis. In our study, diabetic patients were excluded, but the obese individuals may still have insulin resistance, a prediabetic state, which is also a proposed risk factor for periodontitis [32].

In addition to obesity, an unhealthy diet causing weight gain plays a role in the obesity-related inflammatory burden [33–35]. In an experimental rodent model, it was shown that obese rats fed a high-fat and high-carbohydrate diet mimicking the Western diet (known as the "cafeteria diet") caused significantly more advanced alveolar bone loss when compared to non-obese counterparts [34]. In another rodent model, it was observed that a diet enriched with saturated fat was associated with higher inflammatory potential and tissue destruction when compared to a diet high in unsaturated fat in obese mice [34]. Therefore, in future studies regarding obesity and periodontitis in humans, it would be of interest to include the dietary composition of obesity in the analyses.

5. Conclusions

In conclusion, although obese individuals may be prone to have periodontal disease, obesity does not lead to altered cytokine concentrations in saliva. The associations between obesity and salivary cytokine concentrations may be explained by periodontal status and smoking.

Author Contributions: Conceptualization, S.S., U.K.G., and V.S.; data curation, M.G., P.P., A.J., V.S., and P.J.; formal analysis, S.S., U.K.G., M.P., and A.J.; funding acquisition, P.P. and V.S.; methodology, M.G., P.P., M.P., P.J., and E.K.; project administration, U.K.G. and E.K.; resources, V.S. and E.K.; supervision, U.K.G. and E.K.; visualization, S.S.; writing—original draft, S.S. and U.K.G.; writing—review and editing, M.G., P.P., M.P., A.J., V.S., P.J., and E.K.

References

1. NCD Risk Factor Collaboration (NCD-RisC). Trends in adult body-mass index in 200 countries from 1975 to 2014: A pooled analysis of 1698 population-based measurement studies with 19.2 million participants. *Lancet* **2016**, *387*, 1377–1396. [CrossRef]
2. Weisberg, S.P.; McCann, D.; Desai, M.; Rosenbaum, M.; Leibel, R.L.; Ferrante, A.W., Jr. Obesity is associated with macrophage accumulation in adipose tissue. *J. Clin. Invest.* **2003**, *112*, 1796–1808. [CrossRef] [PubMed]
3. Ouchi, N.; Parker, J.L.; Lugus, J.J.; Walsh, K. Adipokines in inflammation and metabolic disease. *Nat. Rev. Immunol.* **2011**, *11*, 85–97. [CrossRef] [PubMed]
4. McArdle, M.A.; Finucane, O.M.; Connaughton, R.M.; McMorrow, A.M.; Roche, H.M. Mechanisms of obesity-induced inflammation and insulin resistance: Insights into the emerging role of nutritional strategies. *Front. Endocrinol.* **2013**, *10*, 52. [CrossRef] [PubMed]
5. Schmidt, F.; Weschenfelder, J.; Sander, C.; Minkwitz, J.; Thormann, J.; Chittka, T.; Mergl, R.; Kirkby, K.; Faßhauer, M.; Stumvoll, M.; et al. Inflammatory cytokines in general and central obesity and modulating effects of physical activity. *PLoS ONE* **2015**, *10*, e0121971. [CrossRef]
6. Azizian, M.; Mahdipour, E.; Mirhafez, S.R.; Shoeibi, S.; Nematy, M.; Esmaily, H.; Ferns, G.; Ghayour-Mobarhan, M. Cytokine profiles in overweight and obese subjects and normal weight individuals matched for age and gender. Ann. *Clin. Biochem.* **2016**, *53*, 663–668. [CrossRef]
7. Chae, J.S.; Paik, J.K.; Kang, R.; Kim, M.; Choi, Y.; Lee, S.H.; Lee, J.H. Mild weight loss reduces inflammatory cytokines, leukocyte count, and oxidative stress in overweight and moderately obese participants treated for 3 years with dietary modification. *Nutr. Res.* **2013**, *33*, 195–203. [CrossRef]

8. Chaffee, B.; Weston, S. Association between chronic periodontal disease and obesity: A systematic review and meta-analysis. *J. Periodontol.* **2010**, *81*, 1708–1724. [CrossRef]
9. Suvan, J.; Petrie, A.; Nibali, L.; Darbar, U.; Rakmanee, T.; Donos, N.; D'Aiuto, F. Association between overweight/obesity and increased risk of periodontitis. *J. Clin. Periodontol.* **2015**, *42*, 733–739. [CrossRef]
10. Keller, A.; Rohde, J.; Raymond, K.; Heitmann, B.L. Association between periodontal disease and overweight and obesity. A systematic review. *J. Periodontol.* **2015**, *86*, 766–776. [CrossRef]
11. Nascimento, G.G.; Leite, F.R.; Do, L.G.; Peres, K.G.; Correa, M.B.; Demarco, F.F.; Peres, M.A. Is weight gain associated with the incidence of periodontitis? A systematic review and meta-analysis. *J. Clin. Periodontol.* **2015**, *42*, 495–505. [CrossRef] [PubMed]
12. Falagas, M.; Kompoti, M. Obesity and infection. *Lancet Infect. Dis.* **2006**, *6*, 438–446. [CrossRef]
13. Van Dyke, T.E.; van Winkelholff, A.J. Infection and inflammation mechanisms. *J. Clin. Periodontol.* **2013**, *40*, S1–S7. [CrossRef] [PubMed]
14. Könönen, E.; Gursoy, M.; Gursoy, U.K. Periodontitis: A Multifaceted Disease of Tooth-Supporting Tissues. *J. Clin. Med.* **2019**, *31*, E1135. [CrossRef]
15. Preshaw, P.M.; Taylor, J.J. How has research into cytokine interactions and their role in driving immune responses impacted our understanding of periodontitis? *J. Clin. Periodontol.* **2011**, *38* (Suppl 11), 60–84. [CrossRef]
16. Kinney, J.; Morelli, T.; Braun, T.; Ramseier, C.; Herr, A.; Sugai, J.; Shelburne, C.; Rayburn, L.; Singh, A.; Giannobile, W. Saliva/pathogen biomarker signatures and periodontal disease progression. *J. Dent. Res.* **2011**, *90*, 752–758. [CrossRef]
17. Gürsoy, U.K.; Könönen, E.; Pussinen, P.; Tervahartiala, T.; Hyvärinen, K.; Suominen, A.; Uitto, V.-J.; Paju, S.; Sorsa, T. Use of host- and bacteria-derived salivary markers in detection of periodontitis: A cumulative approach. *Dis. Markers* **2011**, *30*, 299–306. [CrossRef]
18. Borodulin, K.; Tolonen, H.; Jousilahti, P.; Jula, A.; Juolevi, A.; Koskinen, S.; Kuulasmaa, K.; Laatikainen, T.; Männistö, S.; Peltonen, M.; et al. Cohort profile: The National FINRISK study. *Int. J. Epidemiol.* **2017**, *47*, 696. [CrossRef]
19. Konttinen, H.; Llewellyn, C.; Silventoinen, K.; Joensuu, A.; Männistö, S.; Salomaa, V.; Jousilahti, P.; Kaprio, J.; Perola, M.; Haukkala, A. Genetic predisposition to obesity, restrained eating and changes in body weight: A population-based prospective study. *Int. J. Obes.* **2018**, *42*, 858–865. [CrossRef]
20. Hyvärinen, K.; Laitinen, S.; Paju, S.; Hakala, A.; Suominen-Taipale, L.; Skurnik, M.; Könönen, E.; Pussinen, P. Detection and quantification of five major periodontal pathogens by single copy gene-based real-time PCR. *Innate Immun.* **2009**, *15*, 195–204. [CrossRef]
21. Salminen, A.; Gursoy, U.K.; Paju, S.; Hyvärinen, K.; Mäntylä, P.; Buhlin, K.; Könönen, E.; Nieminen, M.S.; Sorsa, T.; Sinisalo, J. Salivary biomarkers of bacterial burden, inflammatory response, and tissue destruction in periodontitis. *J. Clin. Periodontol.* **2014**, *41*, 442–450. [CrossRef] [PubMed]
22. Gürsoy, U.K.; Pussinen, P.; Salomaa, V.; Syrjäläinen, S.; Könönen, E. Cumulative use of salivary markers with an adaptive design improves detection of periodontal disease over fixed biomarker thresholds. *Acta Odontol. Scand.* **2018**, *76*, 493–496. [CrossRef] [PubMed]
23. Jasim, H.; Olausson, P.; Hedenberg-Magnusson, B.; Ernberg, M.; Ghafouri, B. The proteomic profile of whole and glandular saliva in healthy pain-free subjects. *Sci. Rep.* **2016**, *15*, 39073. [CrossRef] [PubMed]
24. Lehmann-Kalata, A.; Miechowicz, I.; Korybalska, K.; Swora-Cwynar, E.; Czepulis, N.; Łuczak, J.; Orzechowska, Z.; Grzymisławski, M.; Surdacka, A.; Witowski, J. Salivary fingerprint of simple obesity. *Cytokine* **2018**, *110*, 174–180. [CrossRef]
25. Doğusal, G.; Afacan, B.; Bozkurt, E.; Sönmez, I. Gingival crevicular fluid and salivary resistin and tumor necrosis factor-alpha levels in obese children with gingivitis. *J. Periodontol.* **2018**, *89*, 973–982. [CrossRef]
26. Genco, R.; Borgnakke, W. Risk factors for periodontal disease. *Periodontol. 2000* **2013**, *62*, 59–94. [CrossRef]
27. Kern, P.A.; Ranganathan, S.; Li, C.; Wood, L.; Ranganathan, G. Adipose tissue tumor necrosis factor and interleukin-6 expression in human obesity and insulin resistance. *Am. J. Physiol-Endoc. M.* **2001**, *280*, E745–E751. [CrossRef]
28. Wang, P.; Mariman, E.; Renes, J.; Keijer, J. The secretory function of adipocytes in the physiology of white adipose tissue. *J. Cell. Physiol.* **2008**, *216*, 3–13. [CrossRef]

29. Thomson, W.M.; Sheiham, A.; Spencer, A. Sociobehavioral aspects of periodontal disease. *Periodontol. 2000* **2012**, *60*, 54–63. [CrossRef]
30. Laaksonen, M.; Prättälä, R.; Lahelma, E. Sociodemographic determinants of multiple unhealthy behaviours. *Scand. J. Public Healt.* **2003**, *31*, 37–43. [CrossRef]
31. Rezayatmand, R.; Pavlova, M.; Groot, W. Socio-economic aspects of health-related behaviors and their dynamics: A case study for the Netherlands. *Int. J. Health Policy Manag.* **2015**, *5*, 237–251. [CrossRef] [PubMed]
32. Andriankaja, O.; Muñoz-Torres, F.; Vivaldi-Oliver, J.; Leroux, B.; Campos, M.; Joshipura, K.; Pérez, C. Insulin resistance predicts the risk of gingival/periodontal inflammation. *J. Periodontol.* **2018**, *89*, 549–557. [CrossRef] [PubMed]
33. Li, Y.; Lu, Z.; Zhang, X.; Yu, H.; Kirkwood, K.L.; Lopes-Virella, M.F.; Huang, Y. Metabolic syndrome exacerbates inflammation and bone loss in periodontitis. *J. Dent. Res.* **2015**, *94*, 362–370. [CrossRef] [PubMed]
34. Cavagni, J.; de Macedo, I.C.; Gaio, E.J.; Souza, A.; de Molon, R.S.; Cirelli, J.A.; Hoefel, A.L.; Kucharski, L.C.; Torres, I.L.; Rösing, C.K. Obesity and hyperlipidemia modulate alveolar bone loss in wistar rats. *J. Periodontol.* **2016**, *87*, e9–e17. [CrossRef] [PubMed]
35. Muluke, M.; Gold, T.; Kiefhaber, K.; Al-Sahli, A.; Celenti, R.; Jiang, H.; Cremers, S.; Van Dyke, T.; Schulze-Späte, U. Diet-induced obesity and its differential impact on periodontal bone loss. *J. Dent. Res.* **2016**, *95*, 223–229. [CrossRef] [PubMed]

18

Salivary IL-6 mRNA is a Robust Biomarker in Oral Squamous Cell Carcinoma

Ildikó Judit Márton [1,*], József Horváth [2], Péter Lábiscsák [2], Bernadett Márkus [2], Balázs Dezső [3], Adrienn Szabó [4], Ildikó Tar [5], József Piffkó [6], Petra Jakus [6], József Barabás [7], Péter Barabás [7], Lajos Olasz [8], Zsanett Kövér [8], József Tőzsér [2], János Sándor [9], Éva Csősz [2], Beáta Scholtz [2] and Csongor Kiss [10]

1 Department of Operative Dentistry and Endodontics, Faculty of Dentistry, University of Debrecen, 4032 Debrecen, Hungary
2 Department of Biochemistry and Molecular Biology, Faculty of Medicine, University of Debrecen, 4032 Debrecen, Hungary; horvathjozsef21@gmail.com (J.H.); labiscsak.peter@med.unideb.hu (P.L.); jakob.bernadett@med.unideb.hu (B.M.); tozser@med.unideb.hu (J.T.); cseva@med.unideb.hu (É.C.); scholtz@med.unideb.hu (B.S.)
3 Department of Oral Pathology and Microbiology, Faculty of Dentistry and Institute of Pathology, University of Debrecen, 4032 Debrecen, Hungary; dezsob51@gmail.com
4 Department of Maxillofacial Surgery, University of Debrecen, 4032 Debrecen, Hungary; szabo.adrienn@dental.unideb.hu
5 Department of Oral Medicine, Faculty of Dentistry, University of Debrecen, 4032 Debrecen, Hungary; tar.ildiko@dental.unideb.hu
6 Department of Maxillofacial Surgery, University of Szeged, 6720 Szeged, Hungary; piffkojozsef@gmail.com (J.P.); jakus.petra.87@gmail.com (P.J.)
7 Department of Maxillofacial Surgery, Semmelweis University, 1085 Budapest, Hungary; barabas.jozsef@dent.semmelweis-univ.hu (J.B.); dr.barabas.peter@gmail.com (P.B.)
8 Department of Oral and Maxillofacial Surgery, University of Pécs, 7621 Pécs, Hungary; olasz.lajos@pte.hu (L.O.); kover.zsanett@pte.hu (Z.K.)
9 Department of Preventive Medicine, University of Debrecen, 4028 Debrecen, Hungary; sandor.janos@sph.unideb.hu
10 Department of Pediatric Hematology-Oncology, Faculty of Medicine, University of Debrecen, 4032 Debrecen, Hungary; kisscs@med.unideb.hu
* Correspondence: marton.ildiko@dental.unideb.hu

Abstract: Salivary IL-6 mRNA was previously identified as a promising biomarker of oral squamous cell carcinoma (OSCC). We performed a multi-center investigation covering all geographic areas of Hungary. Saliva from 95 patients with OSCC and 80 controls, all Caucasian, were collected together with demographic and clinicopathological data. Salivary IL-6 mRNA was quantified by real-time quantitative PCR. Salivary IL-6 protein concentration was measured by enzyme-linked immune-sorbent assay. IL-6 protein expression in tumor samples was investigated by immunohistochemistry. Normalized salivary IL-6 mRNA expression values were significantly higher ($p < 0.001$) in patients with OSCC (mean ± SE: 3.301 ± 0.885) vs. controls (mean ± SE: 0.037 ± 0.012). Differences remained significant regardless of tumor stage and grade. AUC of the ROC curve was 0.9379 ($p < 0.001$; 95% confidence interval: 0.8973–0.9795; sensitivity: 0.945; specificity: 0.819). Salivary IL-6 protein levels were significantly higher ($p < 0.001$) in patients (mean ± SE: 70.98 ± 14.06 pg/mL), than in controls (mean ± SE: 12.45 ± 3.29). Specificity and sensitivity of IL-6 protein were less favorable than that of IL-6 mRNA. Salivary IL-6 mRNA expression was significantly associated with age and dental status. IL-6 manifestation was detected in tumor cells and tumor-infiltrating leukocytes, suggesting the presence of a paracrine loop of stimulation. Salivary IL-6 mRNA is one of the best performing and clinically relevant biomarkers of OSCC.

Keywords: salivary biomarkers; oral neoplasia; periodontal disease/periodontitis; smoking; ethanol consumption; real-time quantitative PCR; enzyme-linked immune-sorbent assay; immunohistochemistry

1. Introduction

Hungarian males and females exhibit the highest age-standardized rates both for the incidence and the mortality of oral cavity and pharyngeal cancers in Europe without substantial improvements in the last decades [1]. Frequently, oral squamous cell carcinoma (OSCC) is being diagnosed in advanced stages, i.e., stage III and IV, with long-term survival rates around 50% despite considerable progress in surgical methods, radio-, chemo-, and immunotherapy. In contrast, patients with early, i.e., stage I and II lesions, may experience recovery rates up to 80%. Unfortunately, with the exception of the gold standard procedure, tissue biopsy and histopathological analysis, there are no evidence-based, reliable, non-invasive methods for large-scale screening and early detection of OSCC [2,3].

The aim of the present investigation was to study the potential of salivary IL-6 mRNA and IL-6 protein as OSCC-related biomarkers. Saliva was chosen as a complex, informative body-fluid containing biomolecules that originate from multiple sources and may differentiate between healthy subjects and patients with OSCC. Application of advanced molecular methods resulted in the discovery of several candidate salivary proteins, metabolites, mRNAs, miRNAs, and circRNAs associated with OSCC. However, there has been a high degree of variation between results reported by different investigators with respect to the value of these biomolecules as biomarkers detected in patients of different geographic and ethnic backgrounds [4–10]. In addition, salivary levels of inflammatory cytokines, considered as one of the best performing molecular groups of OSCC biomarkers, may be confounded by the presence of oral inflammatory lesions [11–13].

Previously, we applied both targeted and high-throughput molecular methods to identify potentially useful mRNA and protein biomarkers in a small-scale single-institution pilot cohort of patients with OSCC and controls [12,13]. These pilot transcriptomic and proteomic investigations suggested that salivary IL-6 mRNA and protein may prove the best performing biomarkers of OSCC in the Hungarian population. Therefore, we investigated salivary IL-6 mRNA and IL-6 protein in a sample of patients with OSCC covering each geographic area of Hungary. To support the relevance of salivary IL-6 mRNA expression, we were looking for differences in salivary IL-6 protein concentrations of patients and controls and by detecting the expression of IL-6 protein in tumor cells and in tumor-infiltrating leukocytes (TIL). An additional objective was to analyze associations of salivary IL-6 mRNA and protein expression with age, sex, gingival inflammation status, smoking, and ethanol consumption habits in patients with OSCC.

2. Materials and Methods

2.1. Patients and Control Subjects

Between 2 May 2013 and 31 December 2015, 95 adult (>18 years) patients with OSCC, presenting a suitable saliva sample, were enrolled in a multi-centric investigation from four Hungarian sites: Faculty of Dentistry, University of Debrecen, Debrecen ("Debrecen Center"): 26 patients; Faculty of Dentistry, Scientific University of Szeged, Szeged ("Szeged Center"): 24 patients; Faculty of Dentistry, Scientific University of Pécs, Pécs ("Pécs Center"): 25 patients; and Faculty of Dentistry, Semmelweis University, Budapest ("Budapest Center"): 20 patients. Eighty age-matched adult controls, admitted for dental check-ups, were recruited from the same sites. Subjects with previous and present cancer, except for the present OSCC (patients), coexisting diabetes, autoimmune disorders, contagious diseases, and pregnancy were excluded.

The investigation was approved by the Institutional Review Board of the University of Debrecen (No. 3244–8/2011, No. 3722–2012) and by the Scientific and Research Ethics Committee, Medical Research Council, Hungary [(693/PI/12.) 45038-1/2012/EKU]. The Code of Ethics of the World Medical

Association and the ethical standards of the 2000 Revision of the Helsinki Declaration were respected. Signed informed consent was obtained from all participating subjects.

Examination of the oral cavity and the head and neck region was performed by a licensed dental and/or maxillofacial surgeon according to standard methods and criteria of the World Health Organization [14]. Tooth decay was characterized using the DMFT index by calculating the number of decayed (D), missing (M), and filled (F) teeth (T). Periodontal health was characterized by the gingival index (GI) [15]. Suspicious lesions were removed or biopsied, and OSCC was verified by histology investigating the hematoxylin- and eosin-stained slides. The histological differentiation grade of OSCC was defined according to the classification of the World Health Organization (WHO) [16]. The staging was performed according to the 8th edition of the TNM classification of the International Union Against Cancer [17]. Demographic and clinicopathological data, including age, sex, stage, and grade of OSCC, DMFT, and GI indices, were recorded. The stage and grade of OSCC lesions were not available from study subjects of the Pécs Center. Smoking and ethanol consumption habits were recorded from consenting subjects as precisely as possible. Based on the information obtained, we formed two groups in each category. Regarding smoking habits, we distinguished regular smokers and non-smokers/occasional smokers (<10 cigarettes/day). Regarding ethanol consumption habits, we formed two categories: people who consumed ethanol-containing beverages at least once a week vs. those who drank less than once a week.

2.2. *Saliva Collection and Processing*

Unstimulated saliva samples were collected between 9:00 and 11:00 a.m. Patients and controls refrained from eating, drinking, smoking, gum chewing, and performing oral hygiene measures for at least 60 min before sampling. A minimum of 5.0 mL saliva was collected from each participant. Samples were kept on ice throughout collection and processing. Samples were pushed five-times through a 19 g needle then filtered (Millex 25 mm Durapore PVDF 5 μm Sterile, Merck KGaA, Darmstadt, Germany). Three aliquots of 200 μL filtered saliva were mixed with 1 mL PAXgene® reagent in cryotubes, for immediate stabilization of salivary RNA (PAXgene® Blood RNA Tubes, BD Biosciences, Cat.No. 762165, BD Franklin Lakes, NJ, USA). Aliquots of 0.5 mL were pipetted from the remaining saliva filtrate into cryotubes, for ELISA (Cryopure tube, SARSTEDT, Cat.No. 72.380, Nümbrecht, Germany). The PAXgene®-stabilized and proteomic saliva samples were frozen within 60 min from collection and stored at −70 °C until processing.

2.3. *Reverse Transcription and Real-Time Quantitative PCR (qPCR)*

Salivary RNA was isolated with the Direct-zol™ RNA MiniPrep Plus Kit (Zymo research, Cat.No. R2072, Irvine, CA, USA) according to the manufacturer's instructions. RNA sample quality and concentration were characterized by Nanodrop spectrophotometry and by the Agilent 2100 Bioanalyzer system. Expression of IL-6 mRNA and two normalizing genes, GAPDH and ACTB, were quantified using qPCR with TaqMan® assays on a QuantStudio™ 12K Flex Real Time PCR System (Applied Biosystem®, Thermo Fisher Scientific, Waltham, MA, USA). Raw data analysis was performed using the ExpressionSuite Software v1.0.3 (Applied Biosystem®). Samples with a high standard deviation of replicates, or with only one replicate giving a signal in the qPCR assay were categorized as borderline, non-quantifiable-positive ones. Ct values of the latter samples were set uniformly to 39 for the calculations and statistical analysis.

For qPCR efficiency correction, raw Ct values of cDNA serial dilutions (from HeLa total RNA) were used to determine the slope of the assays, using the linear regression function of GraphPad Prism software (GraphPad Software, Inc., CA, USA). PCR efficiency values were calculated, Ct values were corrected, and data were normalized. qPCR efficiencies were as follows: IL-6 = 0.904, GAPDH = 0.814, ACTB = 1.03. Cutoff Ct values (limit of quantitation; LOQ) for each TaqMan® assay were also determined in these experiments. Detailed descriptions of RNA methods were provided as Supplementary data.

2.4. *Enzyme-Linked Immune-Sorbent Assay (ELISA)*

IL-6 protein concentration in saliva samples of patients and controls was determined in duplicates by the sandwich ELISA kit (Human ELISA Kit EK0410, Boster Biological Technology Co., Pleasanton, CA, USA) according to the manufacturer's instructions. Optical density was measured at 450 nm, and concentrations were calculated based on the recorded 7-point calibration curve. LOQ for IL-t6 protein concentration was 4.96 pg/mL.

2.5. *Immunohistochemistry (IHC)*

Sections obtained from 41 preexisting formalin-fixed and paraffin-embedded tissue blocks of patients with proven OSCC from the Debrecen Center were microscopically reviewed by an independent pathologist (BD). Since IHC labeling of preexisting tissue blocks did not interfere with salivary IL-6 mRNA and protein measurements, 15 samples from the previous pilot cohort were co-investigated with the 26 samples collected in the course of the present investigation to increase sample size [12,13]. Serial sections were used for the detection of IL-6 manifestation in tumor cells and TILs by IHC, as described in detail [18]. Briefly, mouse monoclonal antibodies (MoAb, clone 8H12; Invitrogen, Rockford, IL, USA) to IL-6 (8H12; Invitrogen; Thermo Fisher Scientific, Rockford, IL, USA), CD3, CD4, CD20, and CD163 (all from DAKO, Glostrup, Denmark) were used according to manufacturers' instructions. Peroxidase-conjugated anti-mouse secondary immunoglobulin was used with a peroxidase-based detection kit (DAKO, Glostrup, Denmark) and VIP or DAB chromogenic substrates (Vector Labs, Peterborough, UK) for visualization. Stained sections were digitalized using a Panoramic MIDI digital slide scanner (3D-Histech-Zeiss, Budapest, Hungary) equipped with a Hitachi (HV-F22CL) 3CCD camera. Image analysis was performed by the HistoQuant application of Panoramic viewer software 1.15.2 (3D-Histech, Budapest, Hungary) as described [19].

2.6. *Statistical Analysis*

Distribution of demographic characteristics and clinical parameters of patients and controls were described by mean values and standard deviations (SD) for continuous variables. One-way ANOVA for continuous and chi-square test for non-continuous variables were used to check for uneven distribution of patients' parameters between controls and cases. Statistical computation was carried out by IBM SPSS Statistics version 20 (IBM SPSS Statistics for Windows, Version 20.0, Armonk, NY, USA).

In describing the expression of IL-6 mRNA and IL-6 protein, mean values and standard errors (SE) were computed. Differences between patients and controls were assessed with GraphPad Prism, using the Mann-Whitney U-test on the efficiency-corrected, normalized IL-6 mRNA expression values, and IL-6 protein concentration values.

Receiver Operating Characteristic (ROC) curve analysis was carried out on the same data with GraphPad Prism to evaluate the discrimination properties of IL-6 mRNA and IL-6 protein, and the area under the curve (AUC) was determined.

Multivariate linear regression models were applied to investigate the influence of patients' age, sex, DMFT score, GI score, smoking, and ethanol consumption on IL-6 mRNA and IL-6 protein concentrations. Before modeling, IL-6 mRNA and IL-6 protein concentrations were ln-transformed because of these parameters showed right-tailed distribution. The normal distribution of ln transformed values was checked by the Kolmogorov-Smirnov test. Results were described by linear regression coefficients with the corresponding p-values. Statistical computation was carried out by IBM SPSS Statistics version 20.

3. Results

3.1. *Characteristics of Study Participants*

Demographic and clinicopathological characterization of 95 patients with newly diagnosed and histologically-verified OSCC and 80 age-matched controls were summarized in Table 1. There were more males ($N = 60$) than females ($N = 35$) among patients with OSCC, resulting in a significant difference in sex distribution between the patient and control groups. The patient group was characterized by significantly higher DMFT scores than the group of controls. Smoking and ethanol consumption were significantly more frequent among patients than controls. Both IL-6 mRNA and IL-6 protein determination were successfully performed in 53 patient samples. Twenty-one and 21 samples, each, from different patients were suitable for either IL-6 mRNA or IL-6 protein measurements. In the case of the 80 controls, the number of successful salivary analyses were as follows, IL-6 mRNA and IL-6 protein: 55, IL-6 mRNA only: 9, and IL-6 protein: only 16 (Table S1: Demographic, clinicopathological characterization, and IL-6 mRNA and IL-6 protein levels of individual patients with OSCC and controls).

Table 1. Demographic and clinicopathological characterization of patients with oral squamous cell carcinoma (OSCC) and control subjects.

	-	Patients ($N = 95$)	Controls ($N = 80$)	P
Sex	Male	60 (63%)	30 (37%)	0.004 *
	Female	35 (37%)	50 (63%)	
Age	(years; mean ± SD)	61.7 ± 9.8	61.7 ± 9.2	0.982 **
OSCC stage				
N = 70	St I	14 (20%)	–	na ***
	St II	22 (31%)	–	na ***
	St III	13 (19%)	–	na***
	St IV	21 (30%)	–	na ***
Histological grade				
N = 70	G1	17 (24%)	–	na ***
	G2	42 (60%)	–	na ***
	G3	11 (16%)	–	na ***
DMFT	(N; mean ± SD)	64; 27.6 ± 6.4	47; 24.8 ± 6.9	0.011 **
GI	(N; mean ± SD)	36; 0.53 ± 0.49	41; 0.42 ± 0.34	0.79 **
Ethanol consumption	at least once a week	46 (48%)	14 (30%)	0.035 *
	less than once a week	49 (52%)	33 (70%)	
Smoking	regular smoking	62 (65%)	8 (17%)	<0.001 *
	non-smoker or occasional smoker	33 (35%)	40 (83%)	

N = number of patients * chi-square test; ** t-test; *** not applicable.

3.2. *Salivary IL-6 mRNA and IL-6 Protein Expression*

Saliva samples of 74/95 patients and 64/80 controls were suitable for qPCR. The majority of saliva samples from patients were positive for IL-6 mRNA. Initially, there were 18 samples with no quantifiable results. Reverse transcription and qPCR of these cases were repeated, resulting in 71 quantifiable results of 74 IL-6 mRNA samples from patients with OSCC. In contrast, 46 of 64 control samples were non-quantifiable (36 negative, and 10 borderline positive samples) for IL-6 mRNA expression, even in the repeated measurements. Normalized salivary IL-6 mRNA expression values were significantly higher in the group of patients with OSCC than in controls. The difference remained significant when subgroups of patients with different stages and grades were compared with controls (Table 2, Figure 1A). There were no significant differences in IL-6 mRNA expression between subgroups of patients with different stages and grades (data not shown). To test the sensitivity and specificity of salivary IL-6 mRNA as a diagnostic biomarker for OSCC, an ROC curve analysis was performed, and the AUC was calculated. The AUC for IL-6 mRNA was 0.9379 ($p < 0.001$; 95% confidence interval: 0.8973–0.9795; sensitivity: 0.945; specificity: 0.819) (Figure 1C).

Table 2. Differential expression of IL6 mRNA and IL6 protein in the saliva of patients with OSCC and controls.

	IL-6 mRNA Normalized Values				IL-6 Protein [pg/mL]			
Sample	*N*	mean	SE	*p* *	*N*	mean	SE	*p* *
OSCC								
St I-II	31	1.634	0.400	<0.001	30	59.72	18.09	<0.001
St III-IV	23	23.694	19.850	<0.001	28	102.44	28.22	<0.001
G1	9	1.440	0.501	<0.001	16	39.08	10.92	0.005
G2	34	16.327	13.550	<0.001	35	102.56	26.24	<0.001
G3	11	2.505	1.540	<0.001	7	63.58	22.45	0.010
Total	74	3.301	0.885	<0.001	74	70.98	14.06	<0.001
Control	64	0.037	0.012		71	12.45	3.29	

* Statistical comparison (Mann-Whitney U-test) of indicated groups of patient and control samples. There were no significant differences either in IL6 mRNA or IL6 protein expression between different subgroups of patients according to tumor stages and grades.

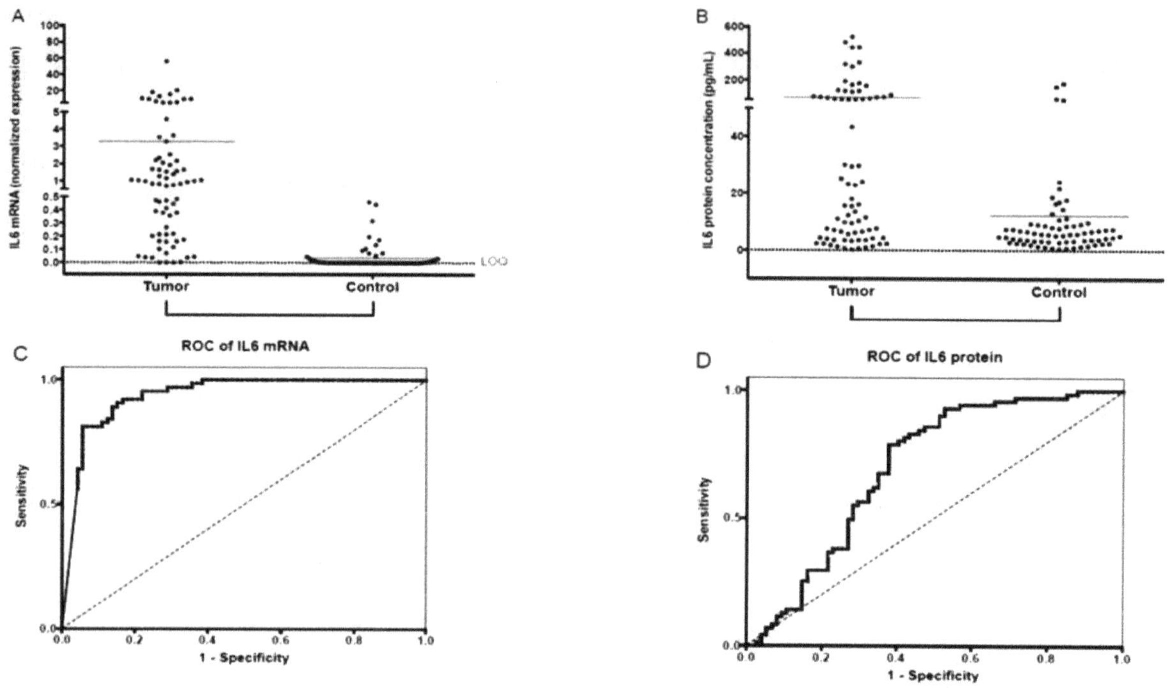

Figure 1. Salivary IL-6 mRNA and IL-6 protein expression. Expression of normalized salivary IL-6 mRNA (**A**) and salivary IL-6 protein (**B**) in patients with OSCC and controls. The horizontal lines indicate the mean. The p values are derived from the Mann-Whitney U test. Differences between Tumor and Control groups proved significant at $p < 0.001$ for both salivary IL-6 mRNA normalized values and for salivary IL-6 protein concentrations ($p < 0.05$ was considered significant). Dotted lines indicate the limit of quantification (LOQ). Receiver operating characteristic (ROC) curves for diagnostic ability of IL-6 mRNA (**C**) and protein (**D**) levels in saliva for OSCC. AUC for IL-6 mRNA = 0.9379 ($p < 0.001$; 95% confidence interval: 0.8973–0.9795; sensitivity: 0.945; specificity: 0.819); AUC for IL-6 protein = 0.6981 ($p < 0.0001$; 95% confidence interval: 0.6105–0.7858; sensitivity: 0.622; specificity: 0.789).

IL-6 protein concentration was measured in 74 suitable salivary samples of 95 patients and in 71/80 controls. Patients with OSCC, both the total patient group and subgroups of patients according to stages and grades, had statistically significantly higher IL-6 concentrations than controls (Table 2, Figure 1B). There were no significant differences in IL-6 protein concentrations of subgroups of patients with different stages and grades. There was a partial overlap between the distribution of the salivary IL-6 protein concentration of the patient and the control groups (Figure 1B). Using ROC analysis, salivary IL-6 protein concentration successfully identified patients with OSCC. The AUC for IL-6 protein was 0.6981 ($p < 0.0001$; 95% confidence interval: 0.6105–0.7858; sensitivity: 0.622; specificity: 0.789) (Figure 1D).

According to the multivariate linear regression analysis, the age and DMFT score had significant associations with ln transformed IL-6 mRNA expression levels. Sex, GI scores, alcohol consumption, and smoking exhibited no statistically significant association either with salivary IL-6 RNA or IL-6 protein expression (Table 3).

Table 3. Associations between demographic variables, gingival inflammation status, ethanol consumption, and smoking habits and ln-transformed salivary levels of IL-6 mRNA and IL-6 protein according to multivariate linear regression analysis.

		ln Transformed IL-6 mRNA		**ln Transformed IL-6 Protein**	
		Adjusted linear regression coefficient	*p*-value	Adjusted linear regression coefficient	*p*-value
Sex	female/male	−0.181	0.1	−0.159	0.11
Age	**Year**	**0.234**	**0.037**	0.174	0.094
DMFT		**0.234**	**0.037**	0.174	0.094
Gingival index		0.094	0.488	0.201	0.1
Alcohol consumption at least once a week/less than once a week		0.561	0.07	−0.1	0.375
Smoking regular smoking non-smoker or Occasional smoker		−0.134	0.232	0.005	0.959

Significant associations are indicated in bold characters.

3.3. *IL-6 Protein Expression in OSCC Tumor Tissue*

We performed an IHC investigation of the neoplastic lesions so as to see if the IL-6 mRNA and protein detected in the saliva of patients with OSCC might be produced by cells in the tumor tissue. We detected a positive IL-6 reaction in 28/41 (68%) samples. In 16/41 samples, neoplastic cells were stained positively, and in 26/41 samples, there were detectable IL-6 protein expression in TILs (Figure 2). TILs consisted mostly of neutrophil granulocytes, CD163-positive macrophages, and CD3-positive T-lymphocytes. Occasionally, CD20-positive B-lymphocytes, plasma cells, and eosinophil granulocytes were found. CD4-positive T-cells predominated over CD8-positive T-cells. The CD4:CD8 ratio was 2:1 in 30/41 (73%) of cases. We noted a CD4:CD8 inversion (CD4:CD8 < 1:2) in 5/41 (12%) cases without signs of tumor cell destruction.

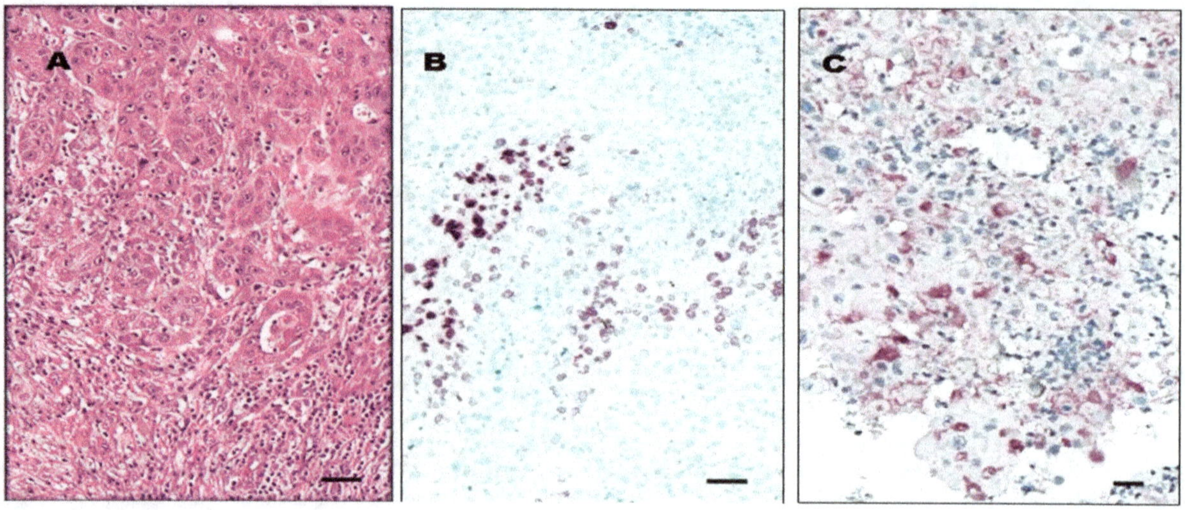

Figure 2. IL-6 protein expression in OSCC tumor tissue. Images from a representative tissue sample exhibiting OSCC with moderate differentiation grade (G2). (**A**) Abundant peri- and intratumoral tumor-infiltrating leukocytes (TILs) surrounding and intermixed with tumor cells (hematoxylin-eosin staining). (**B**) A region of a representative tumor sample showing many IL-6-positive TILs, whereas cancer cells are negative for IL-6 staining. (**C**) Another region of the same representative tumor sample with large squamous carcinoma cells exhibiting IL-6 positivity. Original magnification for all three images is 20×. Horizontal bars indicate 20 μm. Images (B) and (C) represent the immunohistochemistry (IHC) reaction using the peroxidase-based technique with VIP chromogen, as described in Materials and Methods.

4. Discussion

The aim of the present investigation was to validate salivary IL-6 mRNA and protein as a diagnostic biomarker of OSCC. Saliva samples from patients with histologically proven, newly diagnosed OSCC were collected from tertiary treatment centers representing each geographic region of Hungary. The age distribution of patients was similar to previously reported Hungarian regional and nation-wide epidemiologic data. The predominance of female patients with 37% and the prevalence of advanced patients (stage 3 and 4: 62%) in the present investigation was more expressed than observed previously [1,12,20,21]. Although the distribution pattern of histological differentiation grades (G2 > G1 > G3) was similar as that reported in a previous North-Eastern Hungarian cohort, the ratio of less differentiated grades (G2 and G3) was slightly higher but the same as in the preliminary institutional pilot investigation [12,20].

Salivary IL-6 was chosen as the potentially best-performing biomarker from 9 mRNA and 14 protein molecules tested in a small-scale pilot cohort of patients from one of the participating centers (Debrecen) [12,13]. Results on quantitatively determined salivary IL-6 mRNA transcripts have not yet been published prior to our previous pilot cohort and the present multi-center study investigating the largest number of patients with OSCC. Earlier only one study reported on the expression of salivary IL-6 mRNA in patients with OSCC; however, the level of expression was not quantified [22]. We found IL-6 mRNA transcripts by qPCR in 71 of 74 saliva samples of patients with OSCC. In contrast, only 18 of 64 control saliva samples contained quantifiable levels of IL-6 mRNA transcripts, and there was a statistically significant difference in the expression levels of normalized IL-6 mRNA transcripts between patients and controls. With an AUC value of 0.9379 of the ROC curve, IL-6 mRNA is one of the best-performing salivary OSCC biomarkers reported so far [10,23–25].

At the protein level, salivary IL-6 was reported most consistently to distinguish between patients with OSCC and controls with different geographic and ethnic backgrounds. Results with other salivary protein biomarkers were found less coherent [11]. We observed significantly higher IL-6 protein concentrations in the saliva of patients with OSCC vs. controls; however, there was a partial overlap between the distribution of salivary IL-6 concentrations of patients and controls, resulting in a less favorable AUC value of the ROC curve than with salivary IL-6 mRNA. Similar salivary IL-6 concentrations to our results were observed in patients with OSCC by other investigators [4,26–35]. The attempt at normalizing salivary IL-6 protein concentration for salivary total protein concentration abolished the significant difference of salivary IL-6 manifestation observed between patients and controls (data not shown). IL-6 is a low-abundance salivary protein with a concentration in the pg/mL range, whereas salivary total protein concentration is in the mg/mL range and the low signal-to-noise ratio might obscure differences [32]. Moreover, salivary albumin, a high-abundance salivary protein, was reported to correlate with OSCC, similar to IL-6, which may further compromise normalized results [35]. In addition to OSCC, salivary IL-6 protein concentration was investigated in oral premalignant lesions (OPML). The majority of investigators found significantly increased salivary IL-6 protein concentrations in patients with OPML when compared to controls, although the concentration was less excessively elevated in OPML than in OSCC samples [26,34,36,37]. In contrast, Brailo et al. found significantly elevated IL-6 protein concentrations in salivary samples from patients with OSCC but not with OPML [31], suggesting that further studies are requested before establishing a discriminatory role of salivary IL-6 protein between OSCC and OPML. Since data on salivary IL-6 mRNA in patients with OPML are lacking, we can either confirm or refute if salivary IL-6 mRNA, although remarkably sensitive for OSCC, would be proven specific for OSCC as compared to OPML.

Few groups investigated salivary IL-6 expression in association with various tumor stages and differentiation grades. In our study, differences both in salivary IL-6 mRNA and protein expression levels remained significant when comparing subgroups of patients with OSCC according to the stage and grade of their disease with controls, and there were no differences between distinct subgroups of patients. Similar results were reported by Sato et al. and Lisa Cheng et al. [29,32]. Three other groups observed higher salivary IL-6 concentration in patients with advanced lesions [27,32,33].

Conflicting results were reported on the potential influence of age, sex, smoking, and ethanol consumption habits on salivary IL-6 protein concentration in patients with OSCC [27,29,31,33,36]. Using linear regression analysis, we found significant associations between age and DMFT scores and salivary IL-6 mRNA expression confirming the results of our previous pilot studies, suggesting the influence of oral health on salivary OSCC biomarkers [12,13]. Yet, the separation between salivary mRNA levels of patients with and without OSCC is robust enough to maintain its value as an OSCC biomarker. Sex, smoking, and ethanol consumption did not bias the expression of either salivary IL-6 mRNA or IL-6 protein.

In a search for the source of elevated salivary IL-6 levels in patients with OSCC, we investigated the expression of IL-6 protein in the tumor tissue. In the majority of cases, tumor cells, and TILs were positive for IL-6 staining. Similar observations were reported in one publication [38]. These results, together with experimental evidence, suggest that a paracrine loop of stimulation may exist between neoplastic and nonmalignant cells of the tumor microenvironment [39,40]. The positive feedback loop of stimulation may explain the significant upregulation of salivary IL6 expression in patients with OSCC both at the mRNA and protein level when compared to controls. Thus, the IL-6-IL-6 receptor interaction may offer therapeutic targets in OSCC [41].

In conclusion, salivary IL-6 mRNA is a robust biomarker for OSCC in the Hungarian population in comparison with tumor-free control persons. However, caution is warranted before claiming the specificity of this biomarker without investigating salivary IL-6 mRNA in patients with OPML. Further investigations, involving patients from different ethnic groups and geographic regions may prove the value of quantitative salivary IL-6 mRNA expression as a general OSCC biomarker. The relevance of salivary IL-6 mRNA in OSCC was supported by the significantly elevated salivary IL-6 protein concentration in patients with OSCC vs. controls. Moreover, intratumor IL-6 production both by tumor cells and TILs, detected by IHC, may serve as a likely source of salivary IL-6 mRNA and protein in patients with OSCC.

Author Contributions: Conceptualization, I.J.M., J.T., J.S., B.S. and C.K.; data curation, J.S., B.S. and C.K.; formal analysis, P.L., B.M., J.S. and C.K.; funding acquisition, I.J.M.; investigation, I.J.M., J.H., P.L., B.M., B.D., A.S., I.T., J.P., P.J., J.B., P.B., L.O., Z.K., É.C. and C.K.; methodology, I.J.M., J.H., P.L., B.M., B.D., É.C. and B.S.; project administration, I.J.M., É.C., B.S. and C.K.; resources, I.J.M., I.T., J.P., J.B., L.O., J.T., É.C., B.S. and C.K.; software, J.S.; supervision, I.J.M., J.P., J.B. and L.O.; validation, I.J.M. and B.S.; visualization, B.D., É.C. and B.S.; writing—original draft, I.J.M., B.D., J.T., É.C., B.S. and C.K.; writing—review and editing, B.D., É.C., B.S. and C.K.

Acknowledgments: The technical assistance of Hajnalka J. Tóth is acknowledged.

References

1. Diz, P.; Meleti, M.; Diniz-Freitas, M.; Vescovi, P.; Warnakulasuriya, S.; Johnson, N.W.; Kerr, A.R. Oral and pharyngeal cancer in Europe: Incidence, mortality and trends as presented to the Global Oral Cancer Forum. *Trans. Res. Oral Oncol.* **2017**, *2*, 1–13. [CrossRef]
2. Zhang, H.; Dziegielewski, P.T.; Biron, V.L.; Szudek, J.; Al-Qahatani, K.H.; O'Connell, D.A. Survival outcomes of patients with advanced oral cavity squamous cell carcinoma treated with multimodal therapy: A multi-institutional analysis. *J. Otolaryngol. Head Neck Surg.* **2013**, *42*, 30. [CrossRef] [PubMed]
3. Carreras-Torras, C.; Gay-Escoda, C. Techniques for early diagnosis of oral squamous cell carcinoma: Systematic review. *Med. Oral Patol. Oral Cir. Bucal.* **2015**, *20*, e305–e315. [CrossRef] [PubMed]
4. SahebJamee, M.; Eslami, M.; AtarbashiMoghadam, F.; Sarafnejad, A. Salivary concentration of TNFalpha, IL1 alpha, IL6, and IL8 in oral squamous cell carcinoma. *Med. Oral Patol. Oral Cir. Bucal.* **2008**, *13*, E292–E295. [PubMed]
5. Wu, J.Y.; Yi, C.; Chung, H.R.; Wang, D.J.; Chang, W.C.; Lee, S.Y.; Lin, C.T.; Yang, Y.C.; Yang, W.C. Potential biomarkers in saliva for oral squamous cell carcinoma. *Oral Oncol.* **2010**, *46*, 226–231. [CrossRef]
6. Panta, P.; Venna, V.R. Salivary RNA signatures in oral cancer detection. *Anal. Cell. Pathol.* **2014**, *2014*, 450629. [CrossRef]
7. Khan, R.S.; Khurshid, Z.; Akhbar, S.; Faraz Moin, S. Advances of Salivary Proteomics in Oral Squamous Cell Carcinoma (OSCC) Detection: An Update. *Proteomes* **2016**, *4*, 41. [CrossRef]
8. Radhika, T.; Jeddy, N.; Nithya, S.; Muthumeenakshi, R.M. Salivary biomarkers in oral squamous cell carcinoma—An insight. *J. Oral Biol. Craniofac. Res.* **2016**, *6*, S51–S54. [CrossRef]
9. Lohavanichbutr, P.; Zhang, Y.; Wang, P.; Gu, H.; Nagana Gowda, G.A.; Djukovic, D.; Buas, M.F.; Raftery, D.; Chen, C. Salivary metabolite profiling distinguishes patients with oral cavity squamous cell carcinoma from normal controls. *PLoS ONE* **2018**, *13*, e0204249. [CrossRef]
10. Zhao, S.Y.; Wang, J.; Ouyang, S.B.; Huang, Z.K.; Liao, L. Salivary Circular RNAs Hsa_Circ_0001874 and Hsa_Circ_0001971 as Novel Biomarkers for the Diagnosis of Oral Squamous Cell Carcinoma. *Cell. Physiol. Biochem.* **2018**, *47*, 2511–2521. [CrossRef]
11. Sahibzada, H.A.; Khurshid, Z.; Khan, R.S.; Naseem, M.; Siddique, K.M.; Mali, M.; Zafar, M.S. Salivary IL-8, IL-6 and TNF-α as potential diagnostic biomarkers for oral cancer. *Diagnostics* **2017**, *7*, 21. [CrossRef] [PubMed]
12. Horváth, J.; Szabó, A.; Tar, I.; Dezső, B.; Kiss, C.; Márton, I.; Scholtz, B. Oral health may affect the performance of mRNA-based saliva biomarkers for oral squamous cell cancer. *Pathol. Oncol. Res.* **2018**, *24*, 833–842. [CrossRef] [PubMed]
13. Csősz, É.; Lábiscsák, P.; Kalló, G.; Márkus, B.; Emri, M.; Szabó, A.; Tar, I.; Tőzsér, J.; Kiss, C.; Márton, I. Proteomics investigation of OSCC-specific salivary biomarkers in a Hungarian population highlights the importance of identification of population-tailored biomarkers. *PLoS ONE* **2017**, *12*, e0177282. [CrossRef] [PubMed]
14. World Health Organization. *Oral Health Surveys: Basic Methods*, 4th ed.; World Health Organization: Geneva, Switzerland, 1997.
15. Lang, N.P.; Corbet, E.F. Periodontal diagnosis in daily practice. *Int. Dent. J.* **1995**, *45*, 3–15. [PubMed]
16. Pindborg, J.J.; Reichart, P.A.; Smith, C.J.; Van der Waal, I. *Histological Typing of Cancer and Precancer of the Oral Mucosa. WHO International Histological Classification of Tumours*, 2nd ed.; Springer: Berlin, Germany, 1997.
17. Sobin, L.H.; Gospodarowitz, M.K.; Wittekind, C. Head and Neck Tumours: Lip and oral cavity. In *TNM Classification of Malignant Tumours*, 7th ed.; Wiley-Blackwell: Chichester, UK, 2010; pp. 25–29.
18. Tsakiris, I.; Torocsik, D.; Gyongyosi, A.; Dozsa, A.; Szatmari, I.; Szanto, A.; Soos, G.; Nemes, Z.; Igali, L.; Marton, I.; et al. Carboxypeptidase-M is regulated by lipids and CSFs in macrophages and dendritic cells and expressed selectively in tissue granulomas and foam cells. *Lab. Investig.* **2012**, *92*, 345–361. [CrossRef] [PubMed]

19. Szabó, K.; Papp, G.; Dezso, B.; Zeher, M. The histopathology of labial salivary glands in primary Sjögren' syndrome: Focusing on follicular helper T cells in the inflammatory infiltrates. *Mediators Inflamm.* **2014**, *2014*, 631787. [CrossRef]
20. Nemes, J.A.; Redl, P.; Boda, R.; Kiss, C.; Márton, I.J. Oral cancer report from Northeastern Hungary. *Pathol. Oncol. Res.* **2008**, *14*, 85–92. [CrossRef]
21. Németh, Z.; Turi, K.; Léhner, G.; Veres, D.S.; Csurgay, K. The prognostic role of age in oral cancer. A clinical study. *Magy. Onkol.* **2013**, *57*, 166–172. (In Hungarian)
22. St John, M.A.; Li, Y.; Zhou, X.; Denny, P.; Ho, C.M.; Montemagno, C.; Shi, W.; Qi, F.; Wu, B.; Sinha, U.; et al. Interleukin 6 and interleukin 8 as potential biomarkers for oral cavity and oropharyngeal squamous cell carcinoma. *Arch. Otolaryngol. Head Neck Surg.* **2004**, *130*, 929–935. [CrossRef]
23. Brinkmann, O.; Kastratovic, D.A.; Dimitrijevic, M.V.; Konstantinovic, V.S.; Jelovac, D.B.; Antic, J.; Nesic, V.S.; Markovic, S.Z.; Martinovic, Z.R.; Akin, D.; et al. Oral squamous cell carcinoma detection by salivary biomarkers in Serbian population. *Oral Oncol.* **2011**, *47*, 51–55. [CrossRef]
24. Gai, C.; Camussi, F.; Broccoletti, R.; Gambino, A.; Cabras, M.; Molinaro, L.; Carossa, S.; Camussi, G.; Arduino, P.G. Salivary extracellular vesicle-associated miRNAs as potential biomarkers in oral squamous cell carcinoma. *BMC Cancer* **2018**, *18*, 439. [CrossRef] [PubMed]
25. Feng, Y.; Li, Q.; Chen, J.; Yi, P.; Xu, X.; Fan, Y.; Cui, B.; Yu, Y.; Li, X.; Du, Y.; et al. Salivary protease spectrum biomarkers of oral cancer. *Int. J. Oral Sci.* **2019**, *11*, 7. [CrossRef] [PubMed]
26. Rhodus, N.L.; Ho, V.; Miller, C.S.; Myers, S.; Ondrey, F. NF-kappaB dependent cytokine levels in saliva of patients with oral paraneoplastic lesions and oral squamous cell carcinoma. *Cancer Detect. Prev.* **2005**, *29*, 42–45. [CrossRef] [PubMed]
27. Duffy, S.A.; Taylor, J.M.; Terrell, J.E.; Islam, M.; Li, Y.; Wolf, G.T.; Teknos, T.N. Interleukin-6 predicts recurrence and survival among head and neck cancer patients. *Cancer* **2008**, *113*, 750–757. [CrossRef] [PubMed]
28. Katakura, A.; Kamiyama, I.; Takano, N.; Shibahara, T.; Muramatsu, T.; Ishihara, K.; Takagi, R.; Shouno, T. Comparison of salivary cytokine levels in oral cancer patients and healthy subjects. *Bull. Tokyo Dent. Coll.* **2007**, *48*, 199–203. [CrossRef] [PubMed]
29. Sato, J.; Goto, J.; Murata, T.; Kitamori, S.; Yamazaki, Y.; Satoh, A.; Kitagawa, Y. Changes in saliva interleukin-6 levels in patients with oral squamous cell carcinoma. *Oral Surg. Oral Med. Oral Pathol. Oral Radiol. Endod.* **2010**, *110*, 330–336. [CrossRef] [PubMed]
30. Korostoff, A.; Reder, L.; Masood, R.; Sinha, U.K. The role of salivary cytokine biomarkers in tongue cancer invasion and mortality. *Oral Oncol.* **2011**, *47*, 282–287. [CrossRef]
31. Brailo, V.; Vucicevic-Boras, V.; Lukac, J.; Biocina-Lukenda, D.; Zilic-Alajbeg, I.; Milenovic, A.; Balija, M. Salivary and serum interleukin 1 beta, interleukin 6 and tumor necrosis factor alpha in patients with leukoplakia and oral cancer. *Med. Oral Patol. Oral Cir. Bucal* **2012**, *17*, e10–e15. [CrossRef]
32. Lisa Cheng, Y.S.; Jordan, L.; Gorugantula, L.M.; Schneiderman, E.; Chen, H.S.; Rees, T. Salivary interleukin-6 and -8 in patients with oral cancer and patients with chronic oral inflammatory diseases. *J. Periodontol.* **2014**, *85*, 956–965. [CrossRef]
33. Arduino, P.G.; Menegatti, E.; Cappello, N.; Martina, E.; Gardino, N.; Tanteri, C.; Cavallo, F.; Scully, C.; Broccoletti, R. Possible role for interleukins as biomarkers for mortality and recurrence in oral cancer. *Int. J. Biol. Markers* **2015**, *30*, e262–e266. [CrossRef]
34. Panneer Selvam, N.; Sadaksharam, J. Salivary interleukin-6 in the detection of oral cancer and precancer. *Asia. Pac. J. Clin. Oncol.* **2015**, *11*, 236–241. [CrossRef]
35. Rao, M.; Ramesh, A.; Adapa, S.; Thomas, B.; Shetty, J. Correlation of salivary levels of interleukin-6 and albumin with oral squamous cell carcinoma. *J. Health Res. Rev.* **2016**, *3*, 11–14. [CrossRef]
36. Juretic, M.; Cerovic, R.; Belusic-Gobic, M.; Brekalo Prso, I.; Kqiku, L.; Spalj, S.; Pezelj-Ribaric, S. Salivary levels of TNF-α and IL-6 in patients with oral premalignant and malignant lesions. *Folia Biol.* **2013**, *59*, 99–102.
37. Dikova, V.R.; Principe, S.; Bagan, J.V. Salivary inflammatory proteins in patients with oral potentially malignant disorders. *J. Clin. Exp. Dent.* **2019**, *11*, e659–e664. [CrossRef] [PubMed]
38. Jinno, T.; Kawano, S.; Maruse, Y.; Matsubara, R.; Goto, Y.; Sakamoto, T.; Hashiguchi, Y.; Kaneko, N.; Tanaka, H.; Kitamura, R. Increased expression of interleukin-6 predicts poor response to chemoradiotherapy and unfavorable prognosis in oral squamous cell carcinoma. *Oncol. Rep.* **2015**, *33*, 2161–2168. [CrossRef] [PubMed]
39. Yamamoto, T.; Kimura, T.; Ueta, E.; Tatemoto, Y.; Osaki, T. Characteristic cytokine generation patterns in cancer

cells and infiltrating lymphocytes in oral squamous cell carcinomas and the influence of chemoradiation combined with immunotherapy on these patterns. *Oncology* **2003**, *64*, 407–415. [CrossRef]
40. Petruzzi, M.N.; Cherubini, K.; Salum, F.G.; de Figueiredo, M.A. Role of tumour-associated macrophages in oral squamous cells carcinoma progression: An update on current knowledge. *Diagn. Pathol.* **2017**, *12*, 32. [CrossRef]
41. Rossi, J.F.; Lu, Z.Y.; Jourdan, M.; Klein, B. Interleukin-6 as a therapeutic target. *Clin. Cancer Res.* **2015**, *21*, 1248–1257. [CrossRef]

Permissions

All chapters in this book were first published by MDPI; hereby published with permission under the Creative Commons Attribution License or equivalent. Every chapter published in this book has been scrutinized by our experts. Their significance has been extensively debated. The topics covered herein carry significant findings which will fuel the growth of the discipline. They may even be implemented as practical applications or may be referred to as a beginning point for another development.

The contributors of this book come from diverse backgrounds, making this book a truly international effort. This book will bring forth new frontiers with its revolutionizing research information and detailed analysis of the nascent developments around the world.

We would like to thank all the contributing authors for lending their expertise to make the book truly unique. They have played a crucial role in the development of this book. Without their invaluable contributions this book wouldn't have been possible. They have made vital efforts to compile up to date information on the varied aspects of this subject to make this book a valuable addition to the collection of many professionals and students.

This book was conceptualized with the vision of imparting up-to-date information and advanced data in this field. To ensure the same, a matchless editorial board was set up. Every individual on the board went through rigorous rounds of assessment to prove their worth. After which they invested a large part of their time researching and compiling the most relevant data for our readers.

The editorial board has been involved in producing this book since its inception. They have spent rigorous hours researching and exploring the diverse topics which have resulted in the successful publishing of this book. They have passed on their knowledge of decades through this book. To expedite this challenging task, the publisher supported the team at every step. A small team of assistant editors was also appointed to further simplify the editing procedure and attain best results for the readers.

Apart from the editorial board, the designing team has also invested a significant amount of their time in understanding the subject and creating the most relevant covers. They scrutinized every image to scout for the most suitable representation of the subject and create an appropriate cover for the book.

The publishing team has been an ardent support to the editorial, designing and production team. Their endless efforts to recruit the best for this project, has resulted in the accomplishment of this book. They are a veteran in the field of academics and their pool of knowledge is as vast as their experience in printing. Their expertise and guidance has proved useful at every step. Their uncompromising quality standards have made this book an exceptional effort. Their encouragement from time to time has been an inspiration for everyone.

The publisher and the editorial board hope that this book will prove to be a valuable piece of knowledge for researchers, students, practitioners and scholars across the globe.

List of Contributors

Soo Hwan Byun
Department of Oral & Maxillofacial Surgery, Dentistry, Sacred Heart Hospital, Hallym University College of Medicine, Anyang 14068, Korea

Chanyang Min
Hallym Data Science Laboratory, Hallym University College of Medicine, 14068 Anyang, Korea
Graduate School of Public Health, Seoul National University, Seoul 03080, Korea

Yong Bok Kim, Heejin Kim and Seok Jin Hong
Department of Otorhinolaryngology-Head & Neck Surgery, Dongtan Sacred Heart Hospital, Hallym University College of Medicine, Dongtan 18450, Korea

Sung Hun Kang
Department of Biomedical Sciences, College of Medicine, Hallym University, Chuncheon 24252, Korea

Bum Jung Park and Ji Hye Wee
Department of Otorhinolaryngology-Head & Neck Surgery, Sacred Heart Hospital, Hallym University College of Medicine, Anyang 14068, Korea

Hyo Geun Choi
Hallym Data Science Laboratory, Hallym University College of Medicine, 14068 Anyang, Korea
Department of Otorhinolaryngology-Head & Neck Surgery, Sacred Heart Hospital, Hallym University College of Medicine, Anyang 14068, Korea

Fernanda Monedeiro
Department of Environmental Chemistry and Bioanalytics, Faculty of Chemistry, Nicolaus Copernicus University, 87-100 Toruń, Poland
Interdisciplinary Centre of Modern Technologies, Nicolaus Copernicus University, 87-100 Toruń, Poland
Department of Chemistry, Faculty of Philosophy, Science and Letters of Ribeirão Preto, University of São Paulo, Ribeirão Preto CEP 14040-901, Brazil

Paweł Pomastowski, Maciej Milanowski, Tomasz Ligor and Bogusław Buszewski
Department of Environmental Chemistry and Bioanalytics, Faculty of Chemistry, Nicolaus Copernicus University, 87-100 Toruń, Poland
Interdisciplinary Centre of Modern Technologies, Nicolaus Copernicus University, 87-100 Toruń, Poland

Antonino Lo Giudice and Vincenzo Ronsivalle
Department of Medical-Surgical Specialties—Section of Orthodontics, School of Dentistry, University of Catania, Policlinico Universitario "G. Rodolico" Via Santa Sofia 78, 95123 Catania, Italy

Gaetano Isola
Department of Medical-Surgical Specialties, School of Dentistry, University of Catania, Policlinico Universitario "G. Rodolico" Via Santa Sofia 78, 95123 Catania, Italy

Lorenzo Rustico, Marco Portelli and Riccardo Nucera
Department of Biomedical and Dental Sciences and Morphofunctional Imaging, Section of Orthodontics, School of Dentistry, University of Messina, Policlinico Universitario "G. Martino," 98100 Messina, Italy

Yoshiaki Nomura, Ayako Okada, Ryoko Otsuka and Nobuhiro Hanada
Department of Translational Research, Tsurumi University School of Dental Medicine, Kanagawa 230-8501, Japan

Erika Kakuta
Department of Oral bacteriology, Tsurumi University School of Dental Medicine, Kanagawa 230-8501, Japan

Mieko Shimada
Chiba Prefecture University of Health Sciences, Chiba 261-0014, Japan

Yasuko Tomizawa
Department of Cardiovascular Surgery, Tokyo Women's Medical University, Tokyo 162-8666, Japan

Chieko Taguchi and Kazumune Arikawa
Department of Preventive and Public Oral Health, Nihon University School of Dentistry at Matsudo, Matsudo 271-8587, Japan

Hideki Daikoku and Tamotsu Sato
Iwate Dental Association, Morioka 470-2101, Japan

Óscar Rapado-González
Department of Surgery and Medical-Surgical Specialties, Medicine and Dentistry School, Universidade de Santiago de Compostela (USC), 15782 Santiago de Compostela, Spain
Liquid Biopsy Analysis Unit, Translational Medical Oncology (Oncomet), Health Research Institute of Santiago (IDIS), 15706 Santiago de Compostela, Spain
Centro de Investigación Biomédica en Red en Cáncer (CIBERONC), Instituto de Salud Carlos III, 28029 Madrid, Spain

Laura Muinelo-Romay
Liquid Biopsy Analysis Unit, Translational Medical Oncology (Oncomet), Health Research Institute of Santiago (IDIS), 15706 Santiago de Compostela, Spain
Centro de Investigación Biomédica en Red en Cáncer (CIBERONC), Instituto de Salud Carlos III, 28029 Madrid, Spain

Cristina Martínez-Reglero and Ángel Salgado-Barreira
Methodology and Statistics Unit, Galicia Sur Health Research Institute (IISGS), 36312 Vigo, Spain

Almudena Rodríguez-Fernández
Department of Preventive and Public Health, Universidade de Santiago de Compostela (USC), 15782 Santiago de Compostela, Spain

Rafael López-López
Centro de Investigación Biomédica en Red en Cáncer (CIBERONC), Instituto de Salud Carlos III, 28029
Translational Medical Oncology (Oncomet), Health Research Institute of Santiago (IDIS), Complexo Hospitalario Universitario de Santiago de Compostela (SERGAS), 15706 Santiago de Compostela, Spain

Santiago Aguín-Losada and Luis León-Mateos
Translational Medical Oncology (Oncomet), Health Research Institute of Santiago (IDIS), Complexo Hospitalario Universitario de Santiago de Compostela (SERGAS), 15706 Santiago de Compostela, Spain

María Mercedes Suarez-Cunqueiro
Department of Surgery and Medical-Surgical Specialties, Medicine and Dentistry School, Universidade de Santiago de Compostela (USC), 15782 Santiago de Compostela, Spain
Centro de Investigación Biomédica en Red en Cáncer (CIBERONC), Instituto de Salud Carlos III, 28029
Translational Medical Oncology (Oncomet), Health Research Institute of Santiago (IDIS), 15706 Santiago de Compostela, Spain

Mario Dioguardi, Enrica Laneve, Diego Sovereto, Bruna Raddato, Khrystyna Zhurakivska, Filiberto Mastrangelo, Domenico Ciavarella, Lucio Lo Russo and Lorenzo Lo Muzio
Department of Clinical and Experimental Medicine, University of Foggia, Via Rovelli 50, 71122 Foggia, Italy

Vito Crincoli
Department of Basic Medical Sciences, Neurosciences and Sensory Organs, Division of Complex Operating Unit of Dentistry, "Aldo Moro" University of Bari, Piazza G. Cesare 11, 70124 Bari, Italy

Luigi Laino
Multidisciplinary Department of Medical-Surgical and Odontostomatological Specialties, University of Campania "Luigi Vanvitelli", 80121 Naples, Italy

Mario Alovisi
Department of Surgical Sciences, Dental School, University of Turin, 10124 Turin, Italy

Pia Lopez-Jornet
Department Stomatology School of Medicine, Biomedical Research Institute (IMIB-Arrixaca), Faculty of Medicine and Odontology, University of Murcia, 30008 Adv Marques de los Velez s/n, Spain

Candela Castillo Felipe
Department Stomatology School of Medicine, Faculty of Medicine and Odontology, University of Murcia; 30008 Murcia, Spain

Luis Pardo-Marin, Jose J. Ceron and Asta Tvarijonaviciute
Interdisciplinary Laboratory of Clinical Analysis, Interlab-UMU, Regional Campus of International Excellence 'Campus Mare Nostrum', University of Murcia, Espinardo, 30100 Murcia, Spain

Eduardo Pons-Fuster
Biomedical Research Institute (IMIB-Arrixaca), Faculty of Medicine and Odontology, University of Murcia, 30008 Murcia, Spain

Rosa Valletta, Ada Pango, Gregorio Tortora, Roberto Rongo, Gianrico Spagnuolo and Vincenzo D'Antò
Department of Neurosciences, Reproductive Sciences and Oral Sciences, Section of Orthodontics, University of Naples "Federico II", 80131 Naples, Italy

Vittorio Simeon
Department of Mental Health and Preventive Medicine, Medical Statistics Unit, University of Campania "Luigi Vanvitelli", 80138 Napoli, Italy

João Albernaz Neves
Clinical Research Unit (CRU), Centro de Investigação Interdisciplinar Egas Moniz (CiiEM), Egas Moniz, CRL, 2829-511 Caparica, Almada, Portugal

Nathalie Antunes-Ferreira and Alexandre Quintas
Laboratório de Ciências Forenses e Psicológicas Egas Moniz (LCFPEM), Centro de Investigação Interdisciplinar Egas Moniz (CiiEM), Egas Moniz CRL, 2829-511 Caparica, Almada, Portugal
Laboratory of Biological Anthropology and Human Osteology (LABOH), CRIA/FCSH, Universidade NOVA de Lisboa, 1069-061 Lisboa, Portugal

Vanessa Machado, João Botelho, José João Mendes and Ana Sintra Delgado
Orthodontics Department, Egas Moniz Dental Clinic (EMDC), Egas Moniz, CRL, 2829-511 Caparica, Almada, Portugal

Luís Proença
Quantitative Methods for Health Research (MQIS), CiiEM, Egas Moniz, CRL, 2829-511 Caparica, Almada, Portugal

Piero Papi, Andrea Raco, Nicola Pranno, Bianca Di Murro and Giorgio Pompa
Department of Oral and Maxillo-Facial Sciences, "Sapienza" University of Rome, 00161 Rome, Italy

Pier Carmine Passarelli and Antonio D'Addona
Division of Oral Surgery and Implantology, Department of Head and Neck, Oral Surgery, and Implantology Unit, Institute of Clinical Dentistry, Fondazione Policlinico Universitario A. Gemelli IRCCS-Università Cattolica del Sacro Cuore, 00168 Rome, Italy

Maurizio Barbieri
Department of Earth Sciences, "Sapienza" University of Rome, 00161 Rome, Italy

Anna Zalewska and Agnieszka Kossakowska
Experimental Dentistry Laboratory, Medical University of Bialystok, 15-222 Bialystok, Poland

Katarzyna Taranta-Janusz and Anna Wasilewska
Department of Pediatrics and Nephrology, Medical University of Bialystok, 15-222 Bialystok, Poland

Sara Zięba
Students Scientific Club "Biochemistry of Civilization Diseases" at the Department of Hygiene, Epidemiology and Ergonomics, Medical University of Bialystok, 15-222 Bialystok, Poland

Katarzyna Fejfer, Małgorzata Salamonowicz and Paula Kostecka-Sochoń
Conservative Dentistry Department, Medical University of Bialystok, 15-222 Bialystok, Poland

Mateusz Maciejczyk
Department of Hygiene, Epidemiology and Ergonomics, Medical University of Bialystok, 15-222 Bialystok, Poland
Department of Hygiene, Epidemiology and Ergonomics, Medical University of Bialystok, 2c Mickiewicza Street, 15-022 Bialystok, Poland

Emanuela Martina, Anna Campanati, Federico Diotallevi and Annamaria Offidani
Dermatology Clinic, Department of Clinical and Molecular Sciences, Polytechnic Marche University, via Conca 71, 60126 Ancona, Italy

Anna Skutnik-Radziszewska
Experimental Dentistry Laboratory, Medical University of Bialystok, 1 Jana Kilinskiego Street, 15-089 Bialystok, Poland

Iwona Flisiak and Julita Krahel
Department of Dermatology and Venereology, Medical University of Bialystok, 14 Zurawia Street, 15-540 Bialystok, Poland

Urszula Kołodziej and Anna Kotowska-Rodziewicz
Department of Restorative Dentistry, Medical University of Bialystok, 24 A. M. Sklodowskiej-Curie Street, 15-276 Bialystok, Poland

Anna Klimiuk and Anna Zalewska
Experimental Dentistry Laboratory, Medical University of Bialystok, 24 A. M. Sklodowskiej-Curie Street, 15-276 Bialystok, Poland

Alessandro Polizzi, Salvatore Torrisi, Simona Santonocito, Mattia Di Stefano, Francesco Indelicato and Antonino Lo Giudice
Department of General Surgery and Surgical-Medical Specialties, School of Dentistry, University of Catania, AOU Policlinico, Via Plebiscito 628, 95124 Catania, Italy

Dinis Pereira, Vanessa Machado and Ana Sintra Delgado
Orthodontics Department, CRU, CiiEM, Egas Moniz-Cooperativa de Ensino Superior, 2829-511 Almada, Portugal
Clinical Research Unit (CRU), Centro de Investigação Interdisciplinar Egas Moniz (CiiEM), Instituto Universitário Egas Moniz, 2829-511 Almada, Portugal

João Botelho and José João Mendes
Clinical Research Unit (CRU), Centro de Investigação Interdisciplinar Egas Moniz (CiiEM), Instituto Universitário Egas Moniz, 2829-511 Almada, Portugal

Ji Young Hwang
Department of Dentistry, Graduate School, Kyung Hee University, Seoul 02447, Korea

Hyo-Seol Lee, Ok Hyung Nam and Sung Chul Choi
Department of Pediatric Dentistry, School of Dentistry, Kyung Hee University, Seoul 02447, Korea

Jaehyuk Choi
Division of Life Sciences, College of Life Sciences and Bioengineering, Incheon National University, Incheon 22012, Korea

Mi Sun Kim
Department of Pediatric Dentistry, School of Dentistry, Kyung Hee University, Seoul 02447, Korea
Department of Pediatric Dentistry, Kyung Hee University Hospital at Gangdong, Seoul 02447, Korea

Sanna Syrjäläinen, Ulvi Kahraman Gursoy and Mervi Gursoy
Periodontology, Institute of Dentistry, University of Turku, 20520 Turku, Finland

Milla Pietiäinen and Pirkko Pussinen
Oral and Maxillofacial Diseases, University of Helsinki, 00014 Helsinki, Finland

Antti Jula, Veikko Salomaa and Pekka Jousilahti
Finnish Institute for Health and Welfare, 00271 Helsinki, Finland

Eija Könönen
Periodontology, Institute of Dentistry, University of Turku, 20520 Turku, Finland
Oral Health Care,Welfare Division, City of Turku, 20101 Turku, Finland

Ildikó Judit Márton
Department of Operative Dentistry and Endodontics, Faculty of Dentistry, University of Debrecen, 4032 Debrecen, Hungary

József Horváth, Péter Lábiscsák, Bernadett Márkus, József Tőzsér, Éva Csősz and Beáta Scholtz
Department of Biochemistry and Molecular Biology, Faculty of Medicine, University of Debrecen, 4032 Debrecen, Hungary

Balázs Dezső
Department of Oral Pathology and Microbiology, Faculty of Dentistry and Institute of Pathology, University of Debrecen, 4032 Debrecen, Hungary

Adrienn Szabó
Department of Maxillofacial Surgery, University of Debrecen, 4032 Debrecen, Hungary

Ildikó Tar
Department of Oral Medicine, Faculty of Dentistry, University of Debrecen, 4032 Debrecen, Hungary

József Piffkó and Petra Jakus
Department of Maxillofacial Surgery, University of Szeged, 6720 Szeged, Hungary

József Barabás and Péter Barabás
Department of Maxillofacial Surgery, Semmelweis University, 1085 Budapest, Hungary

Lajos Olasz and Zsanett Kövér
Department of Oral and Maxillofacial Surgery, University of Pécs, 7621 Pécs, Hungary

János Sándor
Department of Preventive Medicine, University of Debrecen, 4028 Debrecen, Hungary

Csongor Kiss
Department of Pediatric Hematology-Oncology, Faculty of Medicine, University of Debrecen, 4032 Debrecen, Hungary

Index

www.ingramcontent.com/pod-product-compliance
Lightning Source LLC
LaVergne TN
LVHW081019210926
848485LV00004B/906